Total Pancreatectomy and Islet Auto Transplantation

Srinath Chinnakotla • Melena D. Bellin
Greg J. Beilman
Editors

Total Pancreatectomy and Islet Auto Transplantation

Springer

BYWORD BOOKS™

Editors
Srinath Chinnakotla
Department of Surgery
University of Minnesota Medical School
and University of Minnesota Masonic
Children's Hospital
Minneapolis, MN, USA

Melena D. Bellin
Division of Pediatric Endocrinology,
Department of Pediatrics
University of Minnesota Medical School
Minneapolis, MN, USA

Greg J. Beilman
Department of Surgery
University of Minnesota Medical School
Minneapolis, MN, USA

Co-publishing partnership between Byword Books Private Limited and Springer Nature Singapore Pte Ltd.

ISBN 978-981-92-0017-7 ISBN 978-981-92-0018-4 (eBook)
https://doi.org/10.1007/978-981-92-0018-4

Jointly published with Byword Books.

This Springer imprint is published by the registered company Springer Nature Singapore Pte Ltd.
The registered company address is: 152 Beach Road, #21-01/04 Gateway East, Singapore 189721, Singapore

To all the patients living with chronic pancreatitis—

Your courage in facing daily challenges, your perseverance in moments of pain, and your unwavering hope inspire all of us who care for you.

This work is dedicated to your strength, your resilience, and your journey toward healing.

Foreword

Chronic pancreatitis is a debilitating condition characterized by intractable pain and progressive pancreatic dysfunction. It profoundly affects the quality of life of affected patients. For those suffering from its most severe form, where conventional medical and endoscopic therapies have failed, total pancreatectomy and islet autotransplantation (TPIAT) offers a surgical, albeit complex, solution.

The success of TPIAT results from its ability to address the pain caused by the pancreatic pathology while significantly improving the management of postprocedure diabetes. A substantial majority of patients, approximately 70% to 80%, experience a dramatic reduction in abdominal pain, with many able to discontinue narcotic pain medication. The IAT component aims to preserve endogenous insulin production, and while there is some variation in outcomes depending largely on the duration of symptoms and the presence of calcification, approximately 30% to 40% of patients achieve insulin independence. For the remaining cohort who do require some exogenous insulin, their diabetes is typically far more manageable than the severe, brittle diabetes that would otherwise ensue. This is manifest as minimal insulin requirements and significantly simpler regimens due to the background of endogenous insulin produced by the islet transplant. This comprehensive improvement, addressing both the physical burden of pain and the metabolic challenges, allows individuals to resume a normal daily routine, returning to school or work with a profoundly enhanced quality of life. The holistic restoration of well-being for patients previously incapacitated by their condition includes psychological improvements that are frequently dramatic, especially in the younger patients with gene mutations, many of whom have had symptoms from early childhood.

The procedure's complexity limits its availability to a small number of specialized centers worldwide. The textbook *Total Pancreatectomy and Islet Autotransplantation: Principles and Practice* provides an authoritative and comprehensive exploration of TPIAT, which is only possible due to the legacy of the University of Minnesota Medical Center, widely recognized as the global pioneer of TPIAT. In 1977, David Sutherland and colleagues performed the world's first TPIAT procedure, marking a critical juncture in the management of pancreatic disease. Following the success of these early procedures, the University of Minnesota has developed the largest TPIAT program worldwide with an extraordinary volume of cases, spanning nearly five decades. This experience has resulted in an unparalleled amount of longitudinal data and clinical experience, which provides a unique perspective on long-term outcomes, the evolution of surgical techniques, and the nuances of patient management that is simply not available elsewhere.

The 16 chapters of this book are all authored by leading experts in the field, providing a comprehensive approach to all aspects of TPIAT, beginning with the historical evolution of the procedure and the pathophysiology of chronic pancreatitis. This background is so familiar to the Minneapolis TPIAT group that it facilitates a clear and logical explanation of the clinical indications and necessity for TPIAT. The detailed exploration of patient selection criteria ensures that practitioners can identify suitable candidates, balancing risks and benefits to optimize outcomes. Surgical techniques for total pancreatectomy are described in detail, and the intricacies of islet cell isolation and autotransplantation are explained to highlight the technical requirements needed to maximize the recovered islet cell mass. Postoperative management, a critical aspect of TPIAT, is thoroughly examined, providing guidance on how to address complications including endocrine and exocrine insufficiency. The chapters on outcomes offer a patient-centered perspective, emphasizing the impact of the procedure on quality of life. Long-term follow-up strategies and nutritional considerations are thoughtfully included, acknowledging the lifelong journey of TPIAT patients and the support required from the clinical team. Throughout this textbook, the multidisciplinary nature of TPIAT is stressed, with chapters dedicated to the roles of endocrinologists, gastroenterologists, and pain management colleagues in ensuring holistic care. Ethical considerations and patient counseling are given due attention, recognizing the profound decisions patients face. The book's comprehensive framework is designed to empower clinicians to identify the most appropriate candidates and manage them optimally, thereby realizing the procedure's full potential.

This book represents an indispensable guide for all healthcare professionals involved in the care of patients with complex pancreatic diseases. TPIAT requires technical, laboratory, and research components, all of which are at the frontiers of medical science and which continue to evolve. Continuous refinement of islet isolation techniques and the potential expansion of TPIAT indications to other challenging pancreatic conditions, including certain benign or borderline pancreatic tumors, are areas under consideration and are discussed.

Surgeons, endocrinologists, gastroenterologists, pain specialists, transplant coordinators, researchers, trainees, and patients will find this volume, born from the unparalleled experience of the Minneapolis group, to be the definitive reference work. It is poised to standardize best practice across multidisciplinary teams, shaping clinical practice and fostering continued advances in TPIAT for years to come, thereby elevating the global standard of care and improving patient outcomes worldwide. A fuller understanding of the opportunity provided by TPIAT also offers a perspective for clinical teams in units not presently able to perform TPIAT to understand all the options available for their patients. For units around the world who wish to develop TPIAT programs, the accumulated wisdom in this book will enable them to translate almost five decades of experience into a blueprint for the safe and compassionate treatment of patients with life-changing pancreatic disease.

I am honored to introduce this comprehensive work on TPIAT that serves as a fitting tribute to David Sutherland's legacy. I have no doubt that this textbook will not only educate and inform but also inspire continued innovation and excellence in the treatment of pancreatic diseases.

Ashley R. Dennison

Professor of Hepatobiliary and Pancreatic Surgery, University of Leicester
Leicester, UK

Consultant HPB Surgeon, Glenfield Hospital
University Hospitals of Leicester NHS Trust
Leicester, UK

Tribute to Sutherland

Tribute and Dedication to the Pioneer Who Lit the Path:

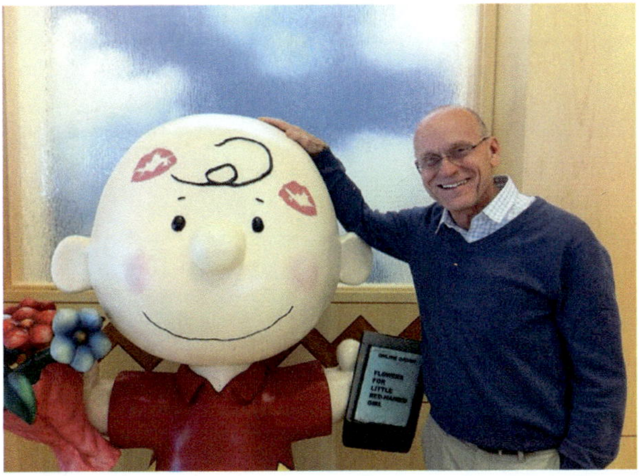

Professor David E. R. Sutherland, MD, PhD (1940–2025), was a transplant surgeon-scientist, pioneer of TPIAT surgery, and mentor whose visionary contributions to pancreas and islet transplantation have transformed the lives of patients with chronic pancreatitis and diabetes and offered hope where little existed before. His long and illustrious career included many firsts in the field of transplantation, including the world's first clinical islet transplants at the University of Minnesota in 1974 and the world's first total pancreatectomy and islet autotransplant (TPIAT) in 1977. This work stands on the foundation he built and is a continuation of the journey he began. Dr. Sutherland's legacy of world-class innovation and compassion lives on in this book, in thousands of patients, in the programs he built, and in the many surgeons he trained around the world.

Preface

Total pancreatectomy with islet autotransplantation (TPIAT) has evolved over the past five decades from a pioneering surgical endeavor, serendipitously discovered in a quest to cure diabetes mellitus with cell therapy, to an established, life-changing treatment for patients with chronic painful pancreatitis that is used when other medical and endoscopic options have failed. What began as a surgical procedure has now become a multidisciplinary therapeutic approach, requiring collaboration among surgeons, endocrinologists, gastroenterologists, pain specialists, radiologists, islet-ologists, and nurse coordinators.

The goal of this textbook is to serve as a comprehensive reference for physicians, surgeons, researchers, and trainees who care for patients with chronic pancreatitis that is refractory to conventional therapies. It aims to describe the latest surgical techniques, perioperative management strategies, advances in islet isolation, and long-term care paradigms. Each chapter reflects the knowledge of experts who have dedicated their careers to improving the outcomes and quality of life for patients facing this complex surgery. It aims not only to provide the latest review of the literature but also the pearls of wisdom learned by the authors in their journeys of caring for these challenging patients.

In addition to surgical techniques, this book emphasizes the importance of patient selection, preoperative counseling, multidisciplinary collaboration, post-operative pain management, and long-term follow-up of diabetes and gastrointestinal issues. It highlights the challenges that remain—expanding the indications to include patients with intraductal papillary mucinous neoplasms and pancreas neoplasms, improving islet yield, enhancing islet engraftment, and managing long-term diabetes risk—and the innovative solutions being developed to address these challenges.

We hope this work will serve as both a practical guide and an inspiration for continued innovation in this important field. Ultimately, our goal is to empower clinicians to offer TPIAT as a safe, effective, and compassionate option to patients with refractory painful chronic pancreatitis.

We are grateful to all the authors for their outstanding contributions, to Dr. Naomi Ruff for editorial support, to Hser Htoo for administrative support, to Dinesh Sinha at Byword Books, and to Springer Publishers for making this book a reality. Last but not least, our heartfelt thanks to the patients whose courage and resilience inspire our work every day.

Minneapolis, MN, USA

Srinath Chinnakotla
Melena D. Bellin
Greg J. Beilman

Contents

About the Editors and Contributors

Editors

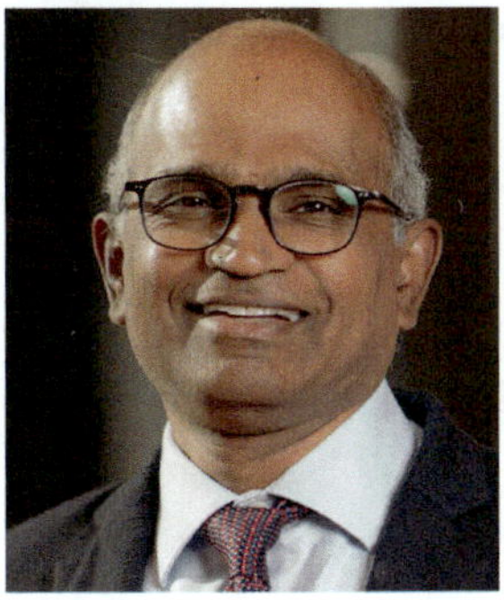

Srinath Chinnakotla is Professor of Surgery and Pediatrics and Surgical Director of Liver and Pediatric Transplantation at the University of Minnesota. He completed medical college at the Jawaharlal Institute of Postgraduate Medical Education & Research, Pondicherry, and surgical residency at JIPMER and AIIMS, New Delhi, India. He was inspired to be an academic surgeon by Prof. N. Ananthakrishnan. He relocated to United States and trained at the University of Nebraska to be a multiorgan transplant surgeon. Srinath is the lead surgeon of the largest TPIAT program in children, which has performed close to 200 TPIAT surgeries and pioneered islet autotransplantation techniques in the smallest children. He is deeply grateful to all his mentors, to his father Dr. C. Sreenivasulu and to his wife Ann Chinnakotla, who supported his pursuit of an academic career in the United States.

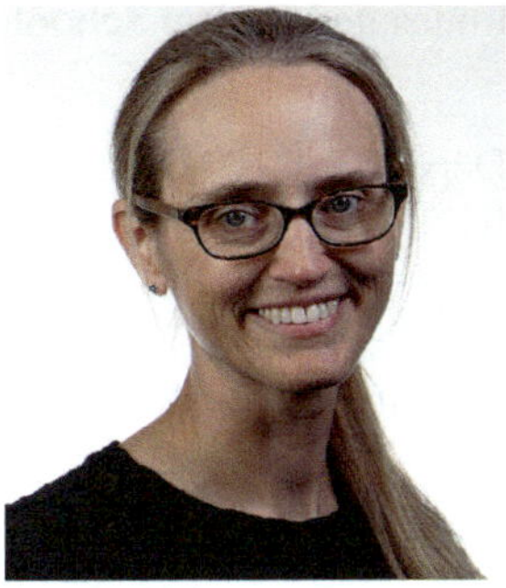

Melena D. Bellin completed her Medical School and Residency and Fellowship training at the University of Minnesota, where she is now a Professor of Pediatrics (Endocrinology) and Surgery, and Co-Director of the TPIAT Program. She has worked in the fields of pancreatitis and cell therapy for diabetes for nearly 20 years, where she has led multiple NIH-funded cohort studies and clinical trials in TPIAT. She has over 200 publications in the field to date and continues to study long-term outcomes as well as strategies to optimize islet engraftment and minimize diabetes risk in this population.

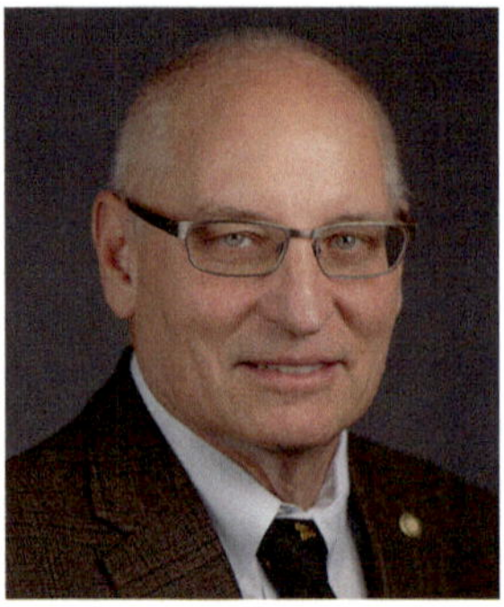

Greg J. Beilman, MD A general surgeon and ICU physician, Greg J. Beilman, MD, currently serves as Interim CEO of the University of Minnesota Physicians at the University of Minnesota Medical School. He is the Owen Wangensteen Research Chair and Professor of Surgery at the University of Minnesota. As a surgeon, Greg has a career-spanning interest in surgical management of acute and chronic pancreatitis. Greg is a retired Colonel in the Army Reserves and has deployed five times. Greg has an active translational research program funded by the Department of Defense, the NIH, and industry. He also has significant experience in Global Health efforts, with his experience in the Army, a decade of patient care and research efforts in Uganda, and recent efforts in Ukraine. Greg served as President of the Surgical Infection Society from 2019–2021.

Contributors

Maisam Abu-El-Haija Cincinnati Children's Hospital Medical Center, Cincinnati, OH, USA

Syed A. Ahmad Division of Surgical Oncology, University of Cincinnati Medical Center, Cincinnati, OH, USA

Francesca Aleotti Pancreatic Surgery Unit, IRCCS Ospedale San Raffaele, Milan, Italy

Appakalai N. Balamurugan Islet Transplantation and Beta Cell Biology, University of Louisville, Norton HealthCare, Louisville, KY, USA

Rosara Bass Nationwide Children's Hospital, OH, USA

Greg J. Beilman Department of Surgery, University of Minnesota Medical School, Minneapolis, MN, USA

Melena D. Bellin Division of Pediatric Endocrinology, Department of Pediatrics, University of Minnesota Medical School, Minneapolis, MN, USA

Louise Berry M Health Fairview, TPIAT Program, Minneapolis, MN, USA

Srinath Chinnakotla Department of Surgery, University of Minnesota Medical School and University of Minnesota Masonic Children's Hospital, Minneapolis, MN, USA

Marie Cook M Health Fairview, Pediatric TPIAT Program, Minneapolis, MN, USA

Elissa M. Downs Division of Pediatric Gastroenterology, Hepatology and Nutrition, University of Minnesota Medical School, Minneapolis, MN, USA

A. Jay Freeman Nationwide Children's Hospital, OH, USA

Martin L. Freeman Division of Gastroenterology, Hepatology and Nutrition, Department of Medicine, University of Minnesota Medical School, Minneapolis, MN, USA

Justin Howard Division of Gastroenterology, Hepatology and Nutrition, Department of Medicine, University of Minnesota Medical School, Minneapolis, MN, USA

Rachel P. Jacobsen M Health Fairview Masonic Children's Hospital, Minneapolis, MN, USA

Aamir Khan Division of Transplantation, Department of Surgery, Virginia Commonwealth University, Richmond, VA, USA

Varvara A. Kirchner Division of Abdominal Transplantation, Stanford University, Palo Alto, CA, USA

Shafahed Kodipad Microbiology and Biotechnology, University of Wolverhampton, Wolverhampton, UK

Jayachandra Kuncha Islet Cell Laboratory, Baylor Scott & White Research Institute, Dallas, TX, USA

Luis F. Lara Division of Digestive Diseases, University of Cincinnati, Cincinnati, OH, USA

Marlon Levy Division of Transplantation, Department of Surgery, Virginia Commonwealth University, Richmond, VA, USA

Bashoo Naziruddin Islet Cell Laboratory, Baylor Scott & White Research Institute, Dallas, TX, USA

Lorenzo Piemonti University "Vita Salute San Raffaele", Milan, Italy

Karthik Ramanathan Department of Surgery, University of Minnesota, Minneapolis, MN, USA

Megan A. Satyadi General Surgery, University of Cincinnati Medical Center, Cincinnati, OH, USA

Emily Scheidecker M Health Fairview, TPIAT Program, Minneapolis, MN, USA

Sarah Jane Schwarzenberg Department of Pediatric Gastroenterology, Hepatology and Nutrition, University of Minnesota, Minneapolis, MN, USA

Guru Trikudanathan Division of Gastroenterology, Hepatology and Nutrition, Department of Medicine, University of Minnesota Medical School, Minneapolis, MN, USA

Petr Vanek Department of Gastroenterology, Masaryk Memorial Cancer Institute, Brno, Czech Republic

Gregory C. Wilson Division of Surgical Oncology, University of Cincinnati College of Medicine, Cincinnati, OH, USA

1 History of Total Pancreatectomy with Islet Autotransplantation

Martin L. Freeman, Melena D. Bellin, Srinath Chinnakotla, and Greg J. Beilman

Abstract

Islet transplantation was first developed as an allogeneic procedure for patients with diabetes mellitus. When the initial allotransplants were unsuccessful, the procedure was attempted in a patient with chronic pancreatitis, undergoing total pancreatectomy using the patient's own islets isolated from the diseased pancreas. The first patient to receive total pancreatectomy (TP) with islet autotransplantation (IAT), in 1977, was cured of a 20-year history of severe pain and remained insulin-free for 6 years until her death from an accident. Subsequently, TPIAT was adopted as a standard procedure for chronic pancreatitis by centers around the world. As of 2025, more than 2000 TPIAT procedures have been performed.

M. L. Freeman
Division of Gastroenterology, Hepatology and Nutrition, Department of Medicine, University of Minnesota Medical School, Minneapolis, MN, USA

M. D. Bellin
Division of Pediatric Endocrinology, Department of Pediatrics, University of Minnesota Medical School, Minneapolis, MN, USA

S. Chinnakotla (✉)
Department of Surgery, University of Minnesota Medical School and University of Minnesota Masonic Children's Hospital, Minneapolis, MN, USA
e-mail: chinni@umn.edu

G. J. Beilman
Department of Surgery, University of Minnesota Medical School, Minneapolis, MN, USA

S. Chinnakotla et al. (eds.), *Total Pancreatectomy and Islet Auto Transplantation*, https://doi.org/10.1007/978-981-92-0018-4_1

Key Points

1. Allogeneic transplantation was first used to treat diabetes mellitus, starting with whole pancreas, then pancreas fragments, and finally isolated islets.
2. Thorough digestion of the pancreas with collagenase and infusion of the isolated islets into the portal vein led to engraftment.
3. Islet autotransplantation (IAT) avoided the immunological rejection that occurred with allotransplantation.
4. Early success with total pancreatectomy with IAT (TPIAT) led to its adoption as a treatment option for painful chronic pancreatitis in patients for whom duct clearance or partial resection was not effective.

1.1 Islet Allotransplantation for Treatment of Diabetes

At the University of Minnesota in early 1968, experiments were ongoing to discover a cure for diabetes. Initial experiments with whole-organ pancreas transplantation in humans were associated with high morbidity and mortality [10]. Attempts to transplant adult pancreatic fragments as free grafts were unsuccessful because the associated exuberant enzymes autodigested the transplanted tissue or injured the host [12]. Therefore, attempts were made to isolate the islets from the pancreas and use them for allotransplantation. The objectives of transplanting the whole pancreas or the islets of Langerhans were the same: to establish normal carbohydrate homeostasis in patients with diabetes mellitus. Techniques for isolation of islets from the pancreas entailed disrupting the exocrine tissue by retrograde perfusion of fluid through the pancreas, mincing the pancreas, and dissociating exocrine and islet tissue with collagenase [13]. Islets are physically less dense than other pancreatic components, so they can be separated from exocrine tissue by centrifugation in a discontinuous density gradient of Ficoll (a polymer of sucrose) [14].

1.2 Identifying the Optimal Site for Transplantation of the Islets

In the initial experiments, isolated islets were transplanted into the peritoneal cavity of rats with drug-induced diabetes [17]. It was noted that the amelioration of diabetes depended on the quantity of islets transplanted. The effectiveness of the islet transplantation was further improved by infusion of islets into the portal vein of the rat [20]: the islets lodged within portal venules without causing deterioration in liver function [20], and the same number of islets that only partially ameliorated the diabetic state when transplanted intraperitoneally would completely normalize plasma glucose levels when transplanted into the portal vein [17]. Further experiments were conducted in pigs, monkeys, and dogs with diabetes induced by either pancreatectomy or streptozotocin [19].

This new technique succeeded for several reasons [20]. First, 90% of exuberant enzyme activity is destroyed during collagenase digestion. Second, collagenase digestion reduces the tissue fragments to a size that allows them to survive by nutrient diffusion until neovascularization occurs. Third, the liver could tolerate the introduction of exuberant tissue, perhaps because its rapid sinusoidal blood flow dilutes or inactivates residual exocrine digestive enzymes [20].

1.3 How the Idea of Islet Autotransplantation Was Initiated

In the first report of human treatment, published in 1977 [16], ten islet transplant procedures were performed in seven patients who had insulin-dependent diabetes mellitus and had undergone kidney transplantation for end-stage diabetic nephropathy 10–36 months earlier. Islet cells for transplantation were procured from infant cadaveric donors. Islet cells were dispersed intraperitoneally in five procedures, implanted in a muscle pocket in one, and infused into the portal vein in four [16]. Although there was initial evidence of graft function and a reduction in insulin requirements in most recipients, there was no significant long-term islet graft function [16]. It was difficult to distinguish graft failure caused by immunological rejection from that caused by inadequate islet mass or technical problems. Dr. David Sutherland discussed these findings with Dr. John Najarian, the chair of surgery at the University of Minnesota at that time, who suggested comparing these outcomes to the outcomes of islet autografts in pancreatectomized patients who could not reject their graft, thus eliminating immunological reaction as a cause of graft failure [20]. This rationale led to the development of islet autotransplantation.

1.4 The Index Case of Human Islet Autotransplantation

The first patient to receive an islet autotransplant was a 39-year-old woman referred to the University of Minnesota Hospital with a 20-year history of repeated episodes of abdominal pain [20]. Peptic ulcer disease had been documented 10 years previously, at which time a combined vagotomy, antrectomy, and gastroduodenostomy were performed. She continued to have abdominal pain, but a recurrent ulcer could not be demonstrated. She was diagnosed with dumping syndrome and underwent a Roux-en-Y gastrojejunostomy. Despite that intervention, she continued to have constant abdominal pain. Although her serum amylase levels were normal, she had lost weight and developed foamy, foul-smelling, waxy stools suggestive of pancreatic insufficiency. She used narcotic analgesics in an attempt to gain pain relief. A clinical diagnosis of chronic pancreatitis was entertained, although the etiology of pancreatitis was obscure. She did not drink alcoholic beverages, but two of her uncles also had a history of pancreatitis, suggesting a familial origin. On physical examination, she was a thin, pale woman with a midline scar and a tender epigastrium. Hematological and blood chemistry results were normal. The estimation of fat in the stool was elevated at 22%, but no other laboratory evidence of malabsorption was found. The results of two glucose tolerance tests were normal. Gastroscopy results were normal. In that era, advanced imaging such as magnetic resonance cholangiopancreatography (MRCP) and even computed tomography (CT) were not available. Because of the previous Roux-en-Y gastrojejunostomy, a retrograde pancreatic ductogram was not possible. Instead, a laparotomy was performed. The preoperative plan was to do a pancreatic ductogram through the tail of the pancreas in order to define the etiology of the pancreatitis and to determine if a pancreatic duct drainage procedure was possible. If not, a near-total pancreatectomy was planned, followed by autotransplantation of the islets. At the time of exploration, the pancreas was fibrotic in appearance. The biopsy of the pancreas confirmed the diagnosis of chronic pancreatitis. A near-total pancreatectomy was performed. The excised portion of the pancreas weighed 42 grams. Immediately upon removal, it was immersed in iced saline and transported to the islet-processing laboratory, where it was rapidly minced in a specially designed mechanical tissue chopper and digested for 20 min with 1440 units of collagenase per gram of tissue in 100 ml of medium 199 at 37 °C. Total tissue insulin content of the pancreas before processing was 17,860 μg; after processing, it was 9877 μg, which meant that 55% of the islet mass was recovered. The suspended tissue containing the patient's own islets was returned to the operating room 1.5 h after the pancreatectomy.

The tissue was slowly infused into the liver via a mesenteric vein. The portal pressure rose from 10 to 14 cm of water during infusion. On the first postoperative day, the plasma glucose levels ranged from 229 to 352 mg/dL. Plasma glucose levels ranged from 140 to 284 mg/dl for the next 4 days and then declined to between 100 and 195 mg/dL for the next 2 weeks. The first week after surgery, the patient received a continuous intravenous infusion of glucose solution, after which she was given oral feedings. Beginning 3 weeks after transplantation, fasting plasma glucose levels ranged from 77 to 204 mg/dL. The patient did not receive insulin at any time after the IAT; the glucose tolerance tests are shown in Fig. 1.1. She was started on pancreatic enzymes. Her liver function tests were mildly elevated, but they

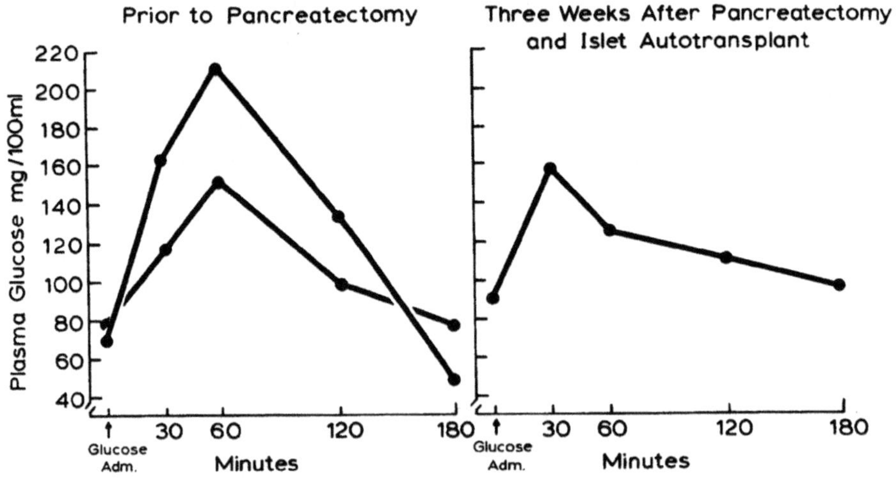

Fig. 1.1 Glucose tolerance test before and after total pancreatectomy in one patient

normalized within 1 month after surgery. The patient was dependent on narcotics for about 6 months after the surgery, but then was successfully withdrawn from narcotic use. She remained pain-free and insulin-free for 6 years after the surgery, when she died after a horseback riding accident [20].

The most important aspect of this case was the establishment of the technical feasibility of islet transplantation in humans [4]. A large quantity of semipurified islet tissue was infused into the portal vein system with no deterioration of liver function, and diabetes was obviated. Thus, if an equal quantity of allogeneic tissue freshly prepared from a cadaveric pancreas failed to ameliorate diabetes after transplantation into a diabetic recipient, failure could be attributed to rejection rather than to technical problems. Because rejection was not an issue with the autotransplant procedure, its success emphasized the need for investigations to focus on the immunological aspects of clinical islet allotransplantation [20].

1.5 Total Pancreatectomy and Islet Transplantation Becomes a Treatment Option for Painful Chronic Pancreatitis

Conventional surgical approaches to chronic pancreatitis include drainage or partial resection procedures. Despite fair success in patients with markedly dilated pancreatic ducts, such operations are not feasible in the majority of patients with chronic pancreatitis, who often have nondilated ducts. Despite technical success, such operations often fail to provide lifelong relief of pain, especially in younger patients with hereditary pancreatitis. Endoscopic therapy has emerged over recent decades as an effective option for patients with chronic pancreatitis, and especially for those with main duct pancreatic stone disease—as long as the duct can be effectively and completely cleared. Complete duct clearance is only possible in about two-thirds of patients using standard endoscopic techniques or extracorporeal shock wave lithotripsy [3, 11] but is now nearly universal with further developments in endoscopic therapy, including pancreatoscopic lithotripsy techniques. Despite all these improvements in nonsurgical techniques, a substantial proportion of patients have intractable pain and may be candidates for total pancreatectomy with islet autotransplantation (TPIAT), especially patients who are younger and without diabetes. As a result of recent progress in both endoscopic therapy and TPIAT, and the fact that traditional drainage operations greatly reduce islet cell yields, an adaptive approach has been adopted at the University of Minnesota to avoid drainage operations in patients who might become candidates for TPIAT [2].

1.6 Adoption of TPIAT Worldwide

Following the success of the Minnesota case, several centers around the United States and the world adopted this procedure (Table 1.1) [1, 2, 5, 8, 15, 23]. In addition to the University of Minnesota, large numbers of islet autotransplants were

Table 1.1 TPIAT procedures worldwide

Authors [ref]	Period	Institution	Number of procedures
Hinshaw et al. [9]	1979–1980	Loma Linda University	5
Rastellini et al. [18]	1990–1996	University of Pittsburgh	5
Wilson et al. [25]	2000–2013	University of Cincinnati	166
Argo et al. [1]	2005–2007	University of Alabama, Birmingham	21
Dixon et al. [6]	1998–2008	Medical University of South Carolina	7
Takita et al. [22]	2006–2009	Baylor University Medical Center	17
Sutherland et al. [21]	1997–2011	University of Minnesota	409
Walsh et al. [24]	2007–2010	Cleveland Clinic	20
Dorlon et al. [7]	2009–2012	Medical University of South Carolina	74
Garcea et al. [8]	1996–2006	University of Leicester	85

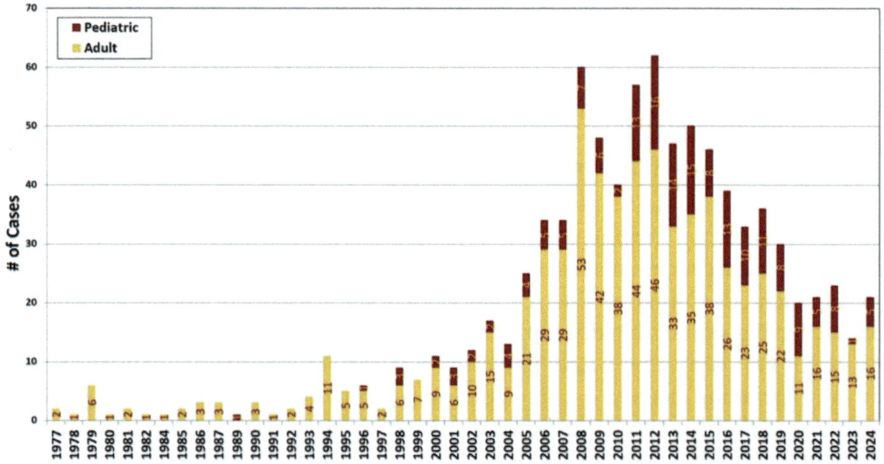

Fig. 1.2 Total pancreatectomy and islet autotransplants performed at the University of Minnesota from the first through 2024

performed at the University of Cincinnati, the University of Leicester, and the University of Geneva early on; together, these centers accounted for approximately 300 patients by the year 2006. The number of centers has continuously expanded worldwide, and, as of 2025, more than 2000 TPIAT procedures have been performed, including 842 at the University of Minnesota (Fig. 1.2).

References

1. Argo JL, Contreras JL, Wesley MM, Christein JD. Pancreatic resection with islet cell autotransplant for the treatment of severe chronic pancreatitis. Am Surg. 2008;74(6):530–6. discussion 6–7
2. Bellin MD, Abu-El-Haija M, Morgan K, Adams D, Beilman GJ, Chinnakotla S, et al. A multicenter study of total pancreatectomy with islet autotransplantation (TPIAT): POST (prospective observational study of TPIAT). Pancreatology. 2018;18(3):286–90. https://doi.org/10.1016/j.pan.2018.02.001.
3. Bick BL, Patel F, Easler JJ, Tong Y, Watkins JL, McHenry L, et al. A comparative study between single-operator pancreatoscopy with intraductal lithotripsy and extracorporeal shock wave lithotripsy for the management of large main pancreatic duct stones. Surg Endosc. 2022;36(5):3217–26. https://doi.org/10.1007/s00464-021-08631-7.
4. Blondet JJ, Carlson AM, Kobayashi T, Jie T, Bellin M, Hering BJ, et al. The role of total pancreatectomy and islet autotransplantation for chronic pancreatitis. Surg Clin North Am. 2007;87(6):1477–501. https://doi.org/10.1016/j.suc.2007.08.014.
5. Coluzzi M, Takita M, Saracino G, Rub Hakim Mohammed A, Darden CM, Testa G, et al. Improved quality of life among chronic pancreatitis patients undergoing total pancreatectomy with islet autotransplantation-single center experience with large cohort of patients. Transpl Int. 2023;36:11409. https://doi.org/10.3389/ti.2023.11409.
6. Dixon J, DeLegge M, Morgan KA, Adams DB. Impact of total pancreatectomy with islet cell transplant on chronic pancreatitis management at a disease-based center. Am Surg. 2008;74(8):735–8. https://doi.org/10.1177/000313480807400812.
7. Dorlon M, Owczarski S, Wang H, Adams D, Morgan K. Increase in postoperative insulin requirements does not lead to decreased quality of life after total pancreatectomy with islet cell autotransplantation for chronic pancreatitis. Am Surg. 2013;79(7):676–80.
8. Garcea G, Weaver J, Phillips J, Pollard CA, Ilouz SC, Webb MA, et al. Total pancreatectomy with and without islet cell transplantation for chronic pancreatitis: a series of 85 consecutive patients. Pancreas. 2009;38(1):1–7. https://doi.org/10.1097/MPA.0b013e3181825c00.
9. Hinshaw DB, Jolley WB, Hinshaw DB, Kaiser JE, Hinshaw K. Islet autotransplantation after pancreatectomy for chronic pancreatitis with a new method of islet preparation. Am J Surg. 1981;142(1):118–22. https://doi.org/10.1016/s0002-9610(81)80020-7.
10. Idezuki Y, Goetz FC, Merkel FK, Najarian JS, Kelly WD, Lillehei RC. Experiences with pancreaticoduodenal allotransplantation. Rev Fr Etud Clin Biol. 1968;13(10):996–9.
11. Issa Y, Kempeneers MA, Bruno MJ, Fockens P, Poley J-W, Ahmed Ali U, et al. Effect of early surgery vs endoscopy-first approach on pain in patients with chronic pancreatitis: the ESCAPE randomized clinical trial. JAMA. 2020;323(3):237–47. https://doi.org/10.1001/jama.2019.20967.
12. Kretschmer GJ. Autotransplantation of pancreatic fragments: investigations in totally pancreatectomized dogs (author's transl). Wien Klin Wochenschr Suppl. 1978;96:3–18.
13. Lacy PE, Kostianovsky M. Method for the isolation of intact islets of Langerhans from the rat pancreas. Diabetes. 1967;16(1):35–9. https://doi.org/10.2337/diab.16.1.35.
14. Lindall A, Steffes M, Sorenson R. Immunoassayable insulin content of subcellular fractions of rat islets. Endocrinology. 1969;85(2):218–23. https://doi.org/10.1210/endo-85-2-218.
15. Morgan KA, Lancaster WP, Owczarski SM, Wang H, Borckardt J, Adams DB. Patient selection for total pancreatectomy with islet autotransplantation in the surgical management of chronic pancreatitis. J Am Coll Surg. 2018;226(4):446–51. https://doi.org/10.1016/j.jamcollsurg.2017.12.018.
16. Najarian JS, Sutherland DE, Matas AJ, Steffes MW, Simmons RL, Goetz FC. Human islet transplantation: a preliminary report. Transplant Proc. 1977;9(1):233–6.
17. Nelken D, Morse SI, Beyer MM, Friedman EA. Prolonged survival of allotransplanted islet of langerhans cells in the rat. Transplantation. 1976;22(1):74–5. https://doi.org/10.1097/00007890-197607000-00013.

18. Rastellini C, Shapiro R, Corry R, Fung JJ, Starzl TE, Rao AS. Treatment of isolated pancreatic islets to reverse pancreatectomy-induced and insulin-dependent type I diabetes in humans: a 6-year experience. Transplant Proc. 1997;29(1–2):746–7. https://doi.org/10.1016/s0041-1345(96)00449-6.
19. Sutherland DE, Steffes MW, Bauer GE, McManus D, Noe BD, Najarian JS. Isolation of human and porcine islets of Langerhans and islet transplantation in pigs. J Surg Res. 1974;16(2):102–11. https://doi.org/10.1016/0022-4804(74)90017-1.
20. Sutherland DE, Matas AJ, Najarian JS. Pancreatic islet cell transplantation. Surg Clin North Am. 1978;58(2):365–82. https://doi.org/10.1016/s0039-6109(16)41489-1.
21. Sutherland DE, Radosevich DM, Bellin MD, Hering BJ, Beilman GJ, Dunn TB, et al. Total pancreatectomy and islet autotransplantation for chronic pancreatitis. J Am Coll Surg. 2012;214(4):409–24; discussion 24–6. https://doi.org/10.1016/j.jamcollsurg.2011.12.040.
22. Takita M, Naziruddin B, Matsumoto S, Noguchi H, Shimoda M, Chujo D, et al. Implication of pancreatic image findings in total pancreatectomy with islet autotransplantation for chronic pancreatitis. Pancreas. 2011;40(1):103–8. https://doi.org/10.1097/MPA.0b013e3181f749bc.
23. Turner KM, Delman AM, Donovan EC, Brunner J, Wahab SA, Dai Y, et al. Total pancreatectomy and islet cell autotransplantation: a 10-year update on outcomes and assessment of long-term durability. HPB (Oxford). 2022;24(11):2013–21. https://doi.org/10.1016/j.hpb.2022.07.001.
24. Walsh RM, Saavedra JRA, Lentz G, Guerron AD, Scheman J, Stevens T, et al. Improved quality of life following total pancreatectomy and auto-islet transplantation for chronic pancreatitis. J Gastrointest Surg. 2012;16(8):1469–77. https://doi.org/10.1007/s11605-012-1914-6.
25. Wilson GC, Sutton JM, Abbott DE, Smith MT, Lowy AM, Matthews JB, et al. Long-term outcomes after total pancreatectomy and islet cell autotransplantation: is it a durable operation? Ann Surg. 2014;260(4):659–65; discussion 65–7. https://doi.org/10.1097/SLA.0000000000000920.

Indications and Patient Selection for Total Pancreatectomy and Islet Autotransplant

2

Greg J. Beilman

It seems unreasonable to tell a patient to wait an indeterminate number of years in the hope of spontaneous subsidence of pain when surgery can offer a 75% success rate. (Andrew Warshaw, 1984)

Abstract

Selecting appropriate candidates for total pancreatectomy and islet autotransplant (TPIAT) is a complex process. The TPIAT procedure is distinctive for several reasons, including the requirement for an experienced surgeon, a specialized islet cell isolation facility, and a committed multidisciplinary team. Islet autotransplantation does not necessitate immunosuppression, but perioperative morbidity remains significant (up to 60%). Patients being considered for TPIAT are best evaluated through a multidisciplinary team approach involving experts in a variety of specialties, utilizing an organized patient-specific treatment algorithm, with care tailored to the individual's needs. The optimal time point for surgery is after issues with lifestyle related to pain or recurrent acute pancreatitis have developed, but before long-term complications from chronic pain arise. Multiple studies have demonstrated that surgery within 24–36 months of the onset of daily pain leads to higher rates of partial or complete pain relief, lower incidence of exocrine insufficiency, and reduced need for further interventions. Patients considered for TPIAT must have confirmed chronic pancreatitis or recurrent acute pancreatitis, significant lifestyle disruption, no reversible underlying cause, failure to improve with medical and endoscopic treatments, and preserved islet cell function. They should not have active cancer, substance abuse, significant heart,

G. J. Beilman (✉)
Department of Surgery, University of Minnesota Medical School, Minneapolis, MN, USA
e-mail: beilman@umn.edu

S. Chinnakotla et al. (eds.), *Total Pancreatectomy and Islet Auto Transplantation*,
https://doi.org/10.1007/978-981-92-0018-4_2

lung, or liver disease, poorly controlled psychiatric conditions, or an inability to support the recovery process.

Key Points
1. The total pancreatectomy and islet autotransplant (TPIAT) procedure requires an experienced surgeon and a specialized islet cell isolation facility.
2. Patients being considered for TPIAT are best evaluated through a multidisciplinary team approach involving experts in a variety of specialties and utilizing an organized patient-specific treatment algorithm, with care tailored to the individual's needs.
3. Islet autotransplantation does not necessitate immunosuppression, but perioperative morbidity remains significant.
4. The optimal time point for surgery is after development of issues with lifestyle related to pain or recurrent acute pancreatitis, but before long-term complications from chronic pain develop; surgery within 24–36 months of onset of daily pain leads to better outcomes.
5. Patients considered for TPIAT must have confirmed chronic pancreatitis or recurrent acute pancreatitis, significant lifestyle disruption, no reversible underlying cause, failure to improve with medical and endoscopic treatments, and preserved islet cell function. They should not have active cancer, substance abuse, significant heart, lung, or liver disease, poorly controlled psychiatric conditions, or an inability to support the recovery process.

2.1 Introduction

Selecting appropriate candidates for total pancreatectomy and islet autotransplant (TPIAT) is a complex process. Although the main objective of the procedure is pain relief, the underlying mechanisms of pain in chronic pancreatitis are not fully understood. Various theories, largely derived from observational studies, attempt to explain its multifactorial nature. In cases with strictures, stones, or disrupted ducts, pain is thought to result from increased pressure within the ducts, interstitial hypertension, and ischemia. The neuropathic theory attributes pain to abnormal nerve growth within the pancreas and heightened perineural inflammation.

Often, the intensity of pain does not correspond with the degree of fibrosis or pancreatic dysfunction, adding another layer of complexity to determining appropriate surgical candidates. A tailored, case-by-case evaluation is essential to match the right therapy to the patient's specific condition. For example, individuals with dilated main ducts or an enlarged pancreatic head may benefit from endoscopic or surgical drainage. Those with localized disease, such as a single stricture, duct disruption, or disease isolated to the pancreatic tail, may respond well to a distal pancreatectomy. However, an increasing number of patients do not qualify for standard surgical or endoscopic treatments and may be appropriate candidates for TPIAT.

In 1977, David Sutherland and colleagues at the University of Minnesota performed the first TPIAT. The procedure was initially conducted to explore the function of isolated pancreatic islets following their transplantation into the portal venous system. Notably, this approach not only alleviated chronic pancreatitis-related pain but also preserved long-term islet cell function [1, 2]. What began as an experimental surgery at a single institution has since expanded to over two dozen centers worldwide, with more than 1000 reported cases [3].

This procedure is distinctive for several reasons. It requires an experienced surgeon to perform one of the more technically demanding operations in modern surgery, as well as a specialized islet cell isolation facility. Additionally, a multidisciplinary team is essential for managing patient care, including addressing diabetes, malnutrition, pain, and exocrine dysfunction, throughout the preoperative evaluation phase, surgery, and recovery. In contrast to most solid organ transplants, IAT does not necessitate immunosuppression, because the patient receives their own tissue. While mortality rates for this surgery remain low (<1% in reported series), perioperative morbidity remains significant, with rates reaching up to 60% following pancreatectomy [4].

2.2 Etiology of Chronic Pancreatitis

One of the challenges in understanding chronic pancreatitis is its often multifactorial origin. The TIGAR-O classification system outlines various risk factors linked to chronic pancreatitis, including toxic-metabolic, idiopathic, genetic, autoimmune, recurrent and severe acute pancreatitis, as well as obstructive causes [5]. Alcohol is the most common contributing factor, playing a role in 40–70% of cases, although fewer than 5% of heavy drinkers develop chronic pancreatitis [6–8]. Smoking is another significant lifestyle factor, both as an independent risk and in combination with alcohol [7, 9].

Certain congenital abnormalities, such as annular pancreas and pancreas divisum, may increase susceptibility to chronic pancreatitis but typically require an additional environmental or genetic risk factor [9]. Advances in DNA sequencing have improved the identification of hereditary pancreatitis, leading to a decline in cases previously labeled as idiopathic. Genetic mutations in *PRSS1, SPINK1, CFTR, CTRC*, and *CASR* have been linked to chronic pancreatitis [10]. Most individuals with a genetic cause of recurrent acute or chronic pancreatitis possess multiple gene variants or experience complex genetic interactions, often in conjunction with environmental stressors [9].

Autoimmune pancreatitis (AIP) is a systemic autoimmune disorder that affects both the pancreas and other organs. It is typically managed with steroids, though sustaining remission can be difficult, and surgical intervention is rarely required [11]. Differentiating AIP from malignancy is crucial, as its presentation can be similar, and unnecessary pancreatic resections have been reported in up to 43% of cases [12].

2.3 Evaluation for Surgery

For patients suspected of having chronic pancreatitis, diagnosis involves a combination of imaging and laboratory assessments. Conducting a thorough patient evaluation is essential for developing a personalized treatment approach (Table 2.1). Functional tests include measuring fecal fat and elastase levels, as well as evaluating pancreatic bicarbonate secretion in response to intravenous secretin. Although diagnosis is often based on clinical symptoms, it should be confirmed through imaging modalities such as endoscopic ultrasound, endoscopic retrograde cholangiopancreatography (ERCP), magnetic resonance cholangiopancreatography, or computed tomography (CT), with a focus on identifying ductal dilation, pancreatic atrophy,

Table 2.1 Evaluation of patients for TPIAT: common components

History:
Drug and alcohol use
Genetic testing
Imaging
Pancreatic interventions
Episodes of pancreatitis
Imaging:
Computed tomography
Magnetic resonance cholangiopancreatography
Endoscopic ultrasound (EUS)
Laboratory:
Fecal elastase
Genetic testing (younger patients, family Hx, no obvious cause)
PEth test
Urine and serum drug screen (selected patients)
CA19–9, CEA
Hemoglobin A1C
Functional testing:
Pancreatic function tests (usually performed at time of EUS)
Mixed meal testing (to evaluate for islet function)

TPIAT total pancreatectomy with islet autotransplant, *PEth* phosphatidylethanol (useful to confirm abstinence from alcohol consumption), *CEA* carcinoembryonic antigen

and calcifications [13]. Diagnostic testing in this setting is further discussed in Chap. 3. Younger patients with no clear underlying cause should undergo genetic counseling and testing. Consulting a medical psychologist is often beneficial as part of the overall evaluation process when determining the most appropriate intervention. For older patients, tumor markers should be evaluated to rule out malignancy as a potential cause of pancreatitis. The use of TPIAT in selected patients with intrapancreatic mucinous neoplasm and other tumors is discussed in Chap. 15. It is critically important to consider other sources of chronic abdominal pain and investigate these as needed.

Once chronic pancreatitis is diagnosed, initial management should focus on medical therapy. This includes lifestyle modifications such as abstaining from alcohol and smoking, along with pain management using non-opioid analgesics like nonsteroidal anti-inflammatory drugs. Opioids should be reserved as a last-line treatment but are often necessary [14]. Additional pain management strategies may involve tricyclic antidepressants, neuromodulating agents such as gabapentin, or interventional techniques like plexus nerve blocks or transcutaneous electrical nerve stimulation. Pancreatic enzyme supplementation may help alleviate pain by regulating feedback mechanisms [15]. As the disease progresses, endocrine dysfunction may require dietary adjustments and supplemental insulin therapy, though these complications typically arise in later stages [13, 14].

However, medical treatment should not continue indefinitely. In recent years, the approach to treating chronic pancreatitis has shifted from prioritizing medical and endoscopic management before considering surgery to a more proactive surgical strategy. Surgery should not be considered a last resort after medical and endoscopic treatments have repeatedly failed. Multiple randomized controlled trials have demonstrated that surgery provides equivalent or superior long-term pain relief compared to endoscopic interventions in selected patient populations [16–20]. According to the 2020 international consensus guidelines [21], both endoscopy and surgery should be considered for patients experiencing severe pain, with surgery recommended following an initial endoscopic attempt. For cases involving pancreatic duct obstruction due to stones or strictures, ERCP may be performed, potentially with pancreatic ductal stenting. Additional endoscopic procedures, such as pancreatic pseudocyst drainage, extracorporeal shock wave lithotripsy for pancreatic stones, endoscopic celiac nerve blocks, or pancreatic sphincterotomy, may also be utilized depending on the patient's specific condition [21, 22].

The primary reason for surgical intervention is persistent, severe pain. Like the fairy tale of the porridge that was just right, performing surgery at just the right time in the disease course is recommended. The optimal time point is after pain or recurrent acute pancreatitis have begun to interfere with lifestyle, but before long-term complications from chronic pain arise [23]. Multiple studies have demonstrated that surgery within 24–36 months of the onset of daily pain leads to higher rates of partial or complete pain relief, lower incidence of exocrine insufficiency, and reduced need for further interventions [17–19, 23–26].

Early surgical intervention may also help prevent ongoing inflammation and fibrosis, which can contribute to neuropathic pain—an especially challenging condition to manage—as well as pancreatic exocrine insufficiency resulting from continued destruction of acinar cells. Additional reasons for surgery include localized complications such as vascular damage, pancreatic fistulas, large pseudocysts, biliary or duodenal strictures, and suspected malignancy [27]. The appropriate surgical intervention depends on patient factors including anatomy, etiology of pancreatitis, and patient's location within the disease process. It is critical to tailor the appropriate surgical intervention based on consideration of these factors.

2.4 Decision-Making Process

At our institution, candidates for TPIAT are evaluated through a multidisciplinary team approach with a weekly meeting involving specialists in gastroenterology, surgery, endocrinology, nursing coordination, health psychology, genetics, nutrition, social work, and pain management. We follow a patient-specific treatment algorithm (Fig. 2.1), with care tailored to the individual's needs. Many patients benefit from medical or endoscopic treatments. For those with pancreatic calcifications and a dilated duct, drainage procedures like the Frey or Beger operations are often recommended, as they typically result in shorter recovery times and favorable long-term outcomes in well-selected patients [28].

Patients who do not respond to medical or endoscopic therapy frequently have small-duct or minimal-change chronic pancreatitis, which involves chronic

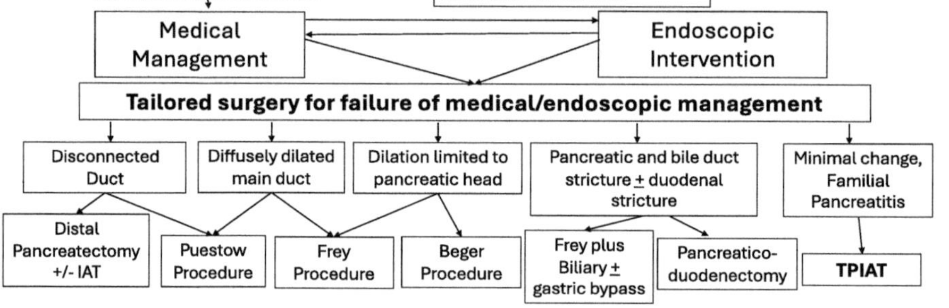

Fig. 2.1 Evaluation and management of patients with chronic pain from pancreatitis. An important concept in the surgical management of patients with pancreatitis is the need for tailored therapy based on patient anatomy and clinical scenario. Total pancreatectomy and islet autotransplantation (TPIAT) is appropriate for a subset of all patients presenting with pancreatitis. *CP*: chronic pancreatitis, *CT*: computed tomography, *EUS*: endoscopic ultrasound, *MRCP*: magnetic resonance cholangiopancreatography

inflammation and damage to the pancreas leading to both exocrine and endocrine dysfunction, as well as ongoing abdominal pain, despite the absence of main duct dilation [29]. In these cases, total pancreatectomy is often the only effective surgical option for pain control [30, 31]. Individuals with genetic or familial forms of the disease are also more likely to experience recurrent or worsening pancreatitis [32].

Eligibility for TPIAT at our institution is based on criteria originally described in 2013 [33]. The *Minnesota criteria* have evolved as research and outcomes from our center and others have allowed tailoring of these factors (Table 2.2). Candidates must have confirmed chronic pancreatitis, significant lifestyle disruption, no reversible underlying cause, failure to improve with medical and endoscopic treatments, and preserved islet cell function. We believe it is important to intervene with surgery at a point when the burden of acute recurrent pancreatitis or chronic pancreatitis is

Table 2.2 University of Minnesota criteria for total pancreatectomy and islet autotransplantation (must fulfill criteria 1–5 and have no active contraindications)

1. Diagnosis of chronic pancreatitis, based on chronic abdominal pain of ≥6-month duration and at least one of the following:
Pancreatic calcifications on computed tomography scan
At least two of the following: ≥4/9 criteria on EUS[a]; compatible ductal or parenchymal abnormalities on secretin MRCP; abnormal endoscopic pancreatic function tests (peak $HCO_3 \leq 80$ mmol/L), abnormal fecal elastase (<200 mcg/g)
Histopathology-confirmed diagnosis of chronic pancreatitis
Compatible clinical history and documented hereditary pancreatitis (e.g., *PRSS1* gene mutation)
History of recurrent acute pancreatitis (more than one episode of characteristic pain associated with imaging diagnostic of acute pancreatitis and/or elevated serum amylase or lipase greater than three times the upper limit of normal)
2. At least one of the following:
Daily narcotic dependence
Pain resulting in impaired quality of life, which may include inability to attend school or work, recurrent hospitalizations, or inability to participate in usual age-appropriate activities
3. Complete evaluation with no reversible cause of pancreatitis present or untreated
4. Failure to respond to appropriate medical and endoscopic therapy
5. Adequate islet cell function (nondiabetic or C-peptide positive on mixed meal test)
Contraindications:
1. Active alcoholism (abstinence for 6 months with documented PEth test prior to surgery).
2. Pancreatic cancer, IPMN[b].
3. End-stage pulmonary disease, cirrhosis, or severe cardiac disease.
4. Poorly controlled psychiatric illness.
5. Inability to comply with postoperative regimen.
6. Illegal drug use (patient must be abstinent for 6 months).

Patients must fulfill each of criteria 1–5

MRCP magnetic resonance cholangiopancreatography, *PEth* phosphatidylethanol

[a]Endoscopic ultrasound criteria of 6/9 or greater are associated with the presence of chronic pancreatitis on surgical pathology in 100% of patients studied [39]

[b]Use of total pancreatectomy and islet autotransplantation in patients with pancreatic cancer or intrapancreatic mucinous neoplasm (IPMN) is discussed further in Chap. 35

creating a significant need to adjust lifestyle (e.g., need for daily narcotics, frequent absences from work, dropping out of school). In our practice, it is not uncommon to see occasional patients before these lifestyle changes have reached a burdensome point. In many such cases, surgical intervention can be delayed until the point where changes have become more burdensome.

Certain factors exclude patients from undergoing this procedure. These include active substance abuse (requiring a minimum of 6 months of sobriety), significant heart or lung disease that increases surgical risk, poorly controlled psychiatric conditions, or an inability to support the sometimes-complicated recovery process [34]. Additionally, pancreatic cancer or widespread pancreatic tumors, as well as existing liver disease such as cirrhosis, portal hypertension, or portal vein thrombosis, are contraindications to major pancreatic surgery or islet transplantation [30, 35]. Patients with diabetes who lack a C-peptide response are also not candidates for islet autotransplantation due to poor islet yield and graft function; however, they may undergo total pancreatectomy alone [36].

It is difficult to overemphasize the importance of multidisciplinary participation and shared decision-making involved in patients with a complex background. In most patients, this discussion yields insights that result in a better care plan for the patient (e.g., recognition of the need for psychological counseling, further diagnostic testing, or medical treatment of a related disease). Certainly, this shared mental model contributes to the patient and family who are better prepared for the major surgery and the significant postoperative lifestyle changes inherent in the procedure.

A number of patients who meet medical criteria will benefit from a delay in surgery to deal with issues to help their recovery; examples include those with dysfunctional pain management, those with ongoing alcohol use or smoking, or those with an unrealistic understanding of the results of surgery. Because surgery is less time-sensitive than for a life-threatening issue like cancer, there is time to help the patient and family be best prepared for this intervention. This is important because the surgery is irreversible, and it is critical to have both patient and family best prepared for this major operation and prolonged recovery.

TPIAT is primarily performed for pain relief. Although it was previously believed that chronic pancreatitis-related pain might resolve on its own over one to two decades, newer research suggests this may not be the case [37]. The timing of surgical intervention remains a topic of ongoing discussion, but data consistently show that better outcomes are achieved when surgery, including TPIAT, is performed within 3 years of the onset of chronic pain [37, 38].

The multidisciplinary team has been critical in helping patients through the many "bumps" inherent in the recovery process after TPIAT, such as problems with pain or diabetes management, or gastrointestinal issues related to abnormal postoperative anatomy. This patient population presents unique challenges, given that chronic pancreatitis is a benign disease and patients will live for decades after this surgery (a very different circumstance than for many patients with pancreatic cancer). Long-term outcomes after TPIAT are further discussed in Chap. 16. In our center, this team approach and ongoing follow-up of these patients has assisted with diagnostic and treatment challenges in this unique population in the years to decades after the operative intervention.

In conclusion, the decision to offer TPIAT to a particular patient is a complex one and should include feedback from a multidisciplinary team with multiple perspectives.

References

1. Najarian JS, Sutherland DE, Baumgartner D, Burke B, Rynasiewicz JJ, Matas AJ, et al. Total or near total pancreatectomy and islet autotransplantation for treatment of chronic pancreatitis. Ann Surg. 1980;192(4):526–42. https://doi.org/10.1097/00000658-198010000-00011.
2. Najarian JS, Sutherland DE, Matas AJ, Steffes MW, Simmons RL, Goetz FC. Human islet transplantation: a preliminary report. Transplant Proc. 1977;9(1):233–6.
3. Lara LF, Bellin MD, Ugbarugba E, Nathan JD, Witkowski P, Wijkstrom M, et al. A study on the effect of patient characteristics, geographical utilization, and patient outcomes for total pancreatectomy alone and total pancreatectomy with islet autotransplantation in patients with pancreatitis in the United States. Pancreas. 2019;48(9):1204–11. https://doi.org/10.1097/MPA.0000000000001405.
4. Nathan JD, Yang Y, Eaton A, Witkowski P, Wijkstrom M, Walsh M, et al. Surgical approach and short-term outcomes in adults and children undergoing total pancreatectomy with islet autotransplantation: a report from the Prospective observational study of TPIAT. Pancreatology. 2022;22(1):1–8. https://doi.org/10.1016/j.pan.2021.09.011.
5. Whitcomb DC, Frulloni L, Garg P, Greer JB, Schneider A, Yadav D, et al. Chronic pancreatitis: an international draft consensus proposal for a new mechanistic definition. Pancreatology. 2016;16(2):218–24. https://doi.org/10.1016/j.pan.2016.02.001.
6. Pezzilli R. Etiology of chronic pancreatitis: has it changed in the last decade? World J Gastroenterol. 2009;15(38):4737–40. https://doi.org/10.3748/wjg.15.4737.
7. Yadav D, Lowenfels AB. The epidemiology of pancreatitis and pancreatic cancer. Gastroenterology. 2013;144(6):1252–61. https://doi.org/10.1053/j.gastro.2013.01.068.
8. Herreros-Villanueva M, Hijona E, Bañales JM, Cosme A, Bujanda L. Alcohol consumption on pancreatic diseases. World J Gastroenterol. 2013;19(5):638–47. https://doi.org/10.3748/wjg.v19.i5.638.
9. Weiss FU, Laemmerhirt F, Lerch MM. Etiology and risk factors of acute and chronic pancreatitis. Visc Med. 2019;35(2):73–81. https://doi.org/10.1159/000499138.
10. Whitcomb DC. Genetic risk factors for pancreatic disorders. Gastroenterology. 2013;144(6):1292–302. https://doi.org/10.1053/j.gastro.2013.01.069.
11. Fan BG, Andrén-Sandberg A. Autoimmune pancreatitis. N Am J Med Sci. 2009;1(4):148–51.
12. Asbun HJ, Conlon K, Fernandez-Cruz L, Friess H, Shrikhande SV, Adham M, et al. When to perform a pancreatoduodenectomy in the absence of positive histology? A consensus statement by the international study Group of Pancreatic Surgery. Surgery. 2014;155(5):887–92. https://doi.org/10.1016/j.surg.2013.12.032.
13. Singh VK, Yadav D, Garg PK. Diagnosis and Management of Chronic Pancreatitis. JAMA. 2019;322(24):2422. https://doi.org/10.1001/jama.2019.19411.
14. Drewes AM, Bouwense SAW, Campbell CM, Ceyhan GO, Delhaye M, Demir IE, et al. Guidelines for the understanding and management of pain in chronic pancreatitis. Pancreatology. 2017;17(5):720–31. https://doi.org/10.1016/j.pan.2017.07.006.
15. Hobbs PM, Johnson WG, Graham DY. Management of pain in chronic pancreatitis with emphasis on exogenous pancreatic enzymes. World J Gastrointest Pharmacol Ther. 2016;7(3):370–86. https://doi.org/10.4292/wjgpt.v7.i3.370.

16. Ali UA, Nieuwenhuijs VB, van Eijck CH, Gooszen HG, van Dam RM, Busch OR, et al. Clinical outcome in relation to timing of surgery in chronic pancreatitis. Arch Surg. 2012;147(10) https://doi.org/10.1001/archsurg.2012.1094.
17. Ahmed Ali U, Pahlplatz JM, Nealon WH, van Goor H, Gooszen HG, Boermeester MA. Endoscopic or surgical intervention for painful obstructive chronic pancreatitis. Cochrane Database Syst Rev. 2015;2015(3):CD007884-CD. https://doi.org/10.1002/14651858.CD007884.pub3.
18. Díte P, Ruzicka M, Zboril V, Novotný I. A prospective, randomized trial comparing endoscopic and surgical therapy for chronic pancreatitis. Endoscopy. 2003;35(7):553–8. https://doi.org/10.1055/s-2003-40237.
19. Cahen DL, Gouma DJ, Nio Y, Rauws EAJ, Boermeester MA, Busch OR, et al. Endoscopic versus surgical drainage of the pancreatic duct in chronic pancreatitis. N Engl J Med. 2007;356(7):676–84. https://doi.org/10.1056/nejmoa060610.
20. Issa Y, Kempeneers MA, Bruno MJ, Fockens P, Poley J-W, Ahmed Ali U, et al. Effect of early surgery vs endoscopy-first approach on pain in patients with chronic pancreatitis: the ESCAPE randomized clinical trial. JAMA. 2020;323(3):237–47. https://doi.org/10.1001/jama.2019.20967.
21. Kitano M, Gress TM, Garg PK, Itoi T, Irisawa A, Isayama H, et al. International consensus guidelines on interventional endoscopy in chronic pancreatitis. Recommendations from the working group for the international consensus guidelines for chronic pancreatitis in collaboration with the International Association of Pancreatology, the American pancreatic association, the Japan pancreas society, and European pancreatic Club. Pancreatology. 2020;20(6):1045–55. https://doi.org/10.1016/j.pan.2020.05.022.
22. Larsen M, Kozarek R. Management of pancreatic ductal leaks and fistulae. J Gastroenterol Hepatol. 2014;29(7):1360–70. https://doi.org/10.1111/jgh.12574.
23. Ke N, Jia D, Huang W, Nunes QM, Windsor JA, Liu X, et al. Earlier surgery improves outcomes from painful chronic pancreatitis. Medicine (Baltimore). 2018;97(19):e0651-e. https://doi.org/10.1097/MD.0000000000010651.
24. Riediger H, Adam U, Fischer E, Keck T, Pfeffer F, Hopt UT, et al. Long-term outcome after resection for chronic pancreatitis in 224 patients. J Gastrointest Surg. 2007;11(8):949–60. https://doi.org/10.1007/s11605-007-0155-6.
25. Yang CJ, Bliss LA, Freedman SD, Sheth S, Vollmer CM, Ng SC, et al. Surgery for chronic pancreatitis. Pancreas. 2015;44(5):819–23. https://doi.org/10.1097/mpa.0000000000000333.
26. Yang CJ, Bliss LA, Schapira EF, Freedman SD, Ng SC, Windsor JA, et al. Systematic review of early surgery for chronic pancreatitis: impact on pain, pancreatic function, and re-intervention. J Gastrointest Surg. 2014;18(10):1863–9. https://doi.org/10.1007/s11605-014-2571-8.
27. Kempeneers MA, Issa Y, Ali UA, Baron RD, Besselink MG, Büchler M, et al. International consensus guidelines for surgery and the timing of intervention in chronic pancreatitis. Pancreatology. 2020;20(2):149–57. https://doi.org/10.1016/j.pan.2019.12.005.
28. Bachmann K, Tomkoetter L, Erbes J, Hofmann B, Reeh M, Perez D, et al. Beger and Frey procedures for treatment of chronic pancreatitis: comparison of outcomes at 16-year follow-up. J Am Coll Surg. 2014;219(2):208–16. https://doi.org/10.1016/j.jamcollsurg.2014.03.040.
29. Strobel O, Büchler MW, Werner J. Surgical therapy of chronic pancreatitis: indications, techniques and results. Int J Surg. 2009;7(4):305–12. https://doi.org/10.1016/j.ijsu.2009.05.011.
30. Sutherland DER, Radosevich DM, Bellin MD, Hering BJ, Beilman GJ, Dunn TB, et al. Total pancreatectomy and islet autotransplantation for chronic pancreatitis. J Am Coll Surg. 2012;214(4):409–26. https://doi.org/10.1016/j.jamcollsurg.2011.12.040.
31. Wilson GC, Sutton JM, Smith MT, Schmulewitz N, Salehi M, Choe KA, et al. Total pancreatectomy with islet cell autotransplantation as the initial treatment for minimal-change chronic pancreatitis. HPB (Oxford). 2015;17(3):232–8. https://doi.org/10.1111/hpb.12341.
32. Sandhu B, Vitazka P, Ferreira-Gonzalez A, Pandya A, Vachhani R, Bouhaidar D, et al. Presence of *SPINK-1* variant alters the course of chronic pancreatitis. J Gastroenterol Hepatol. 2011;26(6):965–9. https://doi.org/10.1111/j.1440-1746.2011.06713.x.

33. Dudeja V, Beilman GJ, Vickers SM. Total Pancreatectomy with islet autotransplantation in patients with malignancy: are we there yet? Ann Surg. 2013;258(2):219–20. https://doi.org/10.1097/SLA.0b013e31829c4a1b.
34. Willner A, Bogner A, Müssle B, Teske C, Hempel S, Kahlert C, et al. Disease duration before surgical resection for chronic pancreatitis impacts long-term outcome. Medicine (Baltimore). 2020;99(44):e22896. https://doi.org/10.1097/MD.0000000000022896.
35. Bellin MD, Freeman ML, Gelrud A, Slivka A, Clavel A, Humar A, et al. Total pancreatectomy and islet autotransplantation in chronic pancreatitis: recommendations from PancreasFest. Pancreatology. 2014;14(1):27–35. https://doi.org/10.1016/j.pan.2013.10.009.
36. Blondet JJ, Carlson AM, Kobayashi T, Jie T, Bellin M, Hering BJ, et al. The role of total pancreatectomy and islet autotransplantation for chronic pancreatitis. Surg Clin North Am. 2007;87(6):1477–501. https://doi.org/10.1016/j.suc.2007.08.014.
37. Vipperla K, Kanakis A, Slivka A, Althouse AD, Brand RE, Phillips AE, et al. Natural course of pain in chronic pancreatitis is independent of disease duration. Pancreatology. 2021;21(3):649–57. https://doi.org/10.1016/j.pan.2021.01.020.
38. Bellin MD, Prokhoda P, Hodges JS, Schwarzenberg SJ, Freeman ML, Dunn TB, et al. Age and disease duration impact outcomes of Total Pancreatectomy and islet autotransplant for PRSS1 hereditary pancreatitis. Pancreas. 2018;47(4):466–70. https://doi.org/10.1097/mpa.0000000000001028.
39. Trikudanathan G, Vega-Peralta J, Malli A, Munigala S, Han Y, Bellin M, et al. Diagnostic performance of endoscopic ultrasound (EUS) for non-calcific chronic pancreatitis (NCCP) based on histopathology. Am J Gastroenterol. 2016;111(4):568–74. https://doi.org/10.1038/ajg.2016.48.

Preoperative Evaluation for Total Pancreatectomy and Islet Autotransplantation (TPIAT) and How to Counsel a Patient

3

Aamir Khan and Marlon Levy

Abstract

Chronic pancreatitis (CP) is a progressive inflammatory disease leading to irreversible pancreatic damage, often causing debilitating pain and exocrine/endocrine dysfunction. For patients with severe, refractory disease, total pancreatectomy with islet autotransplantation (TPIAT) offers a potential solution by alleviating pain and preserving beta-cell function to mitigate brittle diabetes. This chapter outlines a comprehensive, multidisciplinary approach to preoperative evaluation and patient counseling for TPIAT, emphasizing the importance of accurate diagnosis, patient selection, and optimization of outcomes. Key steps include confirming the CP diagnosis, assessing eligibility, optimizing nutritional status, and evaluating endocrine and exocrine pancreatic function. Diagnostic imaging, like magnetic resonance imaging/magnetic resonance cholangiopancreatography and endoscopic ultrasound, plays a critical role in assessing disease severity and anatomy. Patient counseling is essential to set realistic expectations regarding pain relief, diabetes risk, and lifelong enzyme replacement. This chapter highlights the importance of shared decision-making, psychosocial support, and adherence to postoperative care. By integrating evidence-based practices and multidisciplinary collaboration, this approach aims to ensure optimal outcomes and patient satisfaction in TPIAT candidates.

A. Khan (✉) · M. Levy
Division of Transplantation, Department of Surgery, Virginia Commonwealth University, Richmond, VA, USA
e-mail: Aamir.Khan@vcuhealth.org

S. Chinnakotla et al. (eds.), *Total Pancreatectomy and Islet Auto Transplantation*,
https://doi.org/10.1007/978-981-92-0018-4_3

Key Points

- A comprehensive evaluation is needed before pursuing TPIAT to ensure that the patient is a suitable candidate and risks are minimized.
  - Coordinated assessment and care among physicians from multiple disciplines is required.
  - Confirmation of the diagnosis and thorough understanding of medical history and current status is critical.
    Evaluations include clinical assessments, laboratory tests, diagnostic imaging, and assessment of both endocrine and exocrine pancreatic function.
- Patient education and counseling, including psychosocial support, is crucial for managing their expectations and ensuring that they understand the risks and lifelong consequences of the procedure.

3.1 Introduction

Chronic pancreatitis (CP) is a debilitating disease characterized by continuous inflammation, progressive fibrosis, and irreversible damage to the pancreas, often resulting in intractable abdominal pain as well as exocrine and endocrine dysfunction [1, 2]. Diagnosing the disease in its early stages remains challenging. For a subset of patients with severe, medically refractory disease, total pancreatectomy with islet autotransplantation (TPIAT) offers a promising treatment option aimed at alleviating pain and preserving beta-cell function to prevent or mitigate diabetes [2, 3]. This innovative procedure involves the complete removal of the pancreas, followed by isolation and intrahepatic transplantation of the patient's islet cells, which are responsible for insulin production [3].

The decision to pursue TPIAT requires comprehensive evaluation to ensure that candidates are suitable and to address the multifaceted challenges associated with chronic pancreatitis. Despite its benefits, TPIAT is not without challenges; it is a major operation and has lifelong consequences for the patients. Preoperative assessment is essential for optimizing outcomes, minimizing risks, and managing expectations. Furthermore, patient counseling plays a pivotal role in preparing patients and their families for the physical, emotional, and lifestyle changes that accompany the procedure [3, 4]. It is important to understand that this operation is primarily performed to treat intractable pain affecting the quality of life in patients for whom other treatment modalities have failed or are not indicated [2, 3].

The goals of preoperative evaluation for TPIAT are multifaceted, aiming to ensure a thorough and personalized approach to patient care:

1. **Confirm diagnosis:**
   - Establish that the patient's chronic pancreatitis is refractory to medical, endoscopic, or less invasive surgical therapies.
   - Use advanced diagnostic tools such as imaging, genetic testing, and functional assessments, as applicable.

2. **Assess patient eligibility:** Evaluate disease severity, impact on quality of life, and contraindications.
3. **Optimize preoperative status:** Address malnutrition, pain, and comorbidities.
4. **Educate and counsel:** Discuss the surgical procedure, risks, expected outcomes, and lifestyle changes.
5. **Facilitate multidisciplinary collaboration:** Ensure coordinated care among surgeons, radiologists, endocrinologists, nutritionists, pain specialists, and psychologists.

This chapter aims to provide a systematic and detailed approach to evaluating and counseling patients for TPIAT, incorporating evidence-based practices and multidisciplinary approaches. Table 3.1 shows our approach to stepwise evaluation of patients referred for TPIAT at Virginia Commonwealth University (VCU).

Table 3.1 VCU's stepwise protocol for TPIAT evaluation

Step	Evaluation component	Details
Step 1: Initial screening	Referral review	Obtain referral details from primary care physician or specialist Review medical history and indications for TPIAT
	Eligibility criteria assessment	Confirm indications: Chronic pancreatitis (CP), hereditary pancreatitis, or other conditions Exclude contraindications
	Patient education	Provide overview of TPIAT, risks, benefits, and expectations
Step2: Multidisciplinary team consultation	Gastroenterology	Assess the severity of CP and prior interventions
	Endocrinology	Evaluate endocrine function and risk of diabetes after surgery
	Surgery	Assess surgical suitability and discuss the procedure with the patient
	Pain management	Review the current pain regimen and evaluate the need for adjustments
	Nutrition	Assess nutritional status and provide preoperative dietary recommendations
	Psychology/ psychiatry	Evaluate mental health, coping mechanisms, and compliance potential
	Social work	Assess family support, financial readiness, and logistical considerations
Step 3: Diagnostic testing	Imaging	Perform secretin MRI/MRCP, CT scan, or EUS to evaluate pancreatic anatomy and disease severity
	Laboratory tests	Complete metabolic panel, HbA1c, C-peptide, insulin, amylase, and lipase
	Islet function testing	Assess islet cell viability and function (if applicable)

(continued)

Table 3.1 (continued)

Step	Evaluation component	Details
Step 4: Risk assessment and surgical candidacy	Surgical risk	Assess for comorbidities affecting surgical outcomes, e.g., cardiac, pulmonary
	Postoperative diabetes risk	Predict likelihood of insulin dependence after surgery
	Quality of life	Weigh potential improvements in quality of life against surgical risks
Step 5: Patient selection meeting	Multidisciplinary team review	Present case to the TPIAT team for consensus decision-making
Step 6: Preoperative optimization	Pain management optimization	Adjust pain medications to minimize opioid use preoperatively. Referral to addiction medicine if needed
	Nutritional support	Address deficiencies and ensure adequate preoperative nutrition
	Psychological preparation	Address patient concerns, expectations, and provide counseling if necessary
Step 7: Final clearance and scheduling	Informed consent	Review detailed surgical plan and obtain signed consent
	Surgery scheduling	Finalize operative date and preoperative checklist

CT computed tomography, *EUS* endoscopic ultrasound, *MRI* magnetic resonance imaging, *MRCP* magnetic resonance cholangiopancreatography

3.2 Patient Selection and Indications

It is important to understand that not every patient with chronic pancreatitis will be a candidate for TPIAT, because it is a major operation with serious lifelong consequences. Other etiologies for abdominal pain should be ruled out [5]. Therefore, the first step is to identify an appropriate candidate for TPIAT. At VCU, patients who are considered for TPIAT surgery should meet all of the following criteria:

- Diagnosis of chronic pancreatitis (radiological or histological confirmation) or recurrent acute pancreatitis.
- Presence of characteristic refractory abdominal pain affecting quality of life.
- Failure of prior medical and endoscopic treatments.
- Absence of diabetes or C-peptide–positive diabetes.
- Absence of active malignancy confirmed through imaging and, if needed, with pathology.
- Absence of severe untreated cardiac/pulmonary disease or other comorbid conditions precluding safe major surgery.
- No active ongoing substance abuse (e.g., alcohol, drugs) or untreated psychiatric disorders.
- Absence of severe hepatic fibrosis or portal hypertension.
- Ability to comprehend and understand the complexity of the operation and its lifelong consequences.

It is our practice to routinely discuss cases in a multidisciplinary committee composed of radiologists, endoscopists, gastroenterologists/pancreatologists, surgeons, nurse coordinators, and endocrinologists to review patients and approve them for surgery or other interventions. Surgeries are performed once approved by the committee.

3.3 Clinical Assessment and Laboratory Evaluation

A detailed and thorough clinical assessment should be obtained at the time of initial evaluation, and efforts should be made to determine the cause of chronic pancreatitis. With the increasing use of the internet and social media, we have noticed an increasing trend of patient self-referral, as these patients are desperate to find answers for their unrelenting pain and suffering. Patients are often referred to the surgeons with most of their workup already completed, but this should not stop the surgeon from confirming the diagnosis and etiology of chronic pancreatitis. This is important to ensure that no reversible cause of pancreatitis is present or untreated. The revised Version 2 of the toxic-metabolic, idiopathic, genetic, autoimmune, recurrent and severe acute pancreatitis, and obstructive (TIGAR-O) system [6] (Table 3.2) is a helpful guide to risk factors and etiologies that might explain chronic pancreatitis. In cases where there is no clearly identifiable etiology, genetic testing might be warranted, especially in younger patients [6, 7]. Assessing the severity of the disease and any ongoing flares of acute pancreatitis is pivotal to the overall management plan. Evaluation of the duration, frequency, and severity of symptoms, including abdominal pain, pancreatitis episodes, and associated complications (e.g., diabetes, malnutrition), is important. Prior medical, endoscopic, or surgical treatments and their outcomes should be documented. Evaluation of dependence on pain medications, prescribed as well as nonprescribed, especially opioids, is important, as is inquiry into any substance abuse history; this will be important to set up realistic expectations and to work toward prehabilitation for substance abuse. Patients should be screened for prohibitive comorbidities and may sometimes need additional cardiopulmonary testing, determined on an individual, case-by-case basis. A detailed cardiovascular history is mandatory for all patients, and risk factors for coronary artery disease should be sought in the history, because TPIAT is a major surgery with potential for severe complications. We recommend following the American Heart Association/American College of Surgeons (AHA/ACS) guidelines regarding any additional cardiac testing if indicated [8]. Family history is extremely important, as it may give clues to possible genetic mutations (e.g., in *PRSS1, CFTR, SPINK1*) as well as risk of cancer [6, 7]. Nutritional and functional status should be assessed. Patients with alcohol abuse or obesity, in particular, should be evaluated for liver disease and signs of portal hypertension. A transjugular liver biopsy with measurement of hepatic venous pressure gradients may sometimes be needed if there is concern for advanced liver disease on evaluation. Any history of hypercoagulability should be investigated, because this will have implications in the postoperative anticoagulation plan. During physical examination, the

Table 3.2 TIGAR-O Version 2.0: checklist short form [7]

Toxic-metabolic	Alcohol-related (susceptibility and/or progression) 3–4 drinks/day Five or more drinks/day Smoking (if yes, record pack-years) Nonsmoker (<100 cigarettes in lifetime) Past smoker Current smoker Other, NOS (not otherwise specified) Hypercalcemia (total calcium levels >12.0 mg/dL or 3 mmol/L) Hypertriglyceridemia (HTG) HTG risk (fasting >300 mg/dL; nonfasting >500 mg/dL) History of hypertriglyceridemic acute pancreatitis (>500 mg/dL in first 72 h) Medications (name) Toxins, other Chronic kidney disease (CKD)—Stage 5: end-stage renal disease (ESRD) Other, NOS Metabolic, other Diabetes mellitus (with the date of diagnosis if available) Other, NOS
Idiopathic	Early onset (<35 years of age) Late onset (>35 years of age)
Genetic	Suspected; no or limited genotyping available Autosomal dominant (Mendelian inheritance—Single-gene syndrome) *PRSS1* mutations (hereditary pancreatitis) Autosomal recessive (Mendelian inheritance—Single-gene syndrome) *CFTR,* 2 severe variants in *trans* (cystic fibrosis) *CFTR,* <2 severe variants in *trans* (CFTR-RD) *SPINK1,* 2 pathogenic variants in *trans* (*SPINK1*-associated familial pancreatitis) Complex genetics—Non-Mendelian, complex genotypes +/− environment Modifier genes (list pathogenic genetic variants) *PRSS1* locus *CLDN2* locus Others: HTG (list pathogenic genetic variants) Other, NOS
Autoimmune pancreatitis (AIP)/steroid-responsive pancreatitis	AIP type 1—IgG4-related disease AIP type 2

(continued)

Table 3.2 (continued)

Recurrent acute pancreatitis and severe acute pancreatitis	Acute pancreatitis (single episode, including date of event if available) AP etiology—Extra-pancreatic (excluding alcoholic, HTG, hypercalcemia, genetic) Biliary pancreatitis Post-ERCP Traumatic Undetermined or NOS Recurrent acute pancreatitis (number of episodes, frequency, and dates of events if available)
Obstructive	Pancreas divisum Ampullary stenosis Main duct pancreatic stones Widespread pancreatic calcifications Main pancreatic duct strictures Localized mass causing duct obstruction

AP acute pancreatitis, *ERCP* endoscopic retrograde cholangiopancreatography, *HTG* hypertriglyceridemia

focus should be on signs of dehydration, nutritional deficiencies, liver disease, or complications of chronic pancreatitis.

A complete blood count and a full chemistry panel should be obtained, along with a coagulation profile. Blood should be sent for typing and screening. We routinely screen patients for evidence of hepatitis B and C as well as human immunodeficiency virus (HIV). A baseline 12-lead electrocardiogram (EKG) is performed in all patients. Any additional testing is done if needed to look for potential etiologies as per the TIGAR-O V2 system. Other tests like diagnostic imaging, pancreatic function tests, and glucose or mixed-meal tolerance tests are performed to assess the severity of the disease and to determine the islet functional reserve, as discussed below.

3.4 Diagnostic Imaging Studies

A good cross-sectional imaging modality is pivotal in surgical assessment of the pancreas to determine disease severity, any component of ongoing acute pancreatitis, or complications of chronic pancreatitis like pseudocyst which might need to be addressed first. It is also important to understand the anatomy, ductal pathology, and any vascular anatomic aberrations. The diagnosis of advanced chronic pancreatitis with calcifications might be relatively easy with standard imaging, whereas diagnosis of noncalcific chronic pancreatitis in patients with chronic abdominal pain can be quite challenging [9]. Various imaging modalities are available to assess pancreatic disease in chronic pancreatitis.

Most patients would likely have a computed tomography (CT) abdomen done as part of the evaluation of their abdominal pain and other symptoms. CT is helpful to rule out other common etiologies of abdominal pain that might mimic chronic pancreatitis. CT scans are readily available at most places and are helpful to detect morphological changes of advanced chronic pancreatitis. However, they are not useful for detecting early changes of chronic pancreatitis [1, 10].

Contrast-enhanced magnetic resonance imaging (MRI)/MR cholangiopancreatography (MRCP) are essential tools for noninvasive evaluation of the pancreatic ductal system and parenchyma. It will help to evaluate the pancreatic anatomy; degree of fibrosis or atrophy; and presence of ductal strictures, stones, or pseudocysts. It is also useful for detection of subtle changes with early chronic pancreatitis and differentiation between inflammatory changes and malignant lesions [11]. Normal pancreas appears hyperintense on T1-weighted images due to the presence of proteins in the acinar cells [11, 12]. In chronic pancreatitis, there is loss of aqueous proteins in the acini due to inflammation and fibrosis, which shows as hypointensity on T1-weighted images [11, 13]. Addition of other MRI sequences like diffusion-weighted images also increases the diagnostic accuracy for chronic pancreatitis. Adding MRCP to pancreatic MRI significantly improves the assessment of pancreatic and bile ducts and has the benefit of being noninvasive, unlike endoscopic retrograde cholangiopancreatography (ERCP). This has led to ERCP falling out of favor for use in diagnosing chronic pancreatitis.

At our program, we prefer to use MR angiography over CT angiography to define vascular anatomy because it is easier to add those imaging sequences to the regular MRI and it does not involve any ionizing radiation. We also routinely use a secretin-stimulated MRCP, which helps better in the functional and morphological assessment of the pancreas. Conventional MRCP usually fails to demonstrate the side branches. Secretin improves pancreatic duct and side-branch delineation and the detection of anatomic variants like pancreas divisum [14]. It allows monitoring of pancreatic flow dynamics and evaluation of pancreatic exocrine function [14]. Post-secretin dilatation of the pancreatic duct and filling of the duodenum are assessed and graded to quantify pancreatic exocrine insufficiency [15]. It also helps corroborate the pancreatic origin of pain on secretin administration, because patients often report having worsening pain similar to their acute flares.

Transabdominal ultrasound is a useful noninvasive imaging modality that is readily available and does not carry the risk of ionizing radiation. However, it has limited utility in the assessment of the pancreas, which is a retroperitoneal organ, and the overlying bowel gas shadows obscure part or all of the pancreas. It is also difficult to perform in obese individuals. These limitations are overcome by EUS, which is an advanced diagnostic modality for evaluating the pancreas in detail. It is particularly valuable for detecting subtle parenchymal changes, small cystic lesions, and ductal irregularities that may not be apparent on cross-sectional imaging [16]. EUS-guided fine-needle aspiration enables cytological sampling to differentiate benign lesions from malignant lesions. It can also simultaneously be used to perform procedures like celiac plexus block [17] and cyst-gastrostomies, if needed.

Both ultrasound and EUS are operator dependent, and interobserver variability can be a major drawback. Therefore, the Rosemont criteria were developed and are widely used by most endoscopists for diagnosis [18].

There are no major randomized trials comparing imaging modalities for diagnosis of chronic pancreatitis. A meta-analysis by Issa et al. evaluated 43 studies and 3460 patients with suspected chronic pancreatitis [19]. They found that the sensitivity estimates of EUS, MRI, and CT were 81% (95% CI: 70–89%), 78% (95% CI: 69–85%), and 75% (95% CI: 66–83%), respectively, and did not differ significantly from each other. Estimates of specificity were comparable for EUS (90%; 95% CI: 82–95%), ERCP (94%; 95% CI: 87–98%), CT (91%; 95% CI: 81–96%), MRI (96%; 95% CI: 90–98%), and US (98%; 95% CI: 89–100%). A major limitation of this study was heterogeneity across the studies and difficulty of extrapolating the data to early phases of the disease, where newer imaging modalities and techniques might have better sensitivity [19, 20].

3.5 Endocrine and Islet Cell Function Evaluation

Assessing endocrine and islet cell function is an important part of the preoperative evaluation for patients referred for TPIAT surgery. It is important to establish a preoperative baseline for islet functional reserve as well as to predict potential islet yield. This is also important information for discussion with the patient to set up realistic expectations for surgery. Prior pancreatic surgeries and pancreatic fibrosis on MRI result in lower islet yields [21, 22]. To date, islet yield seems to be the best predictor of insulin independence, but it is not known until after the transplant procedure.

The initial basic evaluation should include a fasting blood glucose and HbA1c check [23]. Functional beta-cell mass can be estimated by the response of serum glucose and C-peptide levels during either an oral glucose tolerance test or a mixed-meal tolerance test [24]. These metrics have a modest value in predicting the islet reserve and post-op metabolic outcomes [24–26]. Arginine-stimulated testing is emerging as a safe, reproducible clinical test for predicting islet yield but is not yet routinely available despite its promise. It might be a useful alternative to the mixed-meal tolerance test in young children refusing to consume a liquid test meal [21].

3.6 Pancreatic Function Testing

Pancreatic function testing is vital for assessing exocrine pancreatic function, especially in patients with chronic pancreatitis or suspected exocrine pancreatic insufficiency (EPI). Most patients with chronic pancreatitis, especially in its early stages, do not have clinically significant EPI. Pancreatic function testing should not be used as a definitive test, but rather as an ancillary test in helping with the diagnosis (Table 3.3). Both direct and indirect tests are used in clinical practice.

Table 3.3 Exocrine pancreatic function tests

Direct pancreatic function tests			
Test	Purpose	Pros	Cons
Secretin test [29]	Assesses duct-cell function by measuring bicarbonate and/or volume in response to secretin stimulation via endoscopy	Gold standard for assessing exocrine function	Invasive Expensive Requires specialized equipment Cumbersome
Cholecystokinin (CCK) test [29]	Assesses acinar cell function by measuring enzyme secretion stimulated by CCK, mimicking physiologic conditions	Provides a direct measure of enzyme production	Invasive Cumbersome Requires specialized setup and skilled personnel
Indirect pancreatic function tests			
Fecal elastase-1 [1, 27, 28]	Measures pancreatic enzyme output; low levels indicate exocrine insufficiency	Noninvasive Easy to perform Widely available Useful for screening for exocrine insufficiency	False positives in diarrhea or dilution Limited sensitivity for mild insufficiency
Fecal fat quantification [27]	Measures fat malabsorption: High levels indicate pancreatic exocrine insufficiency	Direct measure of fat absorption Helpful in diagnosing severe EPI	Tedious collection over 72 h Patient compliance issues
^{13}C-mixed triglyceride breath test [23]	Functional assessment of pancreatic lipase activity using labeled substrates	Noninvasive. Reliable and patient-friendly	Limited availability Expensive
Serum trypsinogen [30]	Marker of exocrine function; low levels suggest chronic pancreatic damage	Simple blood test Useful in acute and chronic disease	Not specific for mild exocrine insufficiency
Secretin MRCP [31]	Combines MRCP with secretin stimulation to visualize pancreatic duct response and fluid secretion, giving a good estimate of pancreatic exocrine function	Noninvasive Provides anatomical and functional information Can show early changes of chronic pancreatitis	Requires skilled interpretation Limited availability

Direct pancreatic function tests are considered the traditional gold standard for pancreas function assessment. They require hormonal stimulation and gastroduodenal intubation for collection of pancreatic juice, either using fluoroscopy, endoscopy, or both. They are cumbersome, time-consuming, invasive, and inconvenient to patients and are limited to a few centers. To avoid those problems, a number of indirect pancreatic function tests are available. The 72-hour fecal fat test remains the gold standard for quantification of steatorrhea [27], but since steatorrhea can be found in other gastrointestinal disorders, this test is neither sensitive nor specific for evaluation of EPI. Fecal elastase-1 measurement has gained universal acceptance due to its ease of application and is quite reliable in severe EPI, but results can be inconsistent in mild, early disease. The accuracy of its results also depends on the cutoff chosen. Most laboratories use 200 μg/g as the cutoff for low levels, and levels over 500 are considered normal, but the significance of levels between 200 and 500 μg/g remains unclear. This is especially important for patients who may be having otherwise minimal change early in chronic pancreatitis or who have other coexisting gastrointestinal conditions [28].

3.7 Counseling the Patient

Effective counseling is integral to the success of TPIAT. Patients and families must understand the procedure and its risks, benefits, and long-term implications. Counseling should be patient-centered, empathetic, and thorough. The crux of counseling should be to discuss both the benefits and risks of TPIAT, emphasizing that while improvement in quality of life with pain relief is the primary goal, the risk of diabetes and lifelong dependence on pancreatic enzyme replacement therapy (PERT) and nutritional supplementation [32] are the trade-offs. In our program, we use the concept of shared decision-making by giving all the information to the patients and discussing the management plan with them, including these key elements:

1. **Explain the Procedure and Potential Complications.**
    - Discuss the surgical steps, including total pancreatectomy, islet isolation, and intrahepatic transplantation of islets.
    - Explain the timeline of the surgery, hospitalization, and recovery process.
    - Describe the surgical risks and postoperative complications like bleeding, infection, and anastomotic leaks [3], delayed gastric emptying [33], portal vein thrombosis, and exocrine and endocrine insufficiency.
    - Explain the possibility of aborted surgery, as sometimes the procedure cannot be done safely due to severe inflammation and strong peripancreatic adhesions involving the major vessels. This risk was reviewed in a study of 110 patients in which they found male sex, prior pancreas procedures and stents, and high body mass index (BMI) as risk factors [34].
2. **Set Realistic Expectations.**
    - ***Pain relief:*** Discussion about outcomes related to pain relief is vital to patient understanding and setting up the expectations. Chinnakotla et al. [35] reported in a study of 500 patients that 92.6% achieved pain relief and improved quality of life. At 1 year, only 7.5% of patients had persistent pancreatic pain simi-

lar to preoperative levels, and only 30% of patients were using any narcotics. They also identified risk factors for poor pain outcomes (prolonged postoperative narcotic use) and/or persistent pain after TPIAT that included previous stents (>3), prior narcotic use for >5 years, pancreas divisum, and previous surgical procedures. Pain outcomes are often influenced by preoperative pain management strategies, the duration of chronic pain prior to surgery, and the presence of opioid dependence, but 80–85% of patients report significant pain relief and a subset can discontinue opioid use within a year after TPIAT [5, 36]. Other programs have reported different pain outcomes at 1 year ranging from 23–70% [24].

- ***Risk of post-pancreatectomy diabetes:*** The risk of brittle diabetes and the possibility of lifelong insulin dependence and the need for exogenous enzymes should be discussed. Different studies have reported different insulin independence rates, which mostly depend on the overall islet yield and the duration of follow-up. However, Sutherland et al., in a large series with over 30 years of data, reported that by 3 years, nearly a third were insulin-independent, another third had partial islet function, and slightly more than a third were insulin-dependent; thus, at least two-thirds had some islet function [3]. There is a strong association between islet yield and degree of function, but it is difficult to predict islet yield prior to surgery. Therefore, all patients should be counseled that they must be willing to accept the risk of diabetes as a trade-off for pain relief [3]. Obesity, pancreatic calcifications, EPI, and prior pancreatic surgery are risk factors for the development of diabetes mellitus [37].

3. **Highlight the Importance of Adherence.**

   - Discuss the necessity of lifelong follow-up for managing diabetes, preventing complications, and optimizing transplant outcomes.
   - Stress the importance of adhering to dietary guidelines and enzyme replacement and of monitoring blood glucose levels.
   - Patients must be counseled about lifestyle modifications like frequent small meals, awareness of recognizing symptoms of hypoglycemia, monitoring glucose levels before and after physical activity, and adjusting insulin doses or consuming carbohydrates preemptively to prevent hypoglycemic episodes.

4. **Psychosocial Support and Family Involvement.**

   - Address the emotional and psychological impact of TPIAT, including changes in lifestyle and potential dependency on medical care.
   - Offer support groups or connect patients with individuals who have undergone TPIAT.
   - Engage family members or caregivers in counseling sessions to ensure they understand their role in postoperative care and support.

5. **Discuss Alternative Treatments and Obtain Informed Consent.**
    - Present TPIAT as part of a spectrum of options, including medical management and endoscopic or surgical interventions. Ensure patients understand why TPIAT is being recommended in their case.
    - Encourage questions and ensure the patient has a clear understanding before signing the consent form.

3.8 Conclusion

The preoperative evaluation and counseling process for TPIAT are critical to achieving optimal outcomes and patient satisfaction. A thorough and multidisciplinary approach ensures that the procedure is performed on well-selected patients who are physically and psychologically prepared for the journey ahead. Effective communication, empathy, and education are the cornerstones of this process, laying the groundwork for a successful surgical and postoperative experience.

References

1. Conwell DL, Lee LS, Yadav D, Longnecker DS, Miller FH, Mortele KJ, et al. American pancreatic association practice guidelines in chronic pancreatitis: evidence-based report on diagnostic guidelines. Pancreas. 2014;43(8):1143–62. https://doi.org/10.1097/MPA.0000000000000237.
2. Bellin MD, Freeman ML, Gelrud A, Slivka A, Clavel A, Humar A, et al. Total pancreatectomy and islet autotransplantation in chronic pancreatitis: recommendations from PancreasFest. Pancreatology. 2014;14(1):27–35. https://doi.org/10.1016/j.pan.2013.10.009.
3. DER S, Radosevich DM, Bellin MD, Hering BJ, Beilman GJ, Dunn TB, et al. Total pancreatectomy and islet autotransplantation for chronic pancreatitis. J Am Coll Surg. 2012;214(4):409–26. https://doi.org/10.1016/j.jamcollsurg.2011.12.040.
4. Abu-El-Haija M, Anazawa T, Beilman GJ, Besselink MG, Del Chiaro M, Demir IE, et al. The role of total pancreatectomy with islet autotransplantation in the treatment of chronic pancreatitis: a report from the international consensus guidelines in chronic pancreatitis. Pancreatology. 2020;20(4):762–71. https://doi.org/10.1016/j.pan.2020.04.005.
5. Bellin MD, Freeman ML, Schwarzenberg SJ, Dunn TB, Beilman GJ, Vickers SM, et al. Quality of life improves for pediatric patients after total pancreatectomy and islet autotransplant for chronic pancreatitis. Clin. Gastroenterol. Hepatol. 2011;9(9):793–9. https://doi.org/10.1016/j.cgh.2011.04.024.
6. Whitcomb DC, North American Pancreatitis Study Group. Pancreatitis: TIGAR-O version 2 risk/etiology checklist with topic reviews, updates, and use primers. Clin Transl Gastroenterol. 2019;10(6):e00027-e. https://doi.org/10.14309/ctg.0000000000000027.
7. Whitcomb DC. Hereditary pancreatitis: new insights into acute and chronic pancreatitis. Gut. 1999;45(3):317–22. https://doi.org/10.1136/gut.45.3.317.
8. Thompson A, Fleischmann KE, Smilowitz NR, de las Fuentes L, Mukherjee D, Aggarwal NR, et al. AHA/ACC/ACS/ASNC/HRS/SCA/SCCT/SCMR/SVM guideline for perioperative cardiovascular management for noncardiac surgery: a report of the American College of Cardiology/American Heart Association joint committee on clinical practice guidelines. Circulation. 2024;150(19) https://doi.org/10.1161/cir.0000000000001285.

9. Hernandez LV, Catalano MF. EUS in the diagnosis of early-stage chronic pancreatitis. Best Pract. Res. Clin. Gastroenterol. 2010;24(3):243–9. https://doi.org/10.1016/j.bpg.2010.03.004.
10. Luetmer PH, Stephens DH, Ward EM. Chronic pancreatitis: reassessment with current CT. Radiology. 1989;171(2):353–7. https://doi.org/10.1148/radiology.171.2.2704799.
11. Trikudanathan G, Walker SP, Munigala S, Spilseth B, Malli A, Han Y, et al. Diagnostic performance of contrast-enhanced MRI with secretin-stimulated MRCP for non-calcific chronic pancreatitis: a comparison with histopathology. Am J Gastroenterol. 2015;110(11):1598–606. https://doi.org/10.1038/ajg.2015.297.
12. Balci C. MRI assessment of chronic pancreatitis. Diagn Interv Radiol. 2010; https://doi.org/10.4261/1305-3825.dir.3889-10.0.
13. Kamat R, Gupta P, Rana S. Imaging in chronic pancreatitis: state of the art review. Indian J Radiol Imaging. 2019;29(2):201–10. https://doi.org/10.4103/ijri.IJRI_484_18.
14. Matos C, Cappeliez O, Winant C, Coppens E, Devière J, Metens T. MR imaging of the pancreas: a pictorial tour. Radiographics. 2002;22(1):e2. https://doi.org/10.1148/radiographics.22.1.g02jae2e2.
15. Bian Y, Wang L, Chen C, Lu J-P, Fan J-B, Chen S-Y, et al. Quantification of pancreatic exocrine function of chronic pancreatitis with secretin-enhanced MRCP. World J Gastroenterol. 2013;19(41):7177–82. https://doi.org/10.3748/wjg.v19.i41.7177.
16. Trikudanathan G, Vega-Peralta J, Malli A, Munigala S, Han Y, Bellin M, et al. Diagnostic performance of endoscopic ultrasound (EUS) for non-calcific chronic pancreatitis (NCCP) based on histopathology. Am J Gastroenterol. 2016;111(4):568–74. https://doi.org/10.1038/ajg.2016.48.
17. Sonthalia N, Goenka MK, Patil V, Shah B, Afzalpulkar S. S995 endoscopic ultrasound-guided celiac plexus block for pain relief in chronic pancreatitis is an effective procedure when used judiciously. Am J Gastroenterol. 2021;116(1):S474–S. https://doi.org/10.14309/01.ajg.0000777512.53077.d7.
18. Catalano MF, Sahai A, Levy M, Romagnuolo J, Wiersema M, Brugge W, et al. EUS-based criteria for the diagnosis of chronic pancreatitis: the Rosemont classification. Gastrointest Endosc. 2009;69(7):1251–61. https://doi.org/10.1016/j.gie.2008.07.043.
19. Issa Y, Kempeneers MA, van Santvoort HC, Bollen TL, Bipat S, Boermeester MA. Diagnostic performance of imaging modalities in chronic pancreatitis: a systematic review and meta-analysis. Eur Radiol. 2017;27(9):3820–44. https://doi.org/10.1007/s00330-016-4720-9.
20. Gardner TB, Adler DG, Forsmark CE, Sauer BG, Taylor JR, Whitcomb DC. ACG clinical guideline: chronic pancreatitis. Am J Gastroenterol. 2020;115(3):322–39. https://doi.org/10.14309/ajg.0000000000000535.
21. McEachron KR, Skube ME, Yang Y, Hodges JS, Wilhelm J, Beilman G, et al. Utility of arginine stimulation testing in preoperative assessment of children undergoing total pancreatectomy with islet autotransplantation. Clin Transpl. 2019;33(8):e13647-e. https://doi.org/10.1111/ctr.13647.
22. Morgan KA, Theruvath T, Owczarski S, Adams DB. Total Pancreatectomy with islet autotransplantation for chronic pancreatitis: do patients with prior pancreatic surgery have different outcomes? Am Surg. 2012;78(8):893–6. https://doi.org/10.1177/000313481207800826.
23. Rickels MR, Bellin M, Toledo FGS, Robertson RP, Andersen DK, Chari ST, et al. Detection, evaluation and treatment of diabetes mellitus in chronic pancreatitis: recommendations from PancreasFest 2012. Pancreatology. 2013;13(4):336–42. https://doi.org/10.1016/j.pan.2013.05.002.
24. Yoshimatsu G, Takita M, Haque W, Naziruddin B, Levy MF. Autologous islet cell transplant. In: Contemporary pancreas transplantation. New York: Springer; 2015. p. 1–13.
25. Bellin MD, Blondet JJ, Beilman GJ, Dunn TB, Balamurugan AN, Thomas W, et al. Predicting islet yield in pediatric patients undergoing pancreatectomy and autoislet transplantation for chronic pancreatitis. Pediatr Diabetes. 2010;11(4):227–34. https://doi.org/10.1111/j.1399-5448.2009.00575.x.
26. Lundberg R, Beilman GJ, Dunn TB, Pruett TL, Chinnakotla SC, Radosevich DM, et al. Metabolic assessment prior to total pancreatectomy and islet autotransplant: utility, limitations and potential. Am. J. Transplant. 2013;13(10):2664–71. https://doi.org/10.1111/ajt.12392.

27. Boeck WG, Guido A, Gress TM. Pancreatic function tests: when to choose, what to use. Curr Gastroenterol Rep. 2001;3(2):95–100. https://doi.org/10.1007/s11894-001-0004-9.
28. Mathew A, Fernandes D, Andreyev HJN. What is the significance of a faecal elastase-1 level between 200 and 500μg/g? Frontline Gastroenterol. 2023;14(5):371–6. https://doi.org/10.1136/flgastro-2022-102271.
29. Stevens T, Parsi MA. Update on endoscopic pancreatic function testing. World J Gastroenterol. 2011;17(35):3957–61. https://doi.org/10.3748/wjg.v17.i35.3957.
30. Steinberg WM, Anderson KK. Serum trypsinogen in diagnosis of chronic pancreatitis. Dig Dis Sci. 1984;29(11):988–93. https://doi.org/10.1007/bf01311248.
31. Boraschi P, Donati F, Cervelli R, Pacciardi F. Secretin-stimulated MR cholangiopancreatography: spectrum of findings in pancreatic diseases. Insights Imaging. 2016;7(6):819–29. https://doi.org/10.1007/s13244-016-0517-2.
32. Morgan KA, Lancaster WP, Owczarski SM, Wang H, Borckardt J, Adams DB. Patient selection for total pancreatectomy with islet autotransplantation in the surgical management of chronic pancreatitis. J Am Coll Surg. 2018;226(4):446–51. https://doi.org/10.1016/j.jamcollsurg.2017.12.018.
33. John GK, Singh VK, Pasricha PJ, Sinha A, Afghani E, Warren D, et al. Delayed gastric emptying (DGE) following Total Pancreatectomy with islet auto transplantation in patients with chronic pancreatitis. J Gastrointest Surg. 2015;19(7):1256–61. https://doi.org/10.1007/s11605-015-2848-6.
34. Shahbazov R, Yoshimatsu G, Dabous A, Lawrence MC, Kim PT, Onaca N, et al. The characteristics of aborted procedures in total pancreatectomy with islet autotransplantation for chronic pancreatitis. Pancreas. 2017;46(9):e76–e8. https://doi.org/10.1097/mpa.0000000000000908.
35. Chinnakotla S, Beilman GJ, Dunn TB, Bellin MD, Freeman ML, Radosevich DM, et al. Factors predicting outcomes after a total pancreatectomy and islet autotransplantation lessons learned from over 500 cases. Ann Surg. 2015;262(4):610–22. https://doi.org/10.1097/SLA.0000000000001453.
36. Bellin MD, Beilman GJ, Sutherland DE, Ali H, Petersen A, Mongin S, et al. How durable is total pancreatectomy and intraportal islet cell transplantation for treatment of chronic pancreatitis? J Am Coll Surg. 2019;228(4):329–39. https://doi.org/10.1016/j.jamcollsurg.2018.12.019.
37. Bellin MD, Whitcomb DC, Abberbock J, Sherman S, Sandhu BS, Gardner TB, et al. Patient and disease characteristics associated with the presence of diabetes mellitus in adults with chronic pancreatitis in the United States. Am J Gastroenterol. 2017;112(9):1457–65. https://doi.org/10.1038/ajg.2017.181.

Role of the Transplant Nurse Coordinator for Total Pancreatectomy and Islet Autotransplantation

4

Emily Scheidecker, Louise Berry, and Marie Cook

Abstract

The role of the transplant coordinator in total pancreatectomy with islet autotransplant (TPIAT) is unique and multifaceted. In addition to expert-level skills in nursing assessment, triage, and evaluation, a TPIAT registered nurse care coordinator (RNCC) must possess an in-depth knowledge of pancreatic pathophysiology, pancreatitis and associated complications, abnormal laboratory tests, pertinent imaging, and procedures. Given that pancreatitis affects patients of all ages, the TPIAT RNCC must be capable of providing care to people across the aging spectrum.

Key Points

- The registered nurse care coordinator (RNCC) is the main point of contact for patients and family members, enabling them to navigate the complexity of referral; evaluation; and preoperative, inpatient, and postoperative care.
- The job requires broad knowledge and a wide range of skills to care for patients being evaluated for, undergoing, or recovering from total pancreatectomy with islet autotransplant (TPIAT) surgery.
- Among the core responsibilities of the RNCC are formulating the relevant medical history; working with the financial team to determine financial eligibility; coordinating appointments and testing; and providing clear written and verbal

E. Scheidecker (✉) · L. Berry
M Health Fairview, TPIAT Program, Minneapolis, MN, USA
e-mail: Emily.Scheidecker@Fairview.org; kathryn.berry@pennmedicine.upenn.org

M. Cook
M Health Fairview, Pediatric TPIAT Program, Minneapolis, MN, USA
e-mail: Marie.Cook@fairview.org

S. Chinnakotla et al. (eds.), *Total Pancreatectomy and Islet Auto Transplantation*,
https://doi.org/10.1007/978-981-92-0018-4_4

communication to patients and their families throughout the process, including educating them about the surgery, necessary medical testing, and postsurgical care and regimens that will be required.

- The RNCC is a key liaison between multidisciplinary team (MDT) members, community physicians, pharmacists, home care agencies, and the patient and helps to coordinate care across these domains and ensure continuity of care.
- The RNCC must also be able to provide psychological support with the assistance of a social worker and a health psychologist.

4.1 Overview

Registered nurse care coordinators (RNCC) provide patient care across the care continuum to patients of all ages, both before and after total pancreatectomy with islet autotransplant (TPIAT), including support for patients, families, and caregivers. It is essential that the TPIAT coordinator have expert skills in nursing evaluation, assessment, and triage. Knowledge of pancreatic pathophysiology, pancreatitis and associated complications, abnormal laboratory tests, pertinent imaging, and procedures is critical.

At the time of referral, the coordinator reviews medical records to formulate an accurate history of the pancreatitis. Prior to evaluation, the RNCC collaborates with the finance team to determine financial eligibility. The nurse coordinator must have knowledge of contracts, insurance policies, and financial limitations. Communication with the patient and family must be clear and concise. Interpersonal and team-member skills help to create a positive experience for the medical team and to provide consistent messages to the patient and family. It is important to set expectations up front so there are no unintended consequences or misunderstandings.

The TPIAT care coordinator collaborates with referring providers, doctors, interdisciplinary team members, patients, families, and significant others to evaluate, plan, and manage patient care. In addition, the RNCC serves as a liaison to the multidisciplinary team (MDT) to implement medical management of condition changes, diagnostic test results, and lab results based on knowledge of the patient and the patient's condition, both before and after TPIAT. As a liaison to community physicians, pharmacists, and home care agencies, the TPIAT coordinator helps to ensure the continuity of the care that is provided. Continuity of care helps the health care team to build trust with the patient. Excellent documentation skills and meticulous maintenance of medical records ensure that patient care activities will be seamless. Knowledge of program and protocol development, along with workflow tools such as order sets, provides consistency in direct patient assessment and evaluation and helps the team have a shared understanding and working knowledge of the patient's condition. The TPIAT RNCC works with the medical team to set goals and create a plan for each individual patient.

The TPIAT coordinator will be called upon to provide ongoing education to patients, families, and caregivers who are supporting the patient. Knowledge of teaching and learning theory and a creative approach are needed to accommodate all learning styles and develop unique approaches to assisting transplant patients in the management of their care over the course of a lifetime. In addition to providing professional nursing education, including orienting new staff to the role of transplant coordinator, the coordinator may also serve as a preceptor in student learning situations or provide physician and community education.

Coordinators participate in quality improvement initiatives and help to identify and assist in writing and implementing new policies. Professional development often includes serving on committees. Keeping current with new developments in transplantation through reading, attending seminars, and networking with other coordinators across the nation can improve job satisfaction and promote competency within the role. The transplant TPIAT coordinator provides value to the team and is a role model for how to provide a patient-centered approach to health care.

4.2 Adult Patients Referred for TPIAT

4.2.1 Evaluation of Adults

The RNCC manages the care of the TPIAT patient before, during, and after surgery. They are the main point of contact for patients and family members, enabling them to navigate the complexity of referral; evaluation; and preoperative, inpatient, and postoperative care. The RNCC has the following primary responsibilities:

- Coordinating care across multiple specialties.
- Providing written and verbal education to patients at all time points.
- Providing psychological support with the assistance of a social worker and a health psychologist.
- Reinforcing and explaining any medical testing and/or decisions.

The role of the RNCC following referral of a patient for TPIAT is central to the comprehensive and effective evaluation of appropriate candidates. This begins at the initial patient referral.

Following referral, the RNCC will collect information to assist the multidisciplinary team in determining if a patient should be brought for a full evaluation, usually during a screening call to the patient or review of medical records. The following information should be obtained:

- Demographics.
- Insurance information.
- Location of medical records and imaging.
- Duration and type of pancreatic disease: recurrent acute and/or chronic.
- Investigative or interventional procedures to date.
- Endoscopic ultrasound.
- Endoscopic retrograde pancreatography (ERCP).
- Sphincterotomies.

- Previous abdominal or pancreatic surgeries.
- Magnetic resonance imaging (MRI) or magnetic resonance cholangiopancreatography (MRCP).
- Computed tomography (CT scan).
- Current strategies of pain relief.
- Opioid regimen, including dose and duration of treatments.
- Neuromodulators.
- Topical applications.
- Interventional procedures.
- Nutritional status.
- Weight loss.
- Use of enteral or total parenteral nutrition supplementary feedings.
- Medications.
- Pancreatic enzyme supplementation.
- Proton pump inhibitors.
- Current endocrine and diabetes status.

Once this information is gathered and verified, the RNCC makes an initial presentation to the multidisciplinary team. The team will decide if the patient is a suitable candidate for moving forward with evaluation, and, if so, what specific testing and appointments are most appropriate during the evaluation. A thorough evaluation usually takes place over 2–3 days, depending on necessary testing. It is the responsibility of the RNCC to coordinate all appointments and testing. The RNCC will ensure the patient has a complete understanding of what each appointment entails and why it is needed. Patients are referred for TPIAT when all other interventions to relieve pancreatic pain have been exhausted and they are generally weary of medical appointments, emergency department visits, and hospital stays. They may suffer from medical posttraumatic stress disorder and, as such, the RNCC needs to take special care to ensure they feel understood and validated during these appointments. The RNCC does not necessarily have to accompany the patient to all the appointments but needs to facilitate a smooth flow and minimize the patient's anxiety. There is a lot of important information given and received during the evaluation. The RNCC should encourage the patient to bring a support person with them to appointments as this can be an invaluable tool for retaining knowledge and providing support.

Evaluation appointments may include any of the following as determined by the MDT:

- Gastroenterology: consult or endoscopic intervention.
- Surgical consult.
- Endocrinology.
- Nutritional and endocrinological testing: oral glucose tolerance test or mixed-meal testing.
- Dietitian.
- Social work.

- Health psychology.
- Pain management.
- Physical therapy.
- Laboratory testing.

Once these appointments are complete and all results available, the RNCC will once again bring the patient's case to the multidisciplinary team for review.

Each specialty has a chance to provide information and discuss the results of testing and patient assessments. The RNCC is central to bringing the team together to make an informed, comprehensive, and final decision on treatment options moving forward.

As the team member most familiar with the patient, the RNCC is the one to communicate the decision to the patient and family and should be able to relay this information with compassion and empathy. The care coordinator will also collaborate with the patient's local providers and specialists to update them on the plan of care and to complete any additional testing or procedures necessary prior to scheduling surgery.

As illustrated in Fig. 4.1, the RNCC communicates and coordinates the patient case with all members of the multidisciplinary team.

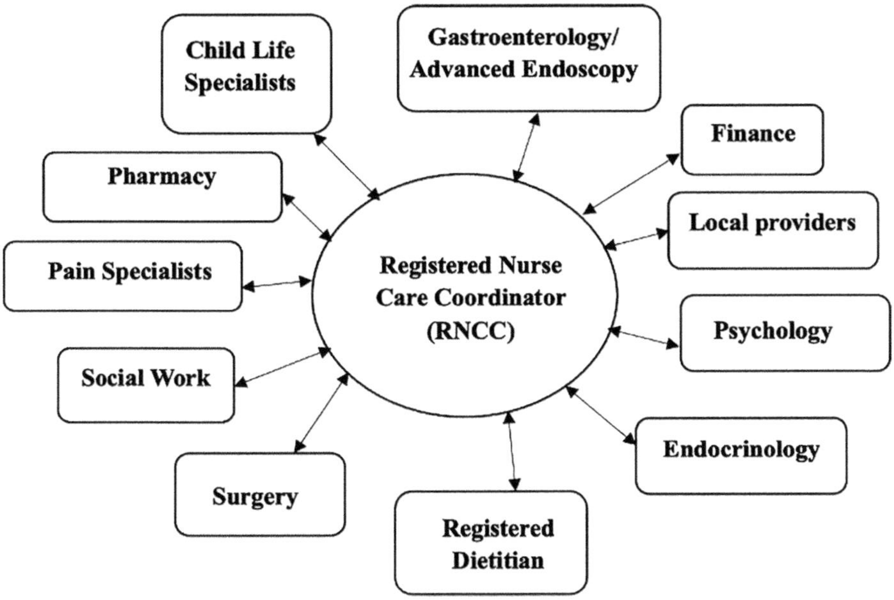

Fig. 4.1 Coordination of multidisciplinary care

4.2.2 Postoperative Coordination of the Adult TPIAT Patient

4.2.2.1 Surgical and Inpatient Care of the Adult TPIAT Patient

During the surgical and inpatient period of the TPIAT care process, the outpatient RNCC remains primarily on the periphery of care, deferring to the expertise and workflows of the inpatient nursing and surgery teams. Patients are initially cared for in an intensive care setting based on care needs such as an intravenous (IV) insulin regimen, continuous enteral feedings via gastrojejunostomy tube, and paravertebral infusion catheters for pain management and patient-controlled analgesia. Generally, nurse-to-patient ratios are lower in intensive care settings, and this allows for closer monitoring of the acute postoperative patient. As patients stabilize and are able to decrease dependency on opioid analgesia, they will transfer to a medical/surgical or transplant specialty care unit. Once transferred, the inpatient team will work to transition patients from intravenous insulin to subcutaneous injections or an insulin pump, will work on both weaning opioid use and transitioning from IV opioid analgesia to oral or enteral formulations, and will assist with advancement of diet and enteral feedings as appropriate. All these specifics are covered in detail in other portions of this work (Chap. 6).

As hospital discharge approaches, the outpatient coordinator will meet with the patient to review medication regimens, reinforce education on tube feeding management and diabetes care, discuss the plan for follow-up care appointments with specialty providers, and verify that patients and caregivers know how and when to contact providers with after-hours concerns.

4.2.2.2 Outpatient Postoperative and Posthospital Care in Adults

The patient will be seen the day after hospital discharge in the specialty infusion center for laboratory tests, general assessment, and hydration therapy as necessary. The RNCC will visit the patient during this visit to verify that all discharge medications were ordered and received appropriately, reinforce diabetes care management, and review appointment schedule.

Following hospital discharge, a home care nurse, separate from the RNCC, will meet with the patient and caregiver at their local address to verify safety with management of enteral feeds and central line care. In addition, the RNCC will be in contact with them daily for status review. Daily status calls will focus on the following:

- Pain Management:
  - Assess if pain is sufficiently managed and work with providers to adjust doses as appropriate.
  - Current daily dosage of medication.
    Verify when the next refill of medications is required and work with pharmacy staff to ensure insurance coverage of medications.
- Bowel Regimen:
  Assess bowel regularity status.

- Adjust bowel regimen medications as necessary to maintain regularity (at least one soft, formed bowel movement daily).
- Exocrine Pancreatic Insufficiency (EPI):
  - Review pancreatic enzyme replacement therapy (PERT) regimen (inline vs. oral).
    Assess for signs and symptoms of EPI and adjust PERT per protocol.
- Endocrine and Islet Transplant:
  - Review diet regimen, food logs, and gastrointestinal (GI) symptoms surrounding any nutritional intake.
  - Review Dexcom continuous glucose monitor (CGM) readings for the previous 24-h period.
    Collaborate with diabetes education and endocrinology providers to adjust insulin regimen or pump settings to maintain tight glycemic control (80–120 mg/dL more than 75% of time).
- Laboratory and Postsurgical Status:
  - Assess wound status: drainage, redness, presence of surgical closure devices.
  - Assess status of lines/drains/etc.: daily gastrostomy-tube output, function of any surgical drains.
  - Weekly to monthly lab draws as required by symptoms:
    - Complete blood count with differential and platelets due to splenectomy.
      Comprehensive metabolic panel to assess efficacy of enteral nutrition regimen.

4.2.3 Long-Term Care and Monitoring of the Adult TPIAT Patient

Following discharge from the hospital and resolution of immediate postoperative needs, long-term care of the TPIAT patient should focus on the following:

1. EPI.
   (a) Patients will need lifelong PERT.
      (i) These need to be Food and Drug Administration (FDA)-approved and not over-the-counter or health-food-store brands.
      (ii) Dosage based on patient's weight and symptoms and as per manufacturer recommendation but not to exceed 2000 lipase units/kg/meal because larger amounts carry a risk of fibrosing colonopathy.
   (b) Proton pump inhibitors may be required in the short term after surgery and possibly for the long term to assist the efficacy of pancreatic enzymes.
   (c) Supplementation of fat-soluble vitamins (A, E, D, and K) in special formulations for the pancreatectomy patient.

   (d) Low-oxalate diet for kidney stone avoidance.
   (e) Nutritional lab surveillance (albumin, vitamin levels, fatty acid levels) immediately; 3, 6, and 12 months postoperatively to ensure stability; then annually.

2. Lifelong management and monitoring of islet function and blood glucose levels.

   (a) Blood sugar monitoring with goal blood sugars of 80–120 mg/dL.
   (b) Use of CGMs and insulin pumps to maintain this range.
   (c) Avoidance of corticosteroids, as these can lead to significantly increased blood sugars that, if uncontrolled, can damage transplanted islets.
   (d) Mixed-meal tolerance testing at 3, 6, and 12 months after islet transplantation to assess islet function.

3. Postsplenectomy immunization status.

   (a) Verify that the patient has MedicAlert identification (jewelry, watch band, tattoo) delineating postsplenectomy status.
   (b) Maintain immunization status with updated vaccinations for postsplenectomy status; guidelines are available via the Centers for Disease Control and Prevention (CDC).
   (c) Provide immediate medical attention for fevers over 101 degrees Fahrenheit with appropriate antibiotic use.

4. Gastrointestinal issues secondary to surgical anastomosis.

   (a) Ulceration at the site of anastomosis—ensure adequate dosing of proton pump inhibitors to help with prevention of this complication.
   (b) Constipation.
   (c) Steatorrhea.
   (d) Small intestinal bacterial overgrowth.
   (e) Potential adhesions.

5. Quality-of-life surveillance—this can be completed per individual institution guidelines and formats such as patient-completed survey or telephone assessment by the RNCC.

4.3 Pediatric Patients Referred for TPIAT

4.3.1 Evaluation

The pancreatitis evaluation includes 12 or more appointments that are scheduled over 3–5 days. A multidisciplinary team approach is key to the evaluation. The evaluation includes a core set of specialist appointments and may include other specialties based on the unique medical history of each child. Each child will meet with all or some of the following:

Specialists:

- Nurse coordinator/pediatric nurse practitioner.
- Gastroenterologist.
- Endocrinologist.
- Transplant surgeon.
- Integrative medicine.
- Pain specialist.
- Physical therapy.
- Health psychology.
- Dietitian.
- Social work.
- Child life specialist.

Additional Testing:

- MRI/MRCP.
- Abdominal ultrasound.
- CT scan of the abdomen and pelvis.
- Endoscopic retrograde cholangiopancreatography (ERCP).
- Endoscopic ultrasound.
- Mixed-meal tolerance test.

4.3.2 Evaluation Goals for the Pediatric Patient, Family, and Primary Health Care Team

The pediatric specialty providers meet as an interdisciplinary team and follow the same protocols to determine evaluation candidacy as above. The primary focus of the evaluation is the overall well-being of the child. Each specialist will make recommendations for care of the child with pancreatitis. The Pain Team and Physical Therapist explore the child's experience with pain and their ability to function normally. It is important that the Pain Team have a complete understanding of the child's emotional and behavioral needs so that the most appropriate recommendations can be made for managing pain. The team seeks to understand how the whole family's life may have been affected by the child's pancreatitis. The Psychologist and Social Worker can provide support that is tailored to each child and family.

Every child is expected to have a comprehensive home care plan in place prior to surgery:

1. Physical Therapy.
   (a) Regular participation in outpatient physical therapy and daily follow-through with the home exercise program provided by our physical therapist or developed through a local physical therapist.
   (b) Ability to walk a mile (not necessarily without pain) before undergoing TPIAT surgery.

2. Integrative Medicine.
   (a) Active strategies such as deep breathing, guided imagery/self-hypnosis, progressive muscle relaxation, and active distraction such as participating in a hobby can help reduce the amount of pain that is felt.
   (b) It is necessary to practice at least one of these active mind-body techniques every day (even when not in pain) for them to be most effective when needed during a pain crisis.
   (c) Passive strategies like massage, essential oils/aromatherapy, watching TV, or using a phone can help but are less effective than the active strategies mentioned above.
3. Psychology.
   (a) Talking with a local therapist is extremely important and standard treatment for every TPIAT candidate. This is necessary to help address possible anxiety and stress around living with a chronic, painful disease and the implications of undergoing a major surgery, exploration of current coping mechanisms (or lack thereof), sleep habits, and any other factors important for preparation and recovery from surgery.
4. Normalization of Life.
   (a) Normal sleep hygiene regimen.
   (b) Normal exercise routine and diet.
   (c) Normal social life with age-matched peers, and not allowing pain to interfere with doing things with friends and/or family.
   (d) Attend school regularly.
      1. Monday through Friday, without exception.
      2. Most importantly, unless in the midst of a pancreatitis episode that requires hospitalization, pain is *not* an acceptable excuse for missing school.
5. Pain Management.
   (a) In many instances, appropriate medications can be helpful.
   (b) Medications alone will not fix the pain disorder.
   (c) The point of analgesic medications is to allow participation in, and to augment, the first four recommendations.
   (d) Patients are required to have a local pain provider who will provide pain management prior to surgery and resume treatment after returning home from surgery. If there is not a local pain team, a primary care provider must be willing to manage pain medications once patients return home.

4.3.3 Postoperative Coordination of the Pediatric TPIAT Patient

Immediately after the surgery, patients are managed in the pediatric intensive care unit by the pediatric intensivists, and the specialty teams are available as consultants. Portal vein thrombosis management includes Doppler ultrasound of the portal vein on days 1 and 7, dextran for 48 h, aspirin 2 mg/kg, and hydroxyurea in addition to a heparin drip 10 U/kg × 7 days.

A near-euglycemic state must be maintained to preserve islet function, which requires the use of an intravenous insulin pump and frequent glucose checks to target glucose levels between 80 and 125 mg/dL. All patients have gastrostomy tubes. Trophic feeds are started and increased to goal as tolerated. An enzyme cartridge is attached to the feedings. Oral feeds are advanced as tolerated over several weeks and then tube feeds are weaned off.

Paravertebral blocks are placed to assist in pain management in addition to the use of patient-controlled analgesic pumps. Patients and families receive diabetes education and learn to manage glucose levels. Closed-loop systems are preferable. The insurance prior authorization process is initiated prior to surgery.

Daily Medication Regimen:

- Multivitamin (ADEK).
- Pancreatic enzymes: 1000–1500 lipase units/kg/meal (half of this dose for snacks).
- Proton pump inhibitor.
- Insulin regimen (pump or subcutaneous injection).
- Prophylactic antibiotic until 1 year after the operation.
- Bowel regimen: stool softeners, MiraLAX, other bulking agents or laxatives.
- Patients have a lifelong requirement for pancreatic enzymes to digest and absorb food. The enzyme dose should not exceed 2000 lipase units/kg/meal and 1000 lipase units/kg/snack OR 10,000 lipase units/kg/day. FDA-approved pancreatic enzyme preparations must be used; enzymes purchased at a health food store are inappropriate. Enzymes must be taken with or just before the first bite of food; they cannot be taken ahead of a meal, even by 5 min. Because there will be some fatty stools even with adequate enzymes, a low-oxalate diet must be followed to prevent oxalate kidney stones.

Fat-soluble vitamins (A, E, D, and K) should be supplemented with special forms that are more absorbable in the intestine of a pancreatic-insufficient patient. If the patient is vegan, adequate intake of animal-derived vitamin B12 is necessary.

Insulin needs will depend on the success of the islet-cell transplant. Goal blood sugars are 80–125 mg/dL in the first 1–2 months posttransplant and subsequently 80–125 mg/dL fasting and < 150 mg/dL postprandial. Goal hemoglobin (Hgb) A1c is <6.5%. Sustained hyperglycemia may result in irreversible islet loss, so glycemic control is tightly maintained in the patients with partial islet function or insulin independence. C-peptide production should be measured by mixed-meal testing at 3 months, 6 months, and then yearly after surgery. Hgb A1c levels should be measured every 3 months. Corticosteroids should be avoided unless medically necessary.

Since part of the TPIAT procedure includes a splenectomy, all pediatric patients will be on daily antibiotic prophylaxis with amoxicillin (or a different antibiotic in the case of penicillin allergy) until 1 year after transplantation. Patients must seek medical attention immediately for oral temperatures greater than 100.5 °F. Patients will need pneumococcal vaccination 5 years after the initial series and quadrivalent meningococcal conjugate vaccine after 3–5 years (3 years if <7 years old at the time of surgery and 5 years if >7 years old) and then every 5 years. Patients aged 10 years and older with asplenia should receive a meningitis B booster dose 1 year after completion of a meningitis B primary series followed by meningitis B booster doses every 2–3 years thereafter. MedicAlert bracelets or necklaces help to ensure health care providers always know the splenectomy status.

Once discharged from the hospital, patients are seen weekly in clinic by the multidisciplinary team to manage nutrition, glucose control, pain, and surgical issues. Patients stay locally for 4 weeks after discharge from the hospital (8 weeks from the surgery date).

At 3, 6, and 12 months postoperatively, a mixed-meal test and laboratory tests are performed. Following TPIAT, nonadherence correlates highly with poor Hgb A1c levels, low vitamin levels, and stool and motility issues.

Laboratory tests include:

- Basic metabolic panel (BMP), complete blood count (CBC), hepatic panel, lipids, iron studies.
- Hgb A1c.
- Timed glucoses and C-peptides.
- Vitamin levels (ADE).
- Essential fatty acids.

4.4 Conclusions

A RN TPIAT clinical coordinator is critical to the success of a TPIAT program. The RN coordinator helps the patients and families navigate the complex multidisciplinary evaluation necessary for TPIAT surgery. The coordinator also helps ensure the patient's adherence to postoperative protocols and helps patients navigate the long-term follow-up care after TPIAT.

Total Pancreatectomy and Islet Autotransplantation: Surgical Approaches

5

Karthik Ramanathan

Abstract

Total pancreatectomy with islet autotransplantation is an emerging surgical technique for management of chronic pancreatitis. By removing the entire root cause of pain, total pancreatectomy allows for a significant reduction, if not outright resolution, of the pain and feeding intolerance associated with chronic pancreatitis, while the islet autotransplant component mitigates the risk of significant brittle diabetes after the pancreatectomy. Preoperative assessment and management of comorbidities, nutritional status, and variations in operative anatomy are critical for limiting peri- and postoperative morbidities. Perioperatively, lines for patient monitoring are placed, including arterial lines for intraoperative monitoring of blood pressure, intravenous catheters for infusions, oro- or nasogastric tubes for decompression, a Foley catheter, and a paravertebral catheter for pain control. Exposure and removal of the pancreas follows a strict procedure so that the blood supply is maintained until the last step to minimize warm ischemia. While the pancreas is processed outside the operating room to isolate the islets, a Roux-en-Y is created. Finally, the isolated islet cells are infused through the stump of the splenic vein or middle colic vein. Although minimally invasive techniques are possible and are associated with shorter hospital stays and less narcotic use, the unpredictable degree of scarring and inflammation due to chronic pancreatitis can increase the difficulty of these procedures.

K. Ramanathan (✉)
Department of Surgery, University of Minnesota, Minneapolis, MN, USA
e-mail: raman120@umn.edu

S. Chinnakotla et al. (eds.), *Total Pancreatectomy and Islet Auto Transplantation*,
https://doi.org/10.1007/978-981-92-0018-4_5

Key Points

1. Total pancreatectomy with islet autotransplantation (TPIAT) represents a surgical approach to management of painful chronic pancreatitis by allowing total removal of the source of pain with preservation of some degree of islet function.
2. Nutritional assessment of patients pre- and postoperatively is of paramount importance, especially given the ever-increasing prevalence of obesity as a comorbid condition.
3. Careful preoperative vascular assessment is critical to understand and ameliorate issues with any aberrant hepatic arterial inflow or portomesenteric venous thrombosis.
4. Although the surgical principles of pancreatectomy have long been established, TPIAT differs from other pancreatectomy techniques in the need to preserve vascular flow to the pancreas until the very end to minimize ischemic injury to the islet cells.
5. Minimally invasive approaches present new opportunities in TPIAT but also require careful consideration of risks involving longer warm ischemic times; economic considerations are also important.

5.1 Introduction

Chronic pancreatitis that is refractory to medical and surgical management can be a challenge for surgeons. A number of surgical techniques have been used in an attempt to ameliorate pain and restore quality of life, including partial resection and drainage procedures such as lateral pancreaticojejunostomy (such as Puestow) or its variants (such as the Frey and Beger procedures). Patients often have transient pain relief, but due to the diffuse nature of the condition and involvement of the entire pancreas, pain eventually recurs in up to 50% of patients [1–6]; exocrine and endocrine insufficiency often develop over time. Total pancreatectomy with islet autotransplantation (TPIAT) is an emerging surgical technique for management of chronic pancreatitis, in which the entire root cause of the pain is removed, providing long-term pain relief [7, 8]. TPIAT allows for a significant reduction, if not outright resolution, of the pain and feeding intolerance associated with chronic pancreatitis while also mitigating the risk of significant postpancreatectomy diabetes [9]. Although TPIAT was previously reserved as a last option and often offered to patients only when surgical resection or drainage procedures had failed, it may now be performed in patients after medical or endoscopic therapy has not achieved the desired results, with excellent long-term outcomes in pain and symptom relief, as well as good preservation of islet function [10–13].

5.2 Preoperative Assessment and Patient Selection

Patient selection for pancreatic surgery requires careful assessment and management of factors that contribute to the risk of adverse outcomes in the intraoperative, perioperative, and postoperative phases [14, 15].

Patients with significant cardiopulmonary risk factors (e.g., smoking) or known heart disease should be assessed for fitness to undergo prolonged anesthesia and surgical stress. Given the elective nature of surgery for chronic pancreatitis, it is best to fully correct medical comorbidities to minimize the risk of adverse outcomes. Patients at very high medical risk due to nonmodifiable conditions should not be considered candidates for TPIAT and should instead be offered less morbid surgery or, more commonly, managed nonsurgically with endoscopy and nerve block techniques as appropriate.

Nutritional assessment is another important consideration. Patients with chronic pancreatitis may present with profound weight loss due to ongoing nausea and pain with eating that leads to food avoidance. This may be true in both lean and obese patients and results in significant protein loss and sarcopenia. In some instances, a feeding tube may be necessary to support patients nutritionally prior to surgery, and close attention should be given to a patient's overall nutritional status throughout the preoperative workup period.

Because obesity is an increasingly common problem generally, it has also become more prevalent in patients with chronic pancreatitis [16]. Assessment of obesity in chronic pancreatitis requires attention to a combination of surgical factors (technical feasibility and complications), nutritional factors (micronutrient deficiency and malnutrition), and, in the case of IAT, the impact of obesity and insulin resistance on islet engraftment and postoperative insulin requirements [16]. Obese patients are generally exposed to higher intraoperative and postoperative surgical risks, including longer operative times and more difficult surgeries, wound infections, hernias, deep venous thrombosis, and more difficult respiratory support. Additionally, the effects of obesity on the body's inflammatory milieu and microbiome can lead to diminished absorption of micronutrients and profound micronutrient deficiencies that also impact wound healing. This malabsorption may be further exacerbated by any concomitant pancreatic exocrine insufficiency that is present preoperatively, while the nature of total pancreatectomy itself requires careful monitoring for steatorrhea and malabsorption postoperatively. This management requires adjustment of pancreatic enzyme replacement dose, potential dietary adjustment, and monitoring of fat-soluble vitamin and micronutrient levels for targeted supplementation. In the preoperative space, consideration should be given to ordering a dietitian consult for optimization prior to surgery. Our group uses a general body mass index (BMI) cutoff of 30 for surgical candidacy, but further study of the effects of sarcopenia, inflammatory milieu, and microbiome on surgical and islet engraftment outcomes across patient BMI ranges may be warranted [16].

A complete preoperative patient assessment should also include contrast-enhanced cross-sectional imaging for full delineation of operative anatomy. It is important to note the hepatic arterial anatomy and any variants of interest (e.g., replaced right or totally replaced hepatic arteries) and their course, either alongside or through the uncinate process and head of the pancreas. In very inflamed, fibrotic fields, identification and preservation of these structures may prove difficult. It is also important to delineate any stenoses/thromboses and collateralization of the portomesenteric and splenic veins. Splenic vein thrombosis with collateralization may increase intraoperative blood loss but is not prohibitive for performance of TPIAT. True portal vein thrombosis with cavernous transformation may prevent safe pancreatic resection or require additional technical modifications.

Our practice is to routinely perform splenectomy with total pancreatectomy. Though some centers have advocated splenic preservation, we have opted for including splenectomy to minimize disruption of blood flow to the body and tail of the pancreas during the procedure, as well as to reduce the risk of resultant splenic vein thrombus and sinistral hypertension. We therefore administer vaccines preoperatively to reduce the risk of postsplenectomy sepsis [17].

Our practice is fortunate to include a colocated islet laboratory, and our typical islet processing time is 5 h. As a result, we typically await the return of cells and infuse prior to case completion. In centers that perform islet processing off-site, up to 24 h may be required to return isolated islets. Various techniques have been described for managing this, including temporary closure with return to the operating room for infusion or completed closure with separate percutaneous access by interventional radiology.

5.3 Perioperative Management

Though these patients do not routinely have significant cardiac disease, they routinely receive arterial lines for intraoperative blood pressure monitoring due to the length of exposure to general anesthesia and the potential for bleeding. They also receive multiple large-bore intravenous catheters or, in the case of difficult access, central venous access. This allows for rapid, large-volume infusion as needed during the procedure. TPIAT patients are unique in terms of fluid requirements during surgery. Long disease duration, inflammatory stimuli of pancreatitis, infusion of an unpurified pancreatic cell preparation, and potential for major blood loss can be challenging for intraoperative fluid management. Over-resuscitation can be associated with dilutional anemia and the need for transfusion, hypoxia (pulmonary edema, supplemental O_2 requirements, and bowel edema [ileus, anastomotic leak]), wound complications (seroma infections), and decreased mobility (pain, swelling, urinary tract infection). Under-resuscitation can be associated with acute kidney injury, risk of portal vein thrombosis after islet cell infusion, and, potentially, islet graft failure. Although TPIAT patients can be resuscitated according to the clinical parameters of standard perioperative fluid therapy, such as blood pressure, central venous pressure, and heart rate, a recent study showed that goal-directed resuscitation therapy using a stroke volume variation monitor can lower transfusion requirements [18]. These patients also routinely have orogastric or nasogastric tubes for intraoperative decompression, as well as a Foley catheter for urine output monitoring, which is maintained for at least one postoperative day. Subcutaneous heparin is typically administered to reduce the risk of intraoperative deep venous thrombosis, and sequential compression devices are also used. Long-acting broad-spectrum antibiotics with suitable enteric pathogen coverage are administered, with selection based on patient allergies [19].

Due to the significant analgesic demands of these patients postoperatively, we generally request our regional pain service to place paravertebral catheters preoperatively [20]. We use these as a mainstay of pain relief following the procedure to help reduce significant narcotic demands. This method is preferred over epidural analgesia due to the need for anticoagulation, both intraoperatively with islet cell infusion as well as postoperatively to reduce the risk of or to treat any resultant portal vein thromboses.

5.4 Surgical Technique: Open

The patient is positioned supine with arms out and all pressure points padded. Lines and devices are placed and secured as described above. The abdomen is prepared appropriately for surgery. Incision options include an upper midline or a left subcostal with a small right extension, based on surgeon preference and abdominal profile. An additional consideration in incision selection is patient surgical history, as some of these patients have undergone abdominal surgery in the past.

Following incision, safe entry into the abdomen is achieved and any adhesions are fully lysed. A surgical retractor is assembled to provide full exposure. The lesser sac is entered through the gastrocolic ligament, and the transverse colon is reflected down through the splenic flexure to fully expose the pancreas. The short gastric arteries are doubly ligated and divided to allow full cephalad retraction of the stomach to expose the spleen and tail of the pancreas. Adhesions between the posterior wall of the stomach and anterior surface of the pancreas should be taken down carefully to avoid injury to the blood vessels and vagus nerves along the lesser curvature..

The spleen is mobilized by dividing the splenorenal and splenocolic ligaments. Using the spleen as a handle, the tail and body of the pancreas are mobilized medially to the level of the superior mesenteric and portal veins. Care is taken to separate the mesocolon from the inferior border of the pancreas and to preserve the middle colic vascular bundle, though this is not always possible in cases of dense inflammation. The tissue around the splenic artery and splenic vein is dissected, taking care to identify and loop the splenic artery on the superior border of the pancreas. The splenic vein is looped distal to the entry of the inferior mesenteric vein. The duodenum is transected 2–4 cm distal to the pylorus, ensuring that the right gastric and gastroepiploic vessels are preserved. The stomach is reflected upward and laterally to expose the head and body of the pancreas. The proximal jejunum is divided 10–20 cm distal to the ligament of Treitz, then freed proximally until the ligament of Treitz has been taken down. The Kocher maneuver is performed to completely mobilize the duodenum and the pancreatic head. The portal triad is isolated and dissected free. The area is carefully examined to identify any aberrant hepatic arteries arising from the superior mesenteric artery. If one exists, it is carefully preserved. The gastroduodenal artery is dissected and looped but not divided.

At this point, the pancreas is attached by the vascular supply, common bile duct, and uncinate process. The bile duct is transected at the superior border of the pancreas. The uncinate process of the pancreas is mobilized off the portal vein by dividing all small tributaries to the portal vein. The vascular structures are divided in the following order: gastroduodenal artery, splenic artery, then splenic vein [17]. The pancreas is then immediately placed in a cold sterile preservative solution and transported to the islet isolation laboratory. The arterial stumps are doubly ligated with suture ligatures. We leave division of the vascular supply of the pancreas to the final step to minimize exposure of the islet tissue to warm ischemia and to support adequate perfusion during the dissection time.

While the islets are being isolated from the pancreas, a Roux-en-Y is created, with each limb of the Roux being 80 cm in length. Both limbs are placed in a retrocolic position through openings in the right and left mesocolon, respectively. An end-to-side choledochojejunostomy is constructed using absorbable sutures. An end-to-side duodenojejunostomy is constructed in a hand-sewn, two-layered fashion, and a gastrojejunostomy tube is placed in the stomach using a Stamm technique, with the tip of the jejunal tube placed in the proximal jejunum. A hand-sewn, two-layered jejunojejunostomy is also constructed, although this may be stapled in accordance with surgeon preference. Mesenteric defects and the ligament of Treitz defect are closed. The Roux limbs are pexied to the mesocolon to close those defects as well.

5.5 Islet Infusion

Once the islet cell preparation is complete, the splenic vein stump or the middle colic vein is cannulated with a 5 French micropuncture kit and attached to pressure tubing with an in-line manometer. The tubing and manometer are all primed with saline and flushed clear of air (Figs. 5.1 and 5.2). The patient receives systemic anticoagulation prior to islet infusion, to a total dose of 70 units per kg [17], and an initial portal pressure measurement is obtained and recorded. The islet preparation is infused by gravity into the portal venous system, with close monitoring of portal pressure (Fig. 5.3). The combination of anticoagulation and increased portal pressure can trigger bleeding in a previously quiescent field, and this is carefully monitored as well. If the pressure is sustained above 25 cm H_2O, infusion is paused and the pressure is allowed time to drop. If it does not, alternative sites for islet placement are considered, such as the peritoneal cavity or omental pocket. If the liver appears diseased or cirrhotic, portal infusion is typically also deferred, and islets are placed intraperitoneally.

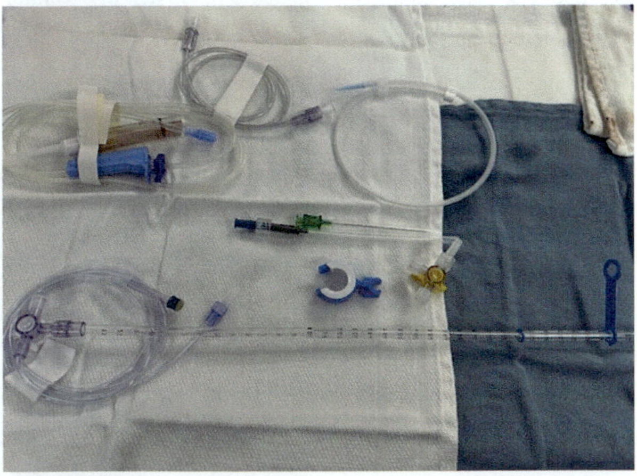

Fig. 5.1 Equipment for islet infusion, including manometer, IV tubing, 3-way stopcock, micropuncture kit, and wire

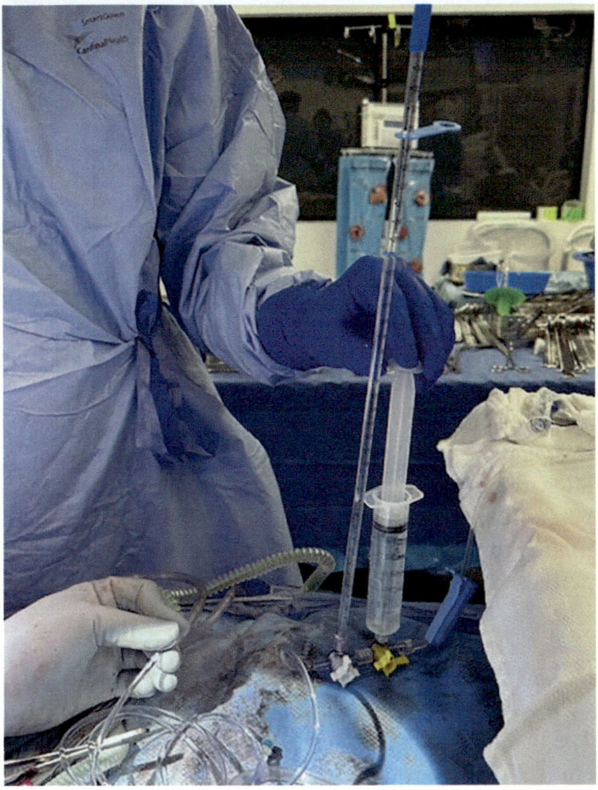

Fig. 5.2 Assembled infusion set with syringe of heparinized saline attached to a stopcock to flush the manometer and lines

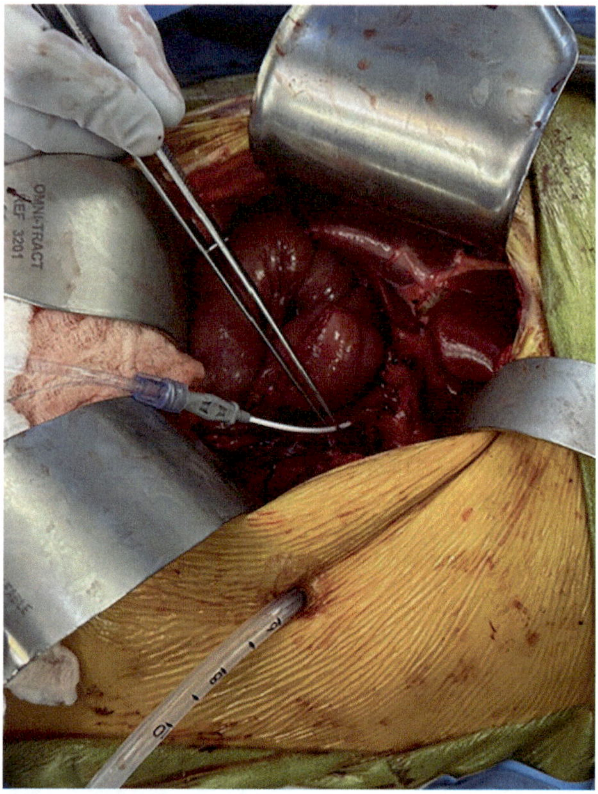

Fig. 5.3 Infusion catheter in the splenic vein stump

5.5.1 Intraperitoneal Technique for Islet Implantation

The islets are gently and uniformly dripped via gravity into the splenic bed, over the liver and the peritoneum. If a surgical drain is placed, it should be occluded for 48 h after transplant to prevent loss of islets. The peritoneum is an easy site to implant but, unlike the liver, the peritoneal cavity is relatively avascular, which can lead to limited oxygen and nutrient diffusion, exposing the transplanted islets to prolonged periods of hypoxia and hindering their survival and function.

5.5.2 Omental Pouch Technique for Islet Implantation

The omentum is an attractive alternative site because it is easily accessible intraoperatively, lacks volume restrictions, and is highly vascularized with portal venous drainage simulating the native pancreatic endocrine pathway. In preparation for omental transplantation, the islets are allowed to settle from their solution to the bottom of the infusion bag before being drawn into a 60-cc syringe. An omentum "bowl" is created by lifting the edges of the omentum from the transverse colon. The islets are dripped into the "bowl," and EVICEL (Johnson & Johnson Wound

Management, Somerville, NJ), a fibrin sealant, is applied over the islets, helping affix them to the omentum to facilitate engraftment. The omental pouch is then closed with a running suture. Stice et al. reported this technique in four patients with no complications and decreasing insulin requirements comparable to those of matched controls who received only islets transplanted intraportally [21].

A surgical drain is typically placed along the pancreatectomy bed and behind the biliary anastomosis to monitor for leaks. The fascia and wound are closed in layers, and all drains and tubes are secured to the skin.

5.6 Surgical Techniques: Minimally Invasive

As minimally invasive surgery grows in prevalence, TPIAT has also been approached both laparoscopically and robotically in selected cases [22–25]. Although early studies were less favorable across a variety of outcomes (morbidity, case duration, and technique differences), these differences have diminished as surgical technique and skill have advanced. In an impressive series from Makary and colleagues [25] spanning 15 robotic, 26 laparoscopic, and 20 open surgeries (with eight open surgeries converted from a minimally invasive approach), no significant differences were found in patient safety, with similar morbidity and no mortality in any of the cohorts. The open surgeries were associated with shorter operative times but more bleeding than either minimally invasive approach. Patients undergoing robotic or laparoscopic TPIAT had shorter hospital stays and lower narcotic utilization over time than the open cohort, though given the significant proportion of open cases resulting from conversion from minimally invasive approaches in the cohort, it is difficult to separate the contributions of underlying disease severity from that of laparotomy [25]. Although conversion from minimally invasive to open was not necessary in most cases, the difficulty of this approach lies in the unpredictable degree of scarring and inflammation associated with chronic pancreatitis and the effect of that change on safe dissection in critical areas. Indeed, the reason for conversion from minimally invasive to open in the majority of cases was difficulty identifying or safely dissecting the portal or superior mesenteric veins, underscoring both the difficulty of safe minimally invasive dissection in the setting of substantial chronic inflammation and the difficulty of preoperative anticipation of this major obstacle to safe conduct of minimally invasive pancreatectomy. Further, one of the identified contraindications to offering a minimally invasive approach was the presence of mesenteritis on cross-sectional imaging, due to the shortened mesentery and difficulty with minimally invasive manipulation, as well as the chronic inflammation detailed above.

There is a notable difference in warm ischemia time between minimally invasive and open approaches, with warm ischemia averaging over 80 min in the robotic cohort, over 50 min in the laparoscopic cohort, and typically only a few minutes with the open approach. Here, warm ischemia is defined as the period between the ligation of the last arterial inflow (gastroduodenal, inferior pancreaticoduodenal, or splenic artery) and the conversion to cold ischemia via preservative flush [25]. This difference is independent of en bloc versus segmental resection technique, because the rates of these approaches were comparable in open surgeries and those with robotic assistance. Though initial reports suggest similar outcomes in islet yield and function, this may need closer follow-up as minimally invasive techniques grow in prevalence. Critically, the authors of this comparative study had access to on-site islet processing, as do we. While other studies have demonstrated minimal effect on islet yield between locally and distantly purified pancreata, it is as yet unknown whether the combination of longer warm and cold ischemia will result in a decrease in islet yield.

5.7 Conclusion

TPIAT remains a radical but very effective surgical approach to management of intractably painful recurrent acute or chronic pancreatitis. It has a well-established record of safety and improved morbidity with refinement in patient management and surgical technique, while also offering the opportunity to ameliorate or prevent postpancreatectomy insulin-dependent diabetes. As surgery expands to include operations on patients with greater obesity and medical comorbidity and benefits from enhanced minimally invasive approaches, TPIAT appears poised for a similar evolution. The nuances of TPIAT, specifically management of perivascular inflammation, warm ischemia, and the effects of insulin resistance on islet functional outcomes, will require a thoughtful approach to managing these new frontiers to preserve and amplify the great impact TPIAT has on treating patients with chronic painful pancreatitis.

References

1. Bradley EL 3rd. Long-term results of pancreatojejunostomy in patients with chronic pancreatitis. Am J Surg. 1987;153(2):207–13.
2. Clifton MS, Pelayo JC, Cortes RA, Grethel EJ, Wagner AJ, Lee H, et al. Surgical treatment of childhood recurrent pancreatitis. J Pediatr Surg. 2007;42(7):1203–7.
3. Gachago C, Draganov PV. Pain management in chronic pancreatitis. World J Gastroenterol. 2008;14(20):3137–48.
4. Holmberg JT, Isaksson G, Ihse I. Long term results of pancreaticojejunostomy in chronic pancreatitis. Surg Gynecol Obstet. 1985;160(4):339–46.
5. Iqbal CW, Moir CR, Ishitani MB. Management of chronic pancreatitis in the pediatric patient: endoscopic retrograde cholangiopancreatography vs operative therapy. J Pediatr Surg. 2009;44(1):139–43. discussion 43
6. Markowitz JS, Rattner DW, Warshaw AL. Failure of symptomatic relief after pancreaticojejunal decompression for chronic pancreatitis. Strategies for salvage. Arch Surg. 1994;129(4):374–9. discussion 9–80.
7. Sutherland DER, Radosevich DM, Bellin MD, Hering BJ, Beilman GJ, Dunn TB, et al. Total pancreatectomy and islet autotransplantation for chronic pancreatitis. J Am Coll Surg. 2012;214(4):409–26.

8. Bellin MD, Freeman ML, Gelrud A, Slivka A, Clavel A, Humar A, et al. Total pancreatectomy and islet autotransplantation in chronic pancreatitis: recommendations from PancreasFest. Pancreatology. 2014;14(1):27–35.
9. Bellin MD, Abu-El-Haija M, Morgan K, Adams D, Beilman GJ, Chinnakotla S, et al. A multicenter study of total pancreatectomy with islet autotransplantation (TPIAT): POST (prospective observational study of TPIAT). Pancreatology. 2018;18(3):286–90.
10. Bellin MD, Eaton A, Ramanathan K, Beilman G, Downs E, Schwarzenberg SJ, et al. Long-term islet graft functional assessments in more than 500 patients undergoing total pancreatectomy with intraportal islet autotransplantation. J Am Coll Surg. 2025;240:405.
11. Chinnakotla S, Beilman GJ, Vock D, Freeman ML, Kirchner V, Dunn TB, et al. Intraportal islet autotransplantation independently improves quality of life after total pancreatectomy in patients with chronic refractory pancreatitis. Ann Surg. 2022;276(3):441–9.
12. Dixon J, DeLegge M, Morgan KA, Adams DB. Impact of total pancreatectomy with islet cell transplant on chronic pancreatitis management at a disease-based center. Am Surg. 2008;74(8):735–8.
13. Wilson GC, Sutton JM, Smith MT, Schmulewitz N, Salehi M, Choe KA, et al. Total pancreatectomy with islet cell autotransplantation as the initial treatment for minimal-change chronic pancreatitis. HPB. 2015;17(3):232–8.
14. Bellin MD, Ramanathan K, Chinnakotla S. Total pancreatectomy with islet auto-transplantation: surgical procedure, outcomes, and quality of life. Adv Surg. 2023;57(1):15–30.
15. Nathan JD, Yang Y, Eaton A, Witkowski P, Wijkstrom M, Walsh M, et al. Surgical approach and short-term outcomes in adults and children undergoing total pancreatectomy with islet autotransplantation: a report from the prospective observational study of TPIAT. Pancreatology. 2022;22(1):1–8.
16. Bellin MD, Eaton A, Ramanathan K, Beilman G, Downs E, Schwarzenberg SJ, et al. Long-term islet graft functional assessment in more than 500 patients undergoing total pancreatectomy with Intraportal islet autotransplantation. J Am Coll Surg. 2025;240(4):405–13.
17. Chinnakotla S, Bellin MD, Schwarzenberg SJ, Radosevich DM, Cook M, Dunn TB, et al. Total pancreatectomy and islet autotransplantation in children for chronic pancreatitis: indication, surgical techniques, postoperative management, and long-term outcomes. Ann Surg. 2014;260(1):56–64.
18. Wagar MK, Magnuson J, Liu PT, Kirchner V, Wilhelm JJ, Freeman ML, et al. The impact of using an intraoperative goal directed fluid therapy protocol on clinical outcomes in patients undergoing total pancreatectomy and islet cell autotransplantation. Pancreatology. 2017;17(4):586–91.
19. Berger MG, Majumder K, Hodges JS, Bellin MD, Schwarzenberg SJ, Gupta S, et al. Microbial contamination of transplant solutions during pancreatic islet autotransplants is not associated with clinical infection in a pediatric population. Pancreatology. 2016;16(4):555–62.
20. Hutchins J, Castro C, Wang Q, Chinnakotla S. Postoperative pain control with paravertebral catheters after pediatric total pancreatectomy and islet autotransplantation: a retrospective cohort study. Paediatr Anaesth. 2016;26(3):315–20.
21. Stice MJ, Dunn TB, Bellin MD, Skube ME, Beilman GJ. Omental pouch technique for combined site islet autotransplantation following Total pancreatectomy. Cell Transplant. 2018;27(10):1561–8.
22. Berger M, Bellin MD, Kirchner V, Schwarzenberg SJ, Chinnakotla S. Laparoscopic-assisted versus open total pancreatectomy and islet autotransplantation: a case-matched study of pediatric patients. J Pediatr Surg. 2020;55(3):558–63.
23. Fan CJ, Hirose K, Walsh CM, Quartuccio M, Desai NM, Singh VK, et al. Laparoscopic total pancreatectomy with islet autotransplantation and intraoperative islet separation as a treatment for patients with chronic pancreatitis. JAMA Surg. 2017;152(6):550.
24. Galvani CA, Rilo HR, Samamé J, Porubsky M, Rana A, Gruessner RWG. Fully robotic-assisted technique for total pancreatectomy with an autologous islet transplant in chronic pancreatitis patients: results of a first series. J Am Coll Surg. 2014;218(3):e73–e8.
25. Kinny-Koster B, Walsh CM, Sun Z, Faghih M, Desai NM, Warren DS, et al. Minimally invasive total pancreatectomy with islet autotransplantation for chronic pancreatitis: the robotic approach. Surg Endosc. 2024;38(7):3948–56.

Islet Isolation Techniques for Total Pancreatectomy with Islet Autotransplantation (TPIAT)

6

Shafahed Kodipad, Jayachandra Kuncha, Bashoo Naziruddin, and Appakalai N. Balamurugan

Abstract

Total pancreatectomy with islet autotransplantation (TPIAT) is a unique procedure that involves close teamwork between transplant surgeons and laboratory technologists. Success, in terms of achieving optimal glycemic control after transplantation, depends on careful selection of patients and the employment of laboratory techniques that will yield high-quality islet mass from the inflamed pancreata. This chapter highlights details on islet isolation technology (Sect. 6.1) and pretransplant assessment of the pancreas for the prediction of improved islet yield and graft function (Sect. 6.2).

Key Points

1. Isolating human islets is a complex and time-critical procedure that necessitates a coordinated effort from a highly trained team.
2. The steps involved in islet isolation are transporting the pancreas, pancreas trimming, ductal cannulation, enzyme perfusion, enzymatic digestion, recombination, purification (if necessary), and final transplant product packaging.

S. Kodipad
Applied Microbiology and Biotechnology, University of Wolverhampton, Wolverhampton, UK

J. Kuncha · B. Naziruddin
Islet Cell Laboratory, Baylor Scott & White Research Institute, Dallas, TX, USA

A. N. Balamurugan (✉)
Islet Transplantation and Beta Cell Biology, University of Louisville, Norton HealthCare, Louisville, KY, USA
e-mail: bala.appakalai@louisville.edu

S. Chinnakotla et al. (eds.), *Total Pancreatectomy and Islet Auto Transplantation*, https://doi.org/10.1007/978-981-92-0018-4_6

3. Each step needs to be adjusted to accommodate the specific case, including the anatomy and condition of the organ, the speed and extent of digestion, and the volume of isolated islets. Frequent sampling during digestion is critical for making any needed adjustments.
4. Many factors affect islet yield and clinical outcomes after TPIAT, including the duration of the chronic pancreatitis; the amount of pancreatic calcification on pre-TPIAT imaging; the levels of certain microRNAs, such as miR-375 and miR-200c; and plasma levels of certain extracellular matrix proteins.

6.1 Islet Cell Isolation

6.1.1 Introduction

Islet autotransplantation (IAT) involves isolating islets from the patient's own removed pancreas and transplanting them into the liver portal vein, with the aim of restoring endogenous insulin production and preventing or alleviating diabetes [1, 2]. While total pancreatectomy (TP) is a relatively common surgical procedure, IAT is not universally available due to the complexity, cost, and need for specialized expertise and facilities compliant with current Good Manufacturing Practices. Recent advancements in islet isolation techniques, including refined collagenase–protease enzyme blends, automated digestion systems, and improved purification methods, are continuously being explored to enhance IAT outcomes and broaden its accessibility [3, 4]. The goal of this chapter is to provide a comprehensive overview of the IAT procedure, emphasizing key factors that contribute to successful clinical outcomes.

Isolating human islets is a complex and time-critical procedure that necessitates a coordinated effort from a highly trained team of typically three to four individuals under the guidance of an experienced supervisor. Adequate preparation of the laboratory environment is crucial and must be completed before the pancreas arrives at the clean-room facility [5]. The steps involved in islet isolation are transporting the pancreas, pancreas trimming, ductal cannulation, enzyme distension, enzymatic digestion, recombination, purification (if necessary), and final transplant product packaging [5, 6]. It is essential to verify that all instrumentation, such as centrifuges, water baths, incubators, microscopes, and thermal probes, are operational, calibrated, and functioning within normal parameters [7].

6.1.2 Pancreas Transport, Trimming, and Cannulation

After the pancreatectomy, the pancreas is immediately immersed in a sterile container filled with chilled preservation solution (University of Wisconsin or histidine-tryptophan-ketoglutarate solution or cold storage) at the surgical site [8]. Upon arrival of the pancreas at the islet isolation facility, the first procedural step is meticulous documentation and quality assessment. A sample of the transport solution is aseptically collected for microbiological analysis to screen for potential contamination (aerobic/fungal, anaerobic, and Gram stain). This is followed by pancreas trimming and cannulation. A trained team member performs an initial brief trim, removing excess fat and connective tissue from around the pancreas but keeping the pancreatic capsule intact to reduce the likelihood of enzyme leakage during ductal perfusion. The choice of catheter for ductal cannulation should be carefully considered and adapted based on the individual anatomy and ductal characteristics of the pancreas encountered during dissection. Once the appropriate catheter is selected and gently inserted into the pancreatic duct, it is crucial to secure it firmly in place to prevent displacement and enzyme backflow during the subsequent perfusion step [5].

6.1.3 Perfusion

6.1.3.1 Collagenase–Protease Enzyme Selection

Enzymatic tissue dissociation is the cornerstone of islet isolation, serving as the critical process to liberate islets from the surrounding exocrine pancreatic tissue [9]. Collagenase is the principal enzyme responsible for breaking down collagen, the most abundant component of the extracellular matrix (ECM) that encases and supports pancreatic tissue. Collagenase preparations, which are derived from *Clostridium histolyticum*, are actually complex mixtures of multiple collagenase isoforms (Class I and Class II) and other enzymatic activities, including neutral proteases, clostripain, and hyaluronidase. Class I collagenases initiate collagen degradation, and Class II collagenases further digest the collagen fragments. Proteases play a synergistic role in ECM digestion by degrading noncollagenous components of the ECM, facilitating islet liberation [10, 11].

The selection of the specific enzyme mixture and its concentration is often tailored based on pancreas weight and donor/organ characteristics to optimize islet release and minimize tissue damage. Most labs use collagenase in combination with neutral protease, thermolysin, or BP-protease. Recently, our group successfully utilized recombinant collagenase in combination with BP-protease for clinical islet autotransplantation [12, 13].

Adjustments to enzyme concentration, digestion temperature, and digestion time may be necessary during the procedure based on real-time monitoring of tissue dissociation and islet liberation, as assessed through frequent digest sampling and microscopic evaluation. The goal is to achieve a balance: sufficient enzymatic activity to effectively dissociate the tissue, but not so aggressive as to damage or overdigest the delicate islets [14].

6.1.3.2 Enzymatic Perfusion of the Pancreas

Enzymatic perfusion serves as the method to deliver the enzyme solution uniformly throughout the pancreatic tissue, initiating the digestion of the ECM and ultimately liberating the islets. During perfusion, the enzyme solution, carefully formulated and dosed as described in the previous section, is administered into the cannulated pancreatic duct [15].

Although ductal perfusion is the standard and most effective method for enzyme delivery in islet isolation, certain challenging pancreatic conditions may render ductal perfusion ineffective or technically infeasible. In these situations, interstitial perfusion, also referred to as tissue injection or direct injection, provides a valuable alternative enzyme-delivery strategy. Interstitial perfusion bypasses the ductal system altogether and involves the direct injection of enzyme solution into the pancreatic parenchyma itself. This technique is typically performed manually, using a needle and syringe to administer the enzyme solution into multiple sites within the pancreas [7].

6.1.3.3 Postdistension Trimming

Successful perfusion of the enzymatic solution results in distension of the pancreas. The next step is postdistension trimming, which involves the meticulous removal of nonpancreatic tissue components to prepare the pancreas for the subsequent digestion and islet liberation stages. Postdistension trimming is performed after the enzyme solution has been perfused throughout the pancreas and initiated ECM digestion, but *before* the mechanical disruption and digestion phases [16], which are described in the next section.

6.1.4 Tissue Digestion: Recirculation Phase

Tissue digestion is the central enzymatic process in islet isolation, where the enzyme solution, now perfused and distributed throughout the trimmed pancreatic tissue, is allowed to actively break down the ECM, ultimately liberating individual islets and small islet clusters from the surrounding exocrine tissue. This digestion phase is typically performed in a specialized digestion vessel, most commonly the Ricordi chamber, which provides a controlled environment for enzymatic reaction, mechanical agitation, and collection of liberated islets [17]. The digestion process is carefully monitored and modulated to achieve efficient tissue dissociation while preserving islet viability and functionality.

The perfused, distended, and trimmed pancreatic tissue is aseptically transferred to the Ricordi chamber, along with any remaining enzyme solution from the perfusion tray or trimming pan, ensuring that all enzyme activity is utilized. The Ricordi chamber is then assembled and connected to a digestion apparatus, which typically consists of a recirculating system with a peristaltic pump, a reservoir for enzyme solution, a heat transfer coil for temperature control, and ports for sampling and solution addition. A critical component of the Ricordi chamber is an internal mesh screen (typically 400–600 μm pore size, often around 500 μm), positioned across the outflow opening. This screen serves to retain undigested tissue fragments within the chamber while allowing liberated islets and smaller tissue particles to pass through and be collected in the recirculating circuit. The digestion process within the Ricordi chamber is typically performed in two phases: Phase 1 (Recirculation) and Phase 2 (Collection) [17].

In Phase 1, the enzyme solution is recirculated through the Ricordi chamber in a closed circuit. The peristaltic pump continuously circulates the enzyme solution, ensuring constant exposure of the pancreatic tissue to the enzymatic activity. Mechanical agitation is applied to the chamber, typically through gentle rocking or shaking, to further promote tissue dissociation and enhance enzyme access to the ECM. The level of mechanical agitation is carefully controlled to be sufficient for tissue disruption but not so vigorous as to damage the islets.

6.1.4.1 Digest Sampling

Digest sampling is an absolutely critical and indispensable component of the islet isolation procedure. It serves as the real-time monitoring and feedback mechanism that guides the entire digestion process, allowing islet isolation teams to assess the progress of tissue dissociation, evaluate islet liberation, and make informed decisions about adjusting digestion parameters.

A systematic microscopic evaluation is performed to assess several key parameters, providing a comprehensive picture of the digestion progress:

- **Quantity of acinar tissue:** The amount of undigested acinar tissue fragments remaining in the sample is assessed. A decreasing amount of acinar tissue over time indicates effective tissue dissociation. Large amounts of intact acinar tissue suggest that digestion is proceeding too slowly or is incomplete.
- **Acinar diameter:** The size and morphology of acinar units are evaluated. As digestion progresses, acinar units should become smaller and more fragmented, indicating ECM breakdown. Again, large, intact acinar units suggest insufficient digestion.
- **Number of islets:** The number of liberated islets visible in the sample is counted or estimated. An increasing number of free islets over time signifies successful islet liberation.
- **Percent free islets:** The proportion of islets that are completely free and unattached to surrounding tissue is estimated. A higher percentage of free islets indicates more advanced digestion.
- **Percent fragmented (overdigested) islets:** Signs of islet fragmentation or overdigestion, such as disrupted islet morphology or dispersed islet cells, are noted. Excessive islet fragmentation suggests overdigestion, potentially due to excessive enzyme dose or prolonged digestion time.
- **Average islet score:** A subjective islet score, based on overall islet morphology, size, and integrity, is often assigned to each digest sample. This score provides a semiquantitative assessment of islet quality throughout digestion.

The information obtained from digest sampling is immediately used to guide adjustments to the digestion process:

- **Sluggish digestion:** If digest samples show minimal tissue dissociation, large amounts of intact acinar tissue, and few free islets, digestion is considered sluggish. In response, the digestion temperature may be increased slightly, or, in some protocols, additional enzyme may be added directly to the recirculation circuit to accelerate digestion.
- **Optimal digestion:** If digest samples show progressive tissue dissociation, decreasing acinar size, increasing numbers of free and intact islets, and minimal islet fragmentation, digestion is considered to be proceeding optimally. In this case, digestion parameters are typically maintained, and the process is allowed to continue.
- **Overdigestion:** If digest samples show excessive islet fragmentation, dispersed islet cells, or a rapid decrease in islet integrity, overdigestion is suspected. In response, the digestion temperature may be lowered, or the digestion process may be transitioned to Phase 2 (collection) earlier than initially planned to halt further enzymatic activity.
- **Transition to Phase 2:** The switch from recirculation to collection is typically triggered when digest sampling indicates a significant increase in the number of free islets and a reduction in large acinar tissue fragments, suggesting that a substantial portion of islets have been liberated and are ready for collection.

6.1.4.2 Digestion of the Severely Fibrotic Pancreas

Several key adaptations in the digestion protocol can be implemented to address the challenges posed by severe fibrosis [7]:

- **Increased enzyme dose:** Fibrotic tissue, with its dense and cross-linked collagen matrix, is inherently more resistant to enzymatic digestion. To overcome this resistance, increasing the enzyme dose, particularly the collagenase component, is often necessary. This may involve increasing the initial enzyme concentration in the perfusion solution or adding supplemental enzyme during the recirculation phase if digestion appears sluggish based on digest sampling. The extent to increase the enzyme dose should be carefully considered and titrated based on the degree of fibrosis and real-time monitoring of the digestion progress.
- **Prolonged digestion time:** Severely fibrotic tissue typically requires longer digestion times to achieve adequate tissue dissociation. Recirculation may be extended beyond the standard duration to allow more time for enzymatic breakdown of the dense ECM. The digestion time extension should be guided by frequent digest sampling and microscopic evaluation. Digestion should be continued until digest samples show reasonable islet liberation, even if it requires significantly longer digestion times than nonfibrotic pancreata.
- **Mechanical disruption strategies:** Enhanced mechanical disruption can aid in enzyme penetration and tissue dissociation in fibrotic pancreata. More forceful shaking or rocking of the Ricordi chamber may be employed, with careful monitoring for any signs of islet damage due to excessive mechanical force. In some protocols, the use of stainless steel marbles within the Ricordi chamber is considered for fibrotic tissue to enhance mechanical disruption.

- **Enzyme recirculation protocol:** For severely fibrotic pancreata that exhibit unusually slow digestion even with increased enzyme dose and prolonged digestion time, an enzyme recirculation protocol can be beneficial [18]. This protocol involves interrupting the standard digestion process after a defined period (e.g., 25 min) and performing an intermediate collection step to recover any free islets liberated early in the digestion. The digestate collected at this intermediate step is centrifuged, and the supernatant, containing active enzyme, is recycled back into the digestion system, effectively increasing the enzyme concentration and extending the enzyme exposure time for the remaining undigested fibrotic tissue. This recirculation step can be repeated multiple times until maximal tissue dissociation is achieved, as assessed by digest sampling.
- **Temperature optimization:** Maintaining the digestion temperature at the higher end of the acceptable range (e.g., 36.5–37°C) can help to intensify enzyme activity and improve digestion efficiency in fibrotic tissue. However, temperature should be carefully monitored and controlled to avoid overheating and potential islet damage.

6.1.5 Tissue Dissection: Collection Phase and Recombination of Islets

Once recirculation is deemed complete, based on digest sampling, the digestion process transitions to collection. The primary objectives of this phase are to efficiently collect the liberated islets, to progressively dilute and inactivate the enzyme solution to prevent overdigestion, and to bring the enzymatic digestion process to a controlled endpoint [16]. The digestate, now containing liberated islets and diluted enzyme solution, is collected in a series of fractions.

The recirculation circuit is switched to an open circuit, diverting the digestate (enzyme solution and liberated islets/tissue fragments) from the Ricordi chamber into a collection vessel. Cold Phase 2 solution (typically chilled Roswell Park Memorial Institute [RPMI] 1640 medium) is added to the digestion circuit to progressively dilute the enzyme concentration and slow down further enzymatic activity, effectively "stopping" the digestion process at the desired endpoint.

Next, the fractions are recombined to consolidate the dispersed digest fractions, which contain free islets in suspension, into a manageable volume in a smaller number of fractions and to prepare them for subsequent purification steps, if necessary, or direct transplantation. This facilitates quality assessment and decision-making regarding purification [5]. Recombination also provides an opportunity to preserve the liberated islets from further enzymatic degradation and transition them into a more protective and stable environment [5].

The fractions are centrifuged and the supernatant is removed, leaving a cell pellet in each conical tube that is carefully examined. Experienced personnel assess the size and appearance of each pellet, noting any visible differences in color, consistency, or the presence of debris. This visual assessment can provide preliminary information about the relative islet content and purity of different fractions.

These pellets, still in multiple conical tubes, represent the "recombined" tissue. They are ready for further processing, such as washing to remove residual enzyme and debris, density gradient purification (if needed), or direct preparation for transplantation if purification is not necessary.

6.1.6 Purification Process: Density Gradient Centrifugation and Fraction Collection

The purification step both reduces the volume of the tissue preparation and, critically, minimizes contamination from exocrine cells and other non-islet components. Although digestion and recombination also concentrate islets, the resulting mixture still contains a substantial proportion of exocrine acinar cells, ductal cells, connective tissue, and cellular debris. Purification, typically through density gradient centrifugation, is often employed to enhance islet purity. This is beneficial in reducing the risk of complications, such as portal hypertension, associated with transplanting large tissue volumes and potentially in improving long-term islet graft function [19].

Isopycnic density gradient centrifugation using the COBE 2991 cell processor is the most established and clinically successful purification method for human islets. This technique exploits the inherent density difference between islets and exocrine tissue. Islets, being less dense than exocrine acinar cells, remain in the lower-density layer when centrifuged through a density gradient, while the denser exocrine tissue sediments into the higher-density layers. The density gradient range for COBE purification widely used by the Clinical Islet Transplantation Consortium is 1.060–1.100 g/cm^3 [19].

After centrifugation, the fraction collection process begins. The first fraction collected from the COBE bag is typically designated as a "waste" fraction and is collected into an empty conical tube. Collection of the purification product fractions begins when the tissue starts to visually appear in the outlet tubing of the COBE bag. The purification product is then collected into a consecutive series of typically 12 conical tubes, each prefilled with 225 mL of cold supplemented Connaught Medical Research Laboratories (CMRL) medium. Each fraction volume collected is typically 25 mL, resulting in a final volume of approximately 250 mL per conical tube (225 mL CMRL +25 mL purification product fraction). The CMRL medium in the collection tubes serves to dilute the density gradient medium and provides a supportive environment for the purified islets.

6.1.7 Transplant Preparation

Although quality control and sterility test results are typically not available until after the islet product is officially released, the islet preparation must be immediately packaged for transplantation once the purification process (if performed) is complete and the product is deemed ready for infusion. If the packed tissue volume of the final islet preparation is greater than 10 mL, the pellet must be divided evenly and loaded into two separate 200-mL transplant bags. This division into two bags is recommended to ensure safe and manageable infusion volumes and to facilitate even distribution of the islet mass during intraportal transplantation. Each transplant bag must be clearly and accurately labeled with the correct patient identification information, including patient name and unique identifiers, and all Food and Drug Administration (FDA)-required labeling information, ensuring proper traceability and regulatory compliance.

The sealed transplant bags are then prepared for transport to the operating room. It is recommended to transport the islet preparation in a room-temperature cooler equipped with validated temperature stabilizers to maintain a consistent and controlled temperature environment during transport, typically around 20–25 °C. This room-temperature transport is preferred to avoid cold-induced apoptosis.

6.1.8 Conclusion

In conclusion, successful islet isolation for autotransplantation from pancreata with pancreatitis is a highly intricate and multifaceted endeavor. It demands meticulous attention to detail, a deep understanding of each procedural step, and the ability to adapt protocols based on real-time assessment of tissue characteristics and digestion progress. From strategic pancreas procurement and preservation to precisely controlled enzymatic digestion and purification, every stage plays a critical role in determining the final islet yield, viability, and functional quality.

6.2 Pretransplant Assessment of Pancreas for Improved Islet Yield and Graft Function

Despite the long history of the total pancreatectomy with islet autotransplantation (TPIAT) procedure, the current results in terms of islet yield and posttransplant graft function need improvement [20]. Multivariate analysis of islet isolation outcomes in TPIAT has shown that transplanting a greater mass of islets directly contributes to improved islet engraftment and posttransplant glycemic control [21]. The following section describes the factors that are helpful in the prediction of islet yield and graft function in TPIAT.

6.2.1 Prediction of Islet Yield and Posttransplant Glycemic Control

6.2.1.1 Duration of Chronic Pancreatitis and Metabolic Screening

Patient selection and assessment of the pancreas with pancreatitis are important for achieving good posttransplant glycemic control in TPIAT. A retrospective consecutive cohort analysis on 76 patients with chronic pancreatitis (CP) who underwent TPIAT showed that the duration of CP plays a major role in islet yield [22]. Patients in this analysis were divided into three groups based on their islet dose: less than 2500 islet equivalents (IEQ)/kg, between 2500 and 5000 IEQ/kg, and more than 5000 IEQ/kg. The length of CP negatively impacted the islet yield and metabolic results. For the entire group, longer illness duration was linked to a lower islet yield (Spearman's correlation = −0.24; $p = 0.04$). A strong correlation was found between higher islet yields and improved metabolic outcomes (HbA1c 7.6% ± 1.1% with <2500 IEQ/kg transplanted vs. 6.6% ± 1.1% with >5000 IEQ/kg; $p = 0.04$). These and similar findings [23] suggest that duration of CP should be factored into the selection of patients for TPIAT.

Another investigation found that islet yield and insulin need after TPIAT are determined by the nature of procedures undergone by the patients before surgery [24]. In this study, patients were divided into four groups: lateral pancreaticojejunostomy (n = 4), distal pancreatectomy (n = 8), Whipple or Beger procedure (n = 14), or transduodenal sphincteroplasty or no prior surgery (n = 50). Patients received transplants of all unpurified islets through portal vein infusion. Measurements were made on insulin demand, viability of cells, islet output, and pancreatic fibrosis. Those with transduodenal sphincteroplasty/no prior surgery or Whipple/Beger procedure had less pancreatic fibrosis and a greater islet yield than those with lateral pancreaticojejunostomy or distal pancreatectomy. Thus, the degree of pancreatic fibrosis, islet yield, and insulin needs in CP patients receiving TPIAT are all strongly associated with prior surgery.

6.2.1.2 Pancreas Imaging Findings and Calcification

Imaging of the pancreas can help to establish the extent of disease markers, such as pancreatic duct status and calcification, and their association with islet yield. Takita et al. [25] examined the implications of pancreatic findings on transabdominal ultrasound and/or abdominal computed tomographic (CT) scan on outcomes of islet isolation and endocrine function after TPIAT. The patients were divided into two groups: the early group (normal or equivocal according to the Cambridge classification) and the advanced group (moderate to marked). The early group's total islet yield per pancreatic weight (6989 ± 659 IEQ/g) and patient body weight (8556 ± 953 IEQ/kg) was considerably higher than the islet yield per pancreatic weight (3567 ± 615 IEQ/g, $p < 0.01$) and body weight (3847 ± 739 IEQ/kg, $p < 0.01$) in the advanced group. Two patients in the advanced group (33%) achieved insulin independence, whereas four patients in the early group (67%) achieved insulin independence. Nevertheless, following transplantation, both groups achieved comparable HbA1c levels and islet graft functionality and outstanding glycemic control, although the early group's islet isolation results were substantially better. Imaging tests like CT and magnetic resonance imaging (MRI) can also measure pancreatic parenchymal degradation through indicators such as reduced pancreatic volume and calcifications, which are strongly linked to decreased islet mass and diabetes outcomes after 1 year [26].

Accurately forecasting postoperative glycemic management in children undergoing the TPIAT procedure is still challenging, but a retrospective analysis suggests that postoperative insulin demand can be predicted from the segmented pancreatic volume obtained from pre-TPIAT images [27]. Postoperative insulin requirements were examined in youngsters (≤18 years old) who received TPIAT. Of 33 recipients, 64% were female (21/33), and the median age was 13 years (IQR: 10–15 years). At 6 months, nine patients (27%) were insulin independent. There was a moderate correlation between total islet equivalents and segmented pancreatic volume (coefficient estimate = 0.34, p = 0.034). Insulin independence was not significantly predicted by multiple regression analysis; however, the total daily dose of insulin per kilogram was significantly predicted by the number of pancreatitis events (estimate = 0.024; p = 0.018) and the segmented pancreas volume by body weight (estimate = −0.71; p < 0.001).

Pancreatic calcification has been associated with low islet yields and insulin dependence after TPIAT. Darden et al. analyzed calcification patterns on CT of the pancreas using a database of 200 consecutive TPIAT procedures [28]. Patterns were classified as no calcification, focal calcification (limited to the head, body, or tail of the pancreas), or diffuse calcification involving more than two sections. Of the three groups, the pancreata with diffuse calcification produced the lowest IEQ yield and IEQ/kg (p < 0.0001), and 12 months after transplant, none of these patients were insulin independent (p < 0.05 compared to the no calcification group). However, 91.7% of the patients in the diffuse calcification group were narcotic-free at 12 months, which was substantially higher than that of those in the no calcification group (p < 0.05). Thus, even individuals with extensive calcification may benefit from TPIAT.

6.2.2 MicroRNA Measurement

Biomarkers for endocrine function following transplantation would aid in the selection of patients well suited for TPIAT. Numerous microRNA (miRNA) families that are controlled by genetic, nutritional, metabolic, and inflammatory stresses coordinate the adaptive responses of β-cells in vivo in diseases like diabetes, obesity, and CP [29–32]. Among numerous miRNAs studied, plasma concentrations of miR-375 before TPIAT are negatively correlated with both postdigestion islet count (r = −0.372, p = 0.04) and C-peptide (r = −0.396, p = 0.03) [33], and miR-29b-3p is inversely associated with postisolation IEQ/kg and islet number/kg (*r* = −0.20, p = 0.02). A multiple regression analysis verified that miR-200c is a negative predictor of endocrine outcomes (coefficient = −7.081, p = 0.001) [34]. miR-375 is likely negatively associated with islet count because it is linked to islet damage during isolation [35]; consistent with this, lower miR-375 is associated with lower hemoglobin A1c (p = 0.04) and a lower insulin demand (p = 0.01) 6 months after TPIAT [35].

6.2.3 Picosirius Red and Laminin Alpha 5 Staining

Picosirius red (PSR) staining is useful for evaluating pancreatic fibrosis alongside other biomarkers. In a retrospective cohort study of 32 CP patients (16 men and 16 women) who underwent TPIAT, the CP tissue showed a considerably larger PSR-positive region ($12.4\% \pm 6.8\%$) than normal pancreatic tissue ($4.0\% \pm 0.5\%$) ($p < 0.05$) [36]. For some forms of collagen quantification, PSR staining with standard polarization microscopy (PSR-POL) may offer both extra and adequate information in a traditional clinical pathology lab. Notably, PSR-POL has a strong correlation with second harmonic generation results despite detecting larger fiber counts, alignment, length, straightness, and width when compared with second harmonic generation images [37].

Plasma levels of the ECM protein laminin alpha 5 (LAMA5) are high in patients with CP, and the peri-islet basal membrane and islet endothelial vascular tissue both overexpress LAMA5 [38]. Elevated LAMA5 expression is suggestive of increasing pancreatic injury and is associated with poor islet yield and poor function of transplanted islets at 3 months.

6.2.4 Assessment of Islet Damage during Isolation

Although stress during the isolation procedure impacts quality and yield, high-quality pancreatic islets are necessary for improved posttransplant endocrine function in TPIAT. Islet injury can be measured throughout isolation using techniques such as morphological evaluation of islet structure, size, fragmentation, islets embedded with acinar tissue, viability, and oxidative stress markers [39] and DNA release [40]. Soluble biomarkers like C-peptide and miRNAs can be used to evaluate islet injury. As noted above, measuring the absolute amount of miRNA-375 and -200c released during islet isolation is effective for predicting islet impairment [35].

Exosomes are extracellular vesicles of 50–200 nm that are released by all cell types to transfer biomolecules and communicate with other cells. Islets secrete exosomes in response to stress conditions such as proinflammatory cytokines and hypoxia [41]. The cargo of the islet exosomes is indicative of the extent of cell damage and may predict posttransplant glycemic control. A recent study [42] showed that exosomes isolated from islet infusion bags of TPIAT recipients ($n = 20$) contained damage-associated molecular pattern (DAMP) proteins, and higher concentrations were correlated with increased insulin requirements ($p = 0.01$) and higher HbA1c after transplant. A deeper exploration of the function of exosomes indicated the activation of inflammatory pathways that may cause damage to islets.

6.2.5 Conclusion

Pretransplant evaluation methods for CP pancreas are beneficial for predicting islet yield before TPIAT. Duration of disease, pancreatic fibrosis, calcification, and inflammation are among the conditions that can affect islet yield and function in patients with CP. Preoperative imaging techniques, such as CT and MRI, can be used to measure pancreatic volume and to spot atrophy or fibrosis, which may be linked to decreased islet yields. Metabolic evaluations, such as insulin secretion assessments, circulating microRNA detection, PSR, and LAMA5 staining of pancreatic sections, may additionally provide information about islet function and possibly forecast islet yield. Monitoring islet damage during isolation using highly sensitive biomarkers will result in modifications of the procedure to minimize cellular damage.

Acknowledgments We extend our deepest gratitude to the courageous families who generously donated their loved ones' organs and tissues for biomedical research. Such important research like this would not be possible without this selfless gift of hope. Thanks to Dr. Appakalai N. Balamurugan's team for processing human pancreases and the organ procurement organizations, Network for Hope (Louisville and Cincinnati) and Lifeline of Ohio, Columbus, for supporting these special families.

And also to Chandrashekhar Bangalore Revanna and Emily Montgomery from Wendy Novak Diabetes Institute, Department of Paediatrics, Paediatric Research Institute, University of Louisville, for their contributions to this book chapter.

References

1. Blondet JJ, Carlson AM, Kobayashi T, Jie T, Bellin M, Hering BJ, et al. The role of total pancreatectomy and islet autotransplantation for chronic pancreatitis. Surg Clin North Am. 2007;87(6):1477–501. x
2. Sutherland DE, Gruessner AC, Carlson AM, Blondet JJ, Balamurugan AN, Reigstad KF, et al. Islet autotransplant outcomes after total pancreatectomy: a contrast to islet allograft outcomes. Transplantation. 2008;86(12):1799–802.
3. Kin T. Islet isolation for clinical transplantation. Adv Exp Med Biol. 2010;654:683–710.
4. Wilhelm JJ, Balamurugan AN, Bellin MD, Hodges JS, Diaz J, Jane Schwarzenberg S, et al. Progress in individualizing autologous islet isolation techniques for pediatric islet autotransplantation after total pancreatectomy in children for chronic pancreatitis. Am J Transplant. 2021;21(2):776–86.
5. Lakey JR, Burridge PW, Shapiro AM. Technical aspects of islet preparation and transplantation. Transpl Int. 2003;16(9):613–32.
6. Kin T, Shapiro AM. Surgical aspects of human islet isolation. Islets. 2010;2(5):265–73.
7. Balamurugan AN, Loganathan G, Bellin MD, Wilhelm JJ, Harmon J, Anazawa T, et al. A new enzyme mixture to increase the yield and transplant rate of autologous and allogeneic human islet products. Transplantation. 2012;93(7):693–702.
8. Hering BJ, Matsumoto I, Sawada T, Nakano M, Sakai T, Kandaswamy R, et al. Impact of two-layer pancreas preservation on islet isolation and transplantation. Transplantation. 2002;74(12):1813–6.
9. Breite AG, Dwulet FE, McCarthy RC. Tissue dissociation enzyme neutral protease assessment. Transplant Proc. 2010;42(6):2052–4.
10. Brandhorst H, Johnson PR, Monch J, Kurfurst M, Korsgren O, Brandhorst D. Comparison of clostripain and neutral protease as supplementary enzymes for human islet isolation. Cell Transplant. 2019;28(2):176–84.
11. Breite AG, McCarthy RC, Dwulet FE. Characterization and functional assessment of Clostridium histolyticum class I (C1) collagenases and the synergistic degradation of

native collagen in enzyme mixtures containing class II (C2) collagenase. Transplant Proc. 2011;43(9):3171–5.
12. Balamurugan AN, Green ML, Breite AG, Loganathan G, Wilhelm JJ, Tweed B, et al. Identifying effective enzyme activity targets for recombinant class I and class II collagenase for successful human islet isolation. Transplant Direct. 2016;2(1):e54.
13. Loganathan G, Subhashree V, Breite AG, Tucker WW, Narayanan S, Dhanasekaran M, et al. Beneficial effect of recombinant rC1rC2 collagenases on human islet function: efficacy of low-dose enzymes on pancreas digestion and yield. Am J Transplant. 2018;18(2):478–85.
14. Anazawa T, Balamurugan AN, Bellin M, Zhang HJ, Matsumoto S, Yonekawa Y, et al. Human islet isolation for autologous transplantation: comparison of yield and function using SERVA/Nordmark versus Roche enzymes. Am J Transplant. 2009;9(10):2383–91.
15. Brandhorst D, Brandhorst H, Johnson PRV. Enzyme development for human islet isolation: five decades of progress or stagnation? Rev Diabet Stud. 2017;14(1):22–38.
16. Ricordi C, Lacy PE, Scharp DW. Automated islet isolation from human pancreas. Diabetes. 1989;38(Suppl 1):140–2.
17. Ricordi C, Goldstein JS, Balamurugan AN, Szot GL, Kin T, Liu C, et al. National Institutes of Health-Sponsored Clinical Islet Transplantation Consortium Phase 3 Trial: manufacture of a complex cellular product at eight processing facilities. Diabetes. 2016;65(11):3418–28.
18. Balamurugan AN, Chang Y, Fung JJ, Trucco M, Bottino R. Flexible management of enzymatic digestion improves human islet isolation outcome from sub-optimal donor pancreata. Am J Transplant. 2003;3(9):1135–42.
19. Anazawa T, Matsumoto S, Yonekawa Y, Loganathan G, Wilhelm JJ, Soltani SM, et al. Prediction of pancreatic tissue densities by an analytical test gradient system before purification maximizes human islet recovery for islet autotransplantation/allotransplantation. Transplantation. 2011;91(5):508–14.
20. Chen ME, Desai CS. Current practices in islet cell autotransplantation. Expert. Rev. Endocrinol. Metab. 2023;18(5):419–25.
21. Mattke J, Eaton A, Wijkstrom M, Witkowski P, Trikudanathan G, Singh VK, et al. Islet isolation outcomes in patients undergoing total pancreatectomy with islet autotransplantation in the POST consortium. Transplantation. 2025;109(1):207–16.
22. Takita M, Lara LF, Naziruddin B, Shahbazov R, Lawrence MC, Kim PT, et al. Effect of the duration of chronic pancreatitis on pancreas islet yield and metabolic outcome following islet autotransplantation. J Gastrointest Surg. 2015;19(7):1236–46.
23. Nanno Y, Wastvedt S, Freeman ML, Trikudanathan G, Schwarzenberg SJ, Downs EM, et al. Metabolic measures before surgery and long-term diabetes outcomes in recipients of total pancreatectomy and islet autotransplantation. Am. J. Transplant. 2021;21(10):3411–20.
24. Wang H, Desai KD, Dong H, Owzarski S, Romagnuolo J, Morgan KA, et al. Prior surgery determines islet yield and insulin requirement in patients with chronic pancreatitis. Transplantation. 2013;95(8):1051–7.
25. Takita M, Naziruddin B, Matsumoto S, Noguchi H, Shimoda M, Chujo D, et al. Implication of pancreatic image findings in total pancreatectomy with islet autotransplantation for chronic pancreatitis. Pancreas. 2011;40(1):103–8.
26. Young MC, Theis JR, Hodges JS, Dunn TB, Pruett TL, Chinnakotla S, et al. Preoperative computerized tomography and magnetic resonance imaging of the pancreas predicts pancreatic mass and functional outcomes after total pancreatectomy and islet autotransplant. Pancreas. 2016;45(7):961–6.
27. Trout AT, Nolan HR, Abu-El-Haija M, Fei L, Lin TK, Elder DA, et al. Imaging prediction of islet yield and post-operative insulin requirement in children undergoing total pancreatectomy with islet autotransplantation. Pancreatology. 2021;21(1):269–74.
28. Darden C, Kumano K, Liu Y, Mohamed A, Mattke J, Lawrence M, et al. Diffuse calcification of pancreas impairs endocrine function and predicts poor outcome in total pancreatectomy with islet autotransplantation. Am J Transplant. 2023;23(11):1781–92.
29. Erener S, Mojibian M, Fox JK, Denroche HC, Kieffer TJ. Circulating miR-375 as a biomarker of β-cell death and diabetes in mice. Endocrinology. 2013;154(2):603–8.

30. LaPierre MP, Stoffel M. MicroRNAs as stress regulators in pancreatic beta cells and diabetes. Mol Metab. 2017;6(9):1010–23.
31. Patel HR, Diaz Almanzar VM, LaComb JF, Ju J, Bialkowska AB. The role of MicroRNAs in pancreatitis development and progression. Int. J. Mol. Sci. 2023;24(2):1057.
32. Belgardt BF, Ahmed K, Spranger M, Latreille M, Denzler R, Kondratiuk N, et al. The microRNA-200 family regulates pancreatic beta cell survival in type 2 diabetes. Nat Med. 2015;21(6):619–27.
33. Yoshimatsu G, Takita M, Kanak MA, Haque WZ, Chang C, Saravanan PB, et al. MiR-375 and miR-200c as predictive biomarkers of islet isolation and transplantation in total pancreatectomy with islet autotransplantation. J. Hepatobiliary Pancreat. Sci. 2016;23(9):585–94.
34. Vasu S, Yang JM, Hodges J, Abu-El-Haija MA, Adams DB, Balamurugan AN, et al. Circulating miRNA in patients undergoing total pancreatectomy and islet autotransplantation. Cell Transplant. 2021;30:963689721999330.
35. Saravanan PB, Kanak MA, Chang CA, Darden C, Yoshimatsu G, Lawrence MC, et al. Islet damage during isolation as assessed by miRNAs and the correlation of miRNA levels with posttransplantation outcome in islet autotransplantation. Am J Transplant. 2018;18(4):982–9.
36. Liu Y, Vasu S, Kumano K, SoRelle JA, Lawrence MC, Naziruddin B. Pancreatic fibrosis assessment using picosirius red staining in chronic pancreatitis patients undergoing total pancreatectomy with islet autotransplantation. J Gastrointest Surg. 2022;26(8):1766–8.
37. Drifka CR, Loeffler AG, Mathewson K, Mehta G, Keikhosravi A, Liu Y, et al. Comparison of picrosirius red staining with second harmonic generation imaging for the quantification of clinically relevant collagen fiber features in histopathology samples. J Histochem Cytochem. 2016;64(9):519–29.
38. Kuncha J, Darden CM, Liu Y, Lawrence M, Sebastian Danobeitia J, Naziruddin B. Correlation of pancreatic laminin alpha 5 expression with clinical outcomes in total pancreatectomy with islet autotransplantation. Cell Transplant. 2025;34:9636897251317048.
39. Avila JG, Tsujimura T, Oberholzer J, Churchill T, Salehi P, Shapiro AMJ, et al. Improvement of pancreatic islet isolation outcomes using glutamine perfusion during isolation procedure. Cell Transplant. 2003;12(8):877–81.
40. Avila JG, Wang Y, Barbaro B, Gangemi A, Qi M, Kuechle J, et al. Improved outcomes in islet isolation and transplantation by the use of a novel hemoglobin-based O2 carrier. Am J Transplant. 2006;6(12):2861–70.
41. Saravanan PB, Kalivarathan J, Khan F, Shah R, Levy MF, Kanak MA. Exosomes in transplantation: role in allograft rejection, diagnostic biomarker, and therapeutic potential. Life Sci. 2023;324:121722.
42. Saravanan PB, Kalivarathan J, McClintock K, Mohammed S, Burch E, Morecock C, et al. Inflammatory and hypoxic stress-induced islet exosomes released during isolation are associated with poor transplant outcomes in islet autotransplantation. Am J Transplant. 2024;24(6):967–82.

Postoperative Pain Management and Pain Outcomes After Total Pancreatectomy and Islet Autotransplantation (TPIAT)

7

Megan A. Satyadi and Syed A. Ahmad

Abstract

Chronic pancreatitis (CP) is a progressive inflammatory condition of the pancreas resulting in irreversible structural damage, exocrine and endocrine dysfunction, and chronic abdominal pain—severely impacting patients' quality of life. Pain, frequently refractory to medical therapy and requiring escalating use of opioids, is the most common and debilitating symptom. For patients with hereditary pancreatitis and for those for whom previous traditional operations have failed, total pancreatectomy with autologous islet cell transplantation may offer improvement or resolution of abdominal pain in over 70% of patients. Resolution of pain after surgery is immediate for a small subset of patients but typically requires multiple months for the majority of patients. Management of pain in the immediate postoperative period and longer term requires the collaboration of a multidisciplinary pain management team including surgeons and pain specialists.

Key Points

1. The physiologic, biochemical, and neuropathic basis of chronic pain in CP is incompletely understood and is multifactorial in nature.
2. TPIAT dramatically reduces or eliminates the need for opiates, with the use of opiates decreasing over time, and improves quality of life.

M. A. Satyadi
General Surgery, University of Cincinnati Medical Center, Cincinnati, OH, USA

S. A. Ahmad (✉)
Division of Surgical Oncology, University of Cincinnati Medical Center, Cincinnati, OH, USA
e-mail: ahmadsy@ucmail.uc.edu

S. Chinnakotla et al. (eds.), *Total Pancreatectomy and Islet Auto Transplantation*,
https://doi.org/10.1007/978-981-92-0018-4_7

3. Which factors predict opiate independence are still unclear.
4. Postoperative pain management needs to be multimodal and balance the treatment of acute and chronic pain.
5. Adjuncts to pain management in CP, such as acupuncture, yoga, mindfulness, and psychological care, are low-risk and potentially helpful.

7.1 Introduction

Chronic pancreatitis (CP) is characterized by progressive inflammation and fibrosis of the pancreas resulting in endocrine and exocrine pancreatic insufficiency. The prevalence of CP varies across different studies; in the United States, it is reported to be between 42 and 73 per 100,000 adults [1–3]. Although CP presents with a variety of local and systemic complications, including malabsorption, nutritional deficiencies, and diabetes mellitus, the most common complaint from patients is abdominal pain [4] because it has a significant impact on quality of life and is unpredictable in nature [5, 6]. Chronic pain in CP is often refractory to medical therapy and can require escalating doses of narcotics in order to achieve adequate pain control [7]. The etiology of CP is multifactorial in nature and can be explained by a combination of physiologic, biochemical, and neuropathic mechanisms.

Managing complications of CP can be a significant burden to the health care system due to frequent hospitalization and utilization of hospital resources [8, 9]. Surgical treatment of CP is warranted in cases of refractory pain, failure of conservative medical and endoscopic management of complications, a known genetic cause of CP, and in cases with concern for malignancy [10]. Traditional surgical approaches to CP are based on the parenchymal and ductal morphology [11–13]. Drainage procedures like the Puestow procedure are used in cases with isolated pancreatic ductal dilatation, whereas formal resections such as the Whipple procedure are performed in cases with significant pancreatic head disease with mass effect on the duodenum or biliary system and concern for malignancy. Combination, duodenal-sparing procedures such as the Frey and Beger procedures are used in patients where pancreatic head disease and ductal dilatation are present.

The final surgical option for patients with CP is the total pancreatectomy with islet autotransplantation (TPIAT). TPIAT consists of resection of the entire gland, isolation of pancreatic islet cells, and autologous transplantation of the islets into the portal system to be taken up by hepatic parenchyma. While TP has historically been avoided unless absolutely necessary owing to the exocrine and endocrine consequences—lifelong reliance on pancreatic enzyme and nutritional supplementation and development of type IIIc diabetes mellitus—TPIAT offers a means for patients to achieve pain relief by removal of the diseased organ while also reducing or eliminating the need for insulin. TPIAT may be performed as an index operation for CP or as completion surgery in patients for whom previous surgical intervention has failed [14–17]. Especially in patients who have already undergone surgery for CP, severe refractory pain is an indication for TPIAT. Additionally, younger patients with hereditary or genetically linked pancreatitis (i.e., *PRSS1*, *SPINK1*, and *CFTR* mutations) are excellent candidates for TPIAT; surgery can be performed at a younger age before significant damage to the pancreas is done and can increase the yield of pancreatic islet cells and the chance of success of autotransplantation [16, 18]. Small-duct disease is also an indication for TPIAT, because decompressive procedures like the Puestow, Frey, and Beger procedures are ineffective for this condition [14, 19].

7.2 Etiology of Pain

The physiologic, biochemical, and neuropathic basis of chronic pain in CP is incompletely understood and is multifactorial in nature.

Local changes produced by the destruction of normal pancreatic parenchyma and replacement with fibrotic connective tissue, as well as pseudocyst formation, offer some explanation for the etiology of abdominal pain. Biliary and duodenal obstruction due to compression by a fibrotic pancreatic head or pancreatic pseudocysts are well-understood causes of abdominal pain, as are digestive issues in CP that are often readily reversible through endoscopic interventions. In cases refractory to less-invasive approaches, one of the surgical approaches discussed above may be appropriate, depending on the patient's specific anatomy. Pancreatic ductal obstruction secondary to fibrosis can also occur, leading to increased secretion and accumulation of pancreatic digestive enzymes that can trigger nociceptive pathways and increased ductal pressures that can trigger stretch-activated neural pathways, producing the classic epigastric pain in CP. Additionally, pancreatic fibrosis may create a compartment-syndrome effect with decreased venous drainage and impaired blood flow, causing local ischemia and tissue acidosis, resulting in severe pain.

Chronic inflammation in CP is associated with upregulation of the profibrotic cytokines platelet-derived growth factor B (PDGFB) and transforming growth factor β1 (TGFβ1), stimulating myofibroblasts and pancreatic stellate cells to synthesize extracellular matrix [20–22]. These chronic changes have been shown to alter the architecture of intrapancreatic nerve fibers. In an experiment described by Bockman et al. looking at tissue samples from patients with alcoholic and autoimmune CP, these nerve fibers exhibited damage to the perineural sheath, with no barrier between the internal neural fibers and surrounding tissue, as well as significant edema [23]. CP has been associated with increased levels of the pro-inflammatory neuropeptides substance P and calcitonin gene-related peptide (CGRP), further perpetuating the hallmark chronic inflammatory and progressively fibrotic state of CP [20, 24]. Substance P primarily acts on the neurokinin 1 (NK1) receptor, which is upregulated in CP. When stimulated, NK1 has vasoconstrictive effects, likely contributing to local ischemia of pancreatic parenchyma and intrapancreatic nerves [25–27].

Several studies have investigated the neuropathologic mechanisms of pain in CP at a central and peripheral level. The majority of nerves carrying afferent pain signals from the pancreas are splanchnic nerves passing through the celiac ganglion [20, 27, 28]. In a chronic inflammatory state, pain receptors in the pancreas are continuously stimulated, producing a sensitizing effect. These pain signals are transmitted to the central nervous system, where the perception of pain is produced and experienced; overactivation and sensitization of the central nervous system create the chronic pain state characteristic of CP [27, 29]. This pattern of hyperexcitability and decreased inhibitory control in CP is demonstrated in other chronic neuropathic pain syndromes.

7.3 A Single-Center Experience with TPIAT for the Management of Refractory Abdominal Pain

TPIAT is not a widely performed procedure in the United States and is offered only in several major centers with well-established TPIAT programs. Our center has been performing TPIAT since 1999 and tracking CP patient outcomes through the prospectively maintained University of Cincinnati Pancreatic Disease Center patient database. TPIAT is used at our institution for the following indications: hereditary pancreatitis, minimal change CP with small-duct disease, recurrent acute pancreatitis, and CP with failure of prior surgical intervention [15, 19, 30, 31].

Between 2000 and 2020, a total of 493 patients underwent 555 operative interventions for CP; 48.5% of the patients underwent TPIAT [30]. In this cohort, 12.0% of patients (n = 59) required additional surgical intervention after their index operation, with 36 of these patients undergoing completion pancreatectomy. Across this cohort for all surgical interventions for CP, not exclusively TPIAT or completion pancreatectomy, 73.1% (n = 331) of patients achieved narcotic independence in the long term, with a median follow-up of 64.5 months. Of the patients still requiring opioids for adequate pain control, the daily morphine equivalent (MEQ) was 60. Overall survival at 1, 5, and 10 years was estimated to be 95.5%, 81.3%, and 63.5%, respectively, with a median follow-up of 83.9 months. On multivariate analysis, persistent narcotic dependence was the only factor associated with worse overall survival.

These results are consistent in TPIAT-only cohorts, as demonstrated in an evaluation of 10-year outcomes of narcotic requirements, endocrine function, and quality-of-life metrics following TPIAT [31]. In a cohort of 142 patients who underwent TPIAT (either as an index operation or after failure of a previous intervention for CP), 71.8% were narcotic dependent preoperatively, with a mean morphine equivalent per day (MEQ/d) of 114.7 ± 14.8. At 1 year follow-up, 66% of patients were narcotic independent, with the rate of independence increasing to 73.3% at 5-year follow-up. This rate remained stable at the 7.5- and 10-year follow-ups, with over 75% of patients achieving opioid independence. The daily requirement of the patients who continued to require narcotics was significantly reduced. At 5-, 7.5-, and 10-year follow-up, MEQ/d decreased to 16.8 ± 4.4, 19.7 ± 5.8, and 10.5 ± 3.8, respectively. Quality-of-life metrics were assessed preoperatively and at follow-up using the SF-36 health survey. Metrics such as bodily pain and physical limitations were assessed on a scale of 0–100, with 100 being the most optimal. Preoperative mean scores for bodily pain and physical limitations were, respectively, 9.3 ± 2.2

and 0.0 ± 0. At 5- and 10-year follow-up, bodily pain quality-of-life scores improved to 57.4 ± 5.5 and 67.7 ± 6.4, respectively. Physical limitation scores improved to 47.2 ± 8.4 and 75.0 ± 6.8 at 5- and 10-year follow-up, respectively. These results suggest that TPIAT has a durable effect on long-term abdominal pain and quality of life, with early narcotic independence being the only predictor of improved long-term quality of life.

Completion pancreatectomy with IAT (CPIAT) in patients who fail traditional decompressive or resection procedures provides improvements in narcotic independence and quality-of-life metrics similar to those of TPIAT at our institution [15]. A study looking at 64 narcotic-dependent patients who underwent CPIAT as a salvage therapy for refractory chronic pancreatitis found that the mean daily requirement decreased from 120.9 MEQ/d preoperatively to 48.5 MEQ/d in patients who continued to require narcotics postoperatively, with a median follow-up of 21.2 months. At follow-up, 52% achieved opioid independence. Based on responses from the SF-36 survey, CPIAT patients also experienced similar improvements in quality-of-life metrics (bodily pain, physical limitations). Bodily pain and physical limitations scores were 7.3 ± 3.4 and 1.8 ± 1.8 preoperatively and improved to 64.7 ± 7.8 and 63.1 ± 10.9, respectively.

Our institution has completed multiple studies examining outcomes after TPIAT and testing the durability of the procedure in terms of pain relief, quality of life, and insulin independence in an attempt to identify factors that predict success in these domains. While we have not yet identified significant factors that predict narcotic independence following TPIAT, higher preoperative daily narcotic requirements are inversely correlated with narcotic independence [32]. We hope to continue investigating these outcomes to guide postoperative management and allow patients to achieve durable pain control.

7.4 Postoperative Pain Management

Weaning narcotics postoperatively after TPIAT is a clinical challenge. For many CP patients, the experience of chronic pain was both a significant physical and psychological challenge [28, 30, 33]. Postoperative management after TPIAT is highly multidisciplinary and consists of tight glucose control, pain management, nutritional and gastrointestinal support, and weaning of pain medications and insulin over the course of months [30, 31]. Balancing the treatment of acute and chronic pain in the setting of recent surgery is highly individualized. Multimodal pain control following surgery is the standard of care at our institution and typically includes opioid patient-controlled analgesia alongside acetaminophen, nonsteroidal anti-inflammatory drugs, and muscle relaxants such as methocarbamol or cyclobenzaprine. Other adjuncts that are commonly used in chronic neuropathic pain syndromes may also be used as continuation of home therapy or based on patient factors and side-effect profiles. These include anticonvulsants such as gabapentin and pregabalin, tricyclic antidepressants (amitriptyline), and selective serotonin and serotonin/norepinephrine reuptake inhibitors (SSRIs and SNRIs).

Our experience would indicate that both narcotic independence, if achieved, and improvement in quality of life can persist for the long term. In addition, a subset of patients not achieving narcotic independence continued to wean their morphine equivalent to a lower basal rate. This finding is not surprising, because the etiology of pain in these patients is often multifactorial and withdrawal from narcotics requires months, if not years, to achieve. In our experience, many patients have a dramatic improvement in their abdominal pain after pancreatectomy, but complete resolution is not immediately achieved. Many of these patients also suffer from narcotic bowel syndrome, and the use of exocrine supplementation can complicate these underlying issues [34]. Therefore, once the pancreatic pain has dissipated, time is required to manage the other underlying causes of abdominal pain.

A multicenter, prospective study is currently in progress: the Individualized Pain Treatment in Chronic Pancreatitis (INPAIN) study aims to understand pain in chronic pancreatitis and to create a tool to help individualize pain management and improve our clinical approach to chronic CP pain [35]. This study seeks to phenotype pain in CP, develop a bedside test panel that clinicians can use to assess pain, and predict which patients will respond well to specific interventions and therapies. This research is very exciting, and we anticipate that the results will have a major impact on our understanding and management of pain in patients with CP and also those who undergo TPIAT.

7.5 Adjuncts to Pain Management in CP

Supportive measures in management of CP are an important aspect of long-term patient care plans. Adjuncts to support digestion and gastrointestinal motility are also commonly utilized. Pancreatic enzyme supplementation to manage acquired pancreatic exocrine insufficiency aids in digestion and can help ameliorate the symptoms associated with malabsorption and indigestion, including abdominal discomfort [36]. Patients should be educated on dietary changes to support their recovery; this includes consuming smaller, frequent meals as well as nutritional supplementation as indicated. Cessation of alcohol and tobacco use is also reinforced [29, 37, 38].

Due to the often debilitating nature of chronic pain in CP, patients may seek adjuncts to conventional methods of pain management to improve quality of life. While few randomized controlled studies have been performed to prove their efficacy, these adjuncts are of relatively low risk to patients and may offer additional therapeutic effects in addition to conventional management.

7.5.1 Acupuncture and Electroacupuncture

Several studies have examined the effects of acupuncture and electroacupuncture on pain relief in patients with acute or chronic pancreatitis. A proof-of-concept randomized controlled study in Denmark demonstrated that acupuncture provided more short-acting pain relief than sham stimulation in CP patients [39]. A similar study in China failed to demonstrate significant pain relief in patients with acute pancreatitis, although improvements in appetite and tolerance of oral intake were noted [40].

7.5.2 Yoga and Mindfulness

A randomized controlled trial as described by Sareen et al. [41, 42] demonstrated that yoga was effective in improving quality of life in CP patients, with reported improvements in overall well-being, mood, and appetite after a 12-week period of biweekly yoga sessions compared to a control group receiving conventional management.

7.5.3 Psychological, Pharmacologic, and Behavioral Interventions

There is also evidence that patients with chronic pain develop secondary mood disorders; patients with CP report a high rate of depression as assessed on hospital screening questionnaires and may benefit from antidepressant therapy. SNRIs such as venlafaxine and duloxetine have a more favorable side-effect profile than tricyclic antidepressants and are often used in patients with concomitant mood disorders and chronic neuropathic pain [29, 33, 43]. While there have been no large-scale clinical trials examining the efficacy of psychological intervention, a small pilot study in 2017 demonstrated that hypnotherapy may reduce pain in CP patients with no adverse effects [44]. Cognitive behavioral therapy may also be an effective, low-risk adjunct in pain management; while no studies have been done specifically in CP patients, cognitive behavioral therapy has been shown to be effective in other chronic pain conditions.

7.6 Summary

TPIAT remains a viable option for the management of refractory abdominal pain in properly selected patients. Based on our experience, over 70% of patients can achieve narcotic independence after the operation. Bellin et al. published recommendations from a consensus conference focusing on the management of TPIAT. This white paper stressed the need for a structured approach for patient evaluation and treatment. A similar structured approach is also necessary for short- and long-term pain management after TPIAT. Most patients cannot be weaned off narcotics immediately and require a multidisciplinary pain team to help them with narcotic cessation over months, if not a year, after surgery. It is also important to rule out other causes of abdominal pain, such as narcotic bowel syndrome, after surgery. Refractory pain despite surgery is poorly understood and is most likely multifactorial. For these patients, adjuncts such as acupuncture, mindfulness, and other integrative interventions may help alleviate the severity of pain and help improve the quality of life.

References

1. Moran RA, Klapheke R, John GK, et al. Prevalence and predictors of pain and opioid analgesic use following total pancreatectomy with islet autotransplantation for pancreatitis. Pancreatology. 2017;17(5):732–7. https://doi.org/10.1016/j.pan.2017.07.005.
2. Cai QY, Tan K, Zhang XL, et al. Incidence, prevalence, and comorbidities of chronic pancreatitis: a 7-year population-based study. World J Gastroenterol. 2023;29(30):4671–84. https://doi.org/10.3748/wjg.v29.i30.4671.
3. Tseng J, Choi EA, Matthews JB. Chronic pancreatitis. In: Shackelford's surgery of the alimentary tract, 2 volume set. Elsevier; 2019. p. 1085–96. https://doi.org/10.1016/B978-0-323-40232-3.00092-3.
4. Braganza JM, Lee SH, McCloy RF, McMahon MJ. Chronic pancreatitis. Lancet. 2011;377(9772):1184–97. https://doi.org/10.1016/S0140-6736(10)61852-1.
5. Mokrowiecka A, Pińkowski D, Małecka-Panas E. Assessment of quality of life in patients with chronic pancreatitis. Med Sci Monit. 2011;17(10):CR583–8. https://doi.org/10.12659/msm.881985.
6. Fitzsimmons D, Kahl S, Butturini G, et al. Symptoms and quality of life in chronic pancreatitis assessed by structured interview and the EORTC QLQ-C30 and QLQ-PAN26. Am J Gastroenterol. 2005;100(4):918–26. https://doi.org/10.1111/j.1572-0241.2005.40859.x.
7. Goulden MR. The pain of chronic pancreatitis: a persistent clinical challenge. Br J Pain. 2013;7(1):8–22. https://doi.org/10.1177/2049463713479230.
8. Olesen SS, Nøjgaard C, Poulsen JL, et al. Chronic pancreatitis is characterized by distinct complication clusters that associate with etiological risk factors. Am J Gastroenterol. 2019;114(4):656–64. https://doi.org/10.14309/ajg.0000000000000147.
9. Ahmed NS, Forbes N, Stukalin I, et al. Population-based trends in healthcare utilization and National Healthcare Spending on pancreatitis in North America. Gastroenterology. 2021;161(5):1698–1701.e5. https://doi.org/10.1053/j.gastro.2021.08.022.
10. Bellin MD, Beilman GJ, Sutherland DE, et al. How durable is Total Pancreatectomy and Intraportal islet cell transplantation for treatment of chronic pancreatitis? J Am Coll Surg. 2019;228(4):329–39. https://doi.org/10.1016/j.jamcollsurg.2018.12.019.
11. Zafar HB. Surgical Management of Chronic Pancreatitis: a systemic review. Cureus. 2023;15(3):e35806. https://doi.org/10.7759/cureus.35806.
12. Bouwense SAW, Kempeneers MA, van Santvoort HC, Boermeester MA, van Goor H, Besselink MG. Surgery in chronic pancreatitis: indication, timing and procedures. Visc Med. 2019;35(2):110–8. https://doi.org/10.1159/000499612.
13. Tez M, Şahingöz E, Martlı HF. Non-pharmacological pain palliation methods in chronic pancreatitis. World J Clin Cases. 2023;11(35):8263–9. https://doi.org/10.12998/wjcc.v11.i35.8263.
14. Morgan KA, Lancaster WP, Owczarski SM, Wang H, Borckardt J, Adams DB. Patient selection for Total Pancreatectomy with islet autotransplantation in the surgical Management of Chronic Pancreatitis. J Am Coll Surg. 2018;226(4):446–51. https://doi.org/10.1016/j.jamcollsurg.2017.12.018.
15. Wilson GC, Sutton JM, Smith MT, et al. Completion pancreatectomy and islet cell autotransplantation as salvage therapy for patients failing previous operative interventions for chronic pancreatitis. Surgery. 2015;158(4):872–8.; discussion 879–880. https://doi.org/10.1016/j.surg.2015.04.045.

16. Bellin MD, Gelrud A, Arreaza-Rubin G, et al. Total pancreatectomy with islet autotransplantation: summary of a National Institute of diabetes and digestive and kidney diseases workshop. Pancreas. 2014;43(8):1163–71. https://doi.org/10.1097/MPA.0000000000000236.
17. Dhar VK, Levinsky NC, Xia BT, et al. The natural history of chronic pancreatitis after operative intervention: the need for revisional operation. Surgery. 2016;160(4):977–86. https://doi.org/10.1016/j.surg.2016.05.030.
18. Bellin MD, Freeman ML, Gelrud A, et al. Total pancreatectomy and islet autotransplantation in chronic pancreatitis: recommendations from PancreasFest. Pancreatology. 2014;14(1):27–35. https://doi.org/10.1016/j.pan.2013.10.009.
19. Wilson GC, Sutton JM, Smith MT, et al. Total pancreatectomy with islet cell autotransplantation as the initial treatment for minimal-change chronic pancreatitis. HPB (Oxford). 2015;17(3):232–8. https://doi.org/10.1111/hpb.12341.
20. Olesen SS, Krauss T, Demir IE, et al. Towards a neurobiological understanding of pain in chronic pancreatitis: mechanisms and implications for treatment. Pain Rep. 2017;2(6):e625. https://doi.org/10.1097/PR9.0000000000000625.
21. Detlefsen S, Sipos B, Feyerabend B, Klöppel G. Fibrogenesis in alcoholic chronic pancreatitis: the role of tissue necrosis, macrophages, myofibroblasts and cytokines. Mod Pathol. 2006;19(8):1019–26. https://doi.org/10.1038/modpathol.3800613.
22. Saloman JL, Li Y, Stello K, et al. Serum biomarkers of nociceptive and neuropathic pain in chronic pancreatitis. J Pain. 2023;24(12):2199–210. https://doi.org/10.1016/j.jpain.2023.07.006.
23. Bockman DE, Buchler M, Malfertheiner P, Beger HG. Analysis of nerves in chronic pancreatitis. Gastroenterology. 1988;94(6):1459–69. https://doi.org/10.1016/0016-5085(88)90687-7.
24. Liu L, Shenoy M, Pasricha PJ. Substance P and calcitonin gene related peptide mediate pain in chronic pancreatitis and their expression is driven by nerve growth factor. JOP. 2011;12(4):389–94.
25. Shrikhande SV, Friess H, di Mola FF, et al. NK-1 receptor gene expression is related to pain in chronic pancreatitis. Pain. 2001;91(3):209–17. https://doi.org/10.1016/S0304-3959(00)00436-X.
26. Fregni F, Pascual-Leone A, Freedman SD. Pain in chronic pancreatitis: a salutogenic mechanism or a maladaptive brain response? Pancreatology. 2007;7(5–6):411–22. https://doi.org/10.1159/000108958.
27. Drewes AM, Krarup AL, Detlefsen S, Malmstrøm ML, Dimcevski G, Funch-Jensen P. Pain in chronic pancreatitis: the role of neuropathic pain mechanisms. Gut. 2008;57(11):1616–27. https://doi.org/10.1136/gut.2007.146621.
28. Talukdar R, Reddy DN. Pain in chronic pancreatitis: managing beyond the pancreatic duct. World J Gastroenterol. 2013;19(38):6319–28. https://doi.org/10.3748/wjg.v19.i38.6319.
29. Drewes AM, Bouwense SAW, Campbell CM, et al. Guidelines for the understanding and management of pain in chronic pancreatitis. Pancreatology. 2017;17(5):720–31. https://doi.org/10.1016/j.pan.2017.07.006.
30. Wilson GC, Turner KM, Delman AM, et al. Long-term survival outcomes after operative Management of Chronic Pancreatitis: two decades of experience. J Am Coll Surg. 2023;236(4):601–10. https://doi.org/10.1097/XCS.0000000000000575.
31. Turner KM, Delman AM, Donovan EC, et al. Total pancreatectomy and islet cell autotransplantation: a 10-year update on outcomes and assessment of long-term durability. HPB (Oxford). 2022;24(11):2013–21. https://doi.org/10.1016/j.hpb.2022.07.001.
32. Ahmad SA, Lowy AM, Wray CJ, et al. Factors associated with insulin and narcotic independence after islet autotransplantation in patients with severe chronic pancreatitis. J Am Coll Surg. 2005;201(5):680–7. https://doi.org/10.1016/j.jamcollsurg.2005.06.268.
33. Maydeo A, Kamat N, Dalal A, Patil G. Advances in the Management of Pain in chronic pancreatitis. Curr Gastroenterol Rep. 2023;25(10):260–6. https://doi.org/10.1007/s11894-023-00898-1.

34. Grunkemeier DMS, Cassara JE, Dalton CB, Drossman DA. The narcotic bowel syndrome: clinical features, pathophysiology, and management. Clin Gastroenterol Hepatol. 2007;5(10):1126–39.; quiz 1121–1122. https://doi.org/10.1016/j.cgh.2007.06.013.
35. Hagn-Meincke R, Dugic A, Agarwal A, et al. Individualized pain treatment in chronic pancreatitis (INPAIN): an international, multicenter, investigator-initiated, prospective, Cohort Study. Pancreas. 2025;54(1):e1–e10. https://doi.org/10.1097/MPA.0000000000002388.
36. Hobbs PM, Johnson WG, Graham DY. Management of pain in chronic pancreatitis with emphasis on exogenous pancreatic enzymes. World J Gastrointest Pharmacol Ther. 2016;7(3):370–86. https://doi.org/10.4292/wjgpt.v7.i3.370.
37. Forsmark CE. Management of Chronic Pancreatitis. Gastroenterology. 2013;144(6):1282–1291. e3. https://doi.org/10.1053/j.gastro.2013.02.008.
38. Jalal M, Campbell JA, Hopper AD. Practical guide to the management of chronic pancreatitis. Frontline Gastroenterol. 2019;10(3):253–60. https://doi.org/10.1136/flgastro-2018-101071.
39. Juel J, Liguori S, Liguori A, et al. Acupuncture for pain in chronic pancreatitis: a single-blinded randomized crossover trial. Pancreas. 2017;46(2):170–6. https://doi.org/10.1097/MPA.0000000000000749.
40. Jang DK, Jung CY, Kim KH, Lee JK. Electroacupuncture for abdominal pain relief in patients with acute pancreatitis: study protocol for a randomized controlled trial. Trials. 2018;19(1):279. https://doi.org/10.1186/s13063-018-2644-1.
41. Sareen S, Kumari V. Yoga for rehabilitation in chronic pancreatitis. Gut. 2006;55(7):1051. https://doi.org/10.1136/gut.2006.093088.
42. Sareen S. Yoga: a tool for improving the quality of life in chronic pancreatitis. WJG. 2007;13(3):391. https://doi.org/10.3748/wjg.v13.i3.391.
43. Nag DS, Swain BP, Anand R, Barman TK, Vatsala. Pain management in chronic pancreatitis. World J Clin Cases. 2024;12(12):2016–22. https://doi.org/10.12998/wjcc.v12.i12.2016.
44. Juel J, Abrahamsen R, Olesen SS, Drewes AM. A pilot-study of hypnotherapy as complementary treatment for pain in chronic pancreatitis. J Complementary and Integrative Medicine. 2018;15(4):20170084. https://doi.org/10.1515/jcim-2017-0084.

Endocrine Management of the Patient Undergoing Total Pancreatectomy with Islet Autotransplantation

8

Melena D. Bellin

Abstract

Total pancreatectomy with islet autotransplantation (TPIAT) is most often performed to reduce pain in patients with disabling forms of recurrent acute and chronic pancreatitis. The IAT portion of the procedure achieves a secondary goal of mitigating postoperative diabetes. Over 80% of patients will have functioning (C-peptide–positive) transplanted islets. Overall, 20–30% of patients will stop insulin entirely, usually between several months to 1 year after TPIAT. Islet mass is the most important predictor of insulin independence, followed by age <2 years. Management of the TPIAT recipient starts with a careful preoperative assessment, screening for diabetes and islet function. Immediately after surgery, glucose is managed with an insulin drip, later transitioned to subcutaneous insulin by multiple daily injections or an insulin pump. Glucose should be strictly targeted to normoglycemia early after transplant to reduce islet loss during the period of islet engraftment. Long-term goals are to maintain HbA1c ≤6.5%. For individuals with islets that function well, insulin can be slowly weaned between 3 months and 1 year after TPIAT. Even patients who are insulin independent will require lifelong monitoring of glucose, as islet attrition occurs after IAT and patients will eventually need to resume insulin. A subset of patients also report hypoglycemia induced by carbohydrate-rich meals or exercise and may need close monitoring, dietary adjustments, and, rarely, pharmacologic management of hypoglycemia.

M. D. Bellin (✉)
Division of Pediatric Endocrinology, Department of Pediatrics, University of Minnesota Medical School, Minneapolis, MN, USA
e-mail: bell0130@umn.edu

S. Chinnakotla et al. (eds.), *Total Pancreatectomy and Islet Auto Transplantation*,
https://doi.org/10.1007/978-981-92-0018-4_8

Key Points

1. Islet autotransplantation will preserve some endogenous beta-cell function in most patients and allow insulin independence in up to 30%.
2. High islet mass and pediatric age are associated with high rates of insulin independence. Insulin independence wanes over time but has been reported even >15 years after TPIAT.
3. Islets are under conditions of hypoxia, inflammation, and mechanical damage at the time of islet infusion. Strictly targeting euglycemia reduces islet loss and optimizes islet engraftment.
4. All patients require lifelong monitoring of glycemia, even if they are not on insulin, since even insulin-independent patients are expected to resume insulin therapy at some point.
5. Some patients report hypoglycemia even off insulin, which may relate to altered intestinal anatomy, increased glucagon-like peptide (GLP)-1 response to meals, and impaired physiologic glucagon response to hypoglycemia.

8.1 Introduction

Total pancreatectomy with islet autotransplantation (TPIAT) is performed with the primary goal of relieving debilitating pain from recurrent acute or chronic pancreatitis and improving quality of life [1, 2]. The goal of the IAT portion of the procedure is to reduce the diabetes burden that results from TP by preserving as much endogenous islet function as possible [3, 4]. Outcomes from the IAT largely depend upon how many islets can be isolated and successfully transplanted from the diseased pancreas [3]. Those individuals with less fibrotic disease tend to have a more successful islet isolation with a greater islet mass transplanted, which, in turn, increases the chance of reaching insulin independence after TPIAT [5–8]. Most patients (80–90%) do have clinically beneficial islet graft function 1 year after TPIAT, and up to 30% achieve insulin independence [3, 9]. Management of the TPIAT recipient after surgery is a factor in the success of the IAT, as hyperglycemia—particularly early after TPIAT—can exacerbate posttransplant islet loss and result in poorer diabetes outcomes [10]. This chapter will review the assessment of the patient before TPIAT, management of diabetes early after TPIAT, and long-term diabetes management including insulin weaning and monitoring of insulin-independent recipients (see Table 8.1). We will also review hypoglycemia occurrence in this population and briefly discuss other endocrine complications of TPIAT surgery including risk for low bone-mineral density.

Table 8.1 Summary of the endocrine management of the TPIAT recipient before and after TPIAT

Management	Peritransplant (within 1 week of TPIAT)	Early (<3 months) after TPIAT	Long-term (>3 months) after TPIAT
Diabetes pharmacologic management	Intravenous insulin drip (transition to subcutaneous ~4–7 days postoperatively)	Subcutaneous insulin therapy with multiple daily injections or insulin pump. All or nearly all patients are treated with insulin during this time of islet revascularization and engraftment	Subcutaneous insulin therapy with multiple daily injections or an insulin pump, if needed. Wean to maintain glucose goals Non-insulin medications are nonstandard but may be considered on a case-by-case basis
Blood glucose monitoring	Hospital-calibrated meter for insulin dosing, +/– continuous glucose monitoring (CGM)	CGM is usually preferred in the outpatient setting, but a glucometer is needed as backup, due to possible false readings (particularly with hydroxyurea use)	Insulin-dependent patients: CGM usually preferred, with glucometer as backup Insulin-independent patients: Intermittent CGM (at least 10–15 days/month) *or* glucose meter checks 3–4 days per week) fasting and nonfasting)
Blood glucose targets	80–125 mg/dl	70–140 mg/dl on CGM for most of the day, or premeal BG 80–125 mg/dl	Minimum of 75% time in target range 70–180 mg/dl on CGM; achieving ≥75% in the tighter target of 70–140 mg/dl is optimal in insulin-independent patients
Laboratory monitoring	As needed (usually limited to hospital glucose readings)	At 3 months: HbA1c and mixed-meal tolerance test with fasting and stimulated glucose and C-peptide	At 6 months, 12 months, and then yearly: HbA1c and mixed-meal tolerance test with fasting and stimulated glucose and C-peptide

(continued)

Table 8.1 (continued)

Management	Peritransplant (within 1 week of TPIAT)	Early (<3 months) after TPIAT	Long-term (>3 months) after TPIAT
Non-diabetes endocrine considerations			Monitor for hypoglycemia (insulin-dependent and insulin-independent patients) Check vitamin D with routine labs; periodic DEXA scans for bone health Consider low-dose ACTH stimulation test if there are signs of adrenal insufficiency, especially in patients on opioids (risk of hypothalamic-pituitary-adrenal axis suppression)

ACTH adrenocorticotropic hormone, *DEXA* dual-energy X-ray absorptiometry, *BG* blood glucose

8.2 Endocrine Assessment of the Patient Being Considered for TPIAT

As reviewed in Chap. 2, TPIAT is performed most often for patients who have recurrent acute and/or chronic pancreatitis. Patients with pancreatitis are at risk for prediabetes and diabetes, resulting primarily from defects in insulin secretion from inflammatory damage and fibrotic loss of beta cells, but, in some cases, also complicated by insulin resistance [11]. In those with chronic pancreatitis, the prevalence of pancreatogenic diabetes is around 40% in adults and 6% in children [12–15]. The American Diabetes Association recommends yearly monitoring with, at minimum, fasting glucose and hemoglobin A1c for patients with chronic pancreatitis [16].

Because of this known high risk for pancreatogenic diabetes (sometimes also called type 3c diabetes or post-pancreatitis diabetes), it is important that any patient being considered for TPIAT is screened before surgery for metabolic function, at minimum with fasting glucose and hemoglobin A1c to evaluate diabetes status [17]. At our center, we also recommend assessment of baseline islet function (specifically beta-cell function) by performing a simple mixed-meal test where the patient consumes a standard physiologic meal replacement beverage (we use Boost High Protein, 6 ml/kg to a maximum of 360 ml), and glucose and C-peptide are measured fasting before the nutritional shake and at 30- to 60-min intervals after the beverage for 2 h [18]. This provides a baseline assessment of insulin secretion for later follow-up. Because we have observed some patients in our population with presymptomatic type 1 diabetes, we also recommend testing beta-cell autoantibodies as part of the evaluation process [19–21]. Continuous glucose monitoring is being evaluated as a preoperative evaluation tool (and, as noted later, is used routinely postoperatively) [22–24].

Patients who have known diabetes or are newly diagnosed with diabetes upon evaluation may still be candidates for TPIAT if there is sufficient insulin secretory capacity to try to preserve islet function [25]. We have previously demonstrated that about 50% of these individuals will maintain C-peptide positivity after TPIAT. Among patients with diabetes at evaluation, those who have low C-peptide before TPIAT and rare patients with type 1 diabetes autoantibodies tend to lose all islet function and may be less likely to benefit from IAT [19, 21]. However, currently, there is no standard cutoff for when to perform IAT in patients with pancreatogenic diabetes, so this decision is made on a case-by-case basis. It is important to note that IAT does not *reverse* diabetes, and ultimately some islets are lost during transplantation, so all patients who have preexisting diabetes need to know that they will be insulin-dependent after IAT, and the only purpose of IAT is to try to retain some of the endogenous islet function to reduce glycemic lability and ease diabetes management.

In the U.S. literature, 90% of individuals who underwent TPIAT did not have diabetes at the time of TPIAT. These patients were on a spectrum ranging from normoglycemia to prediabetes. Individuals with prediabetes can reach insulin independence, but it is less common than in those individuals who have normal glycemic testing preoperatively [17, 26]. In general, preoperative hemoglobin A1c is strongly associated with diabetes outcomes after surgery, including insulin independence, glycemic control, and islet graft function [17]. Pre-TPIAT C-peptide is most strongly predictive of islet graft function but is more variable in predicting insulin independence. Other factors that have been associated with lower rates of insulin independence include high body mass index (overweight/obese) and prior lateral pancreaticojejunostomy or distal pancreatectomy [8, 9]. In contrast, young childhood age is associated with very robust insulin independence, and sustained islet function is reported for preadolescent children [1, 8, 18, 27, 28].

A critically important part of the evaluation and pre-TPIAT process is counseling patients with realistic expectations of diabetes after surgery. Even for a patient who has normal metabolic testing, there is a 100% chance of temporary insulin use and a high likelihood of needing some exogenous insulin lifelong. All patients undergoing TPIAT must be willing to accept and manage diabetes as a trade-off for reducing pancreatic pain. The diabetes education process starts before TPIAT and continues after the operation [4].

8.3 Management of Diabetes in the Peritransplant and Early Posttransplant Period

Following pancreatectomy, islets are isolated as described in Chap. 9 and infused intraportally. In the native pancreas, islets are richly vascularized and—despite being only 1–2% of the total pancreas mass—receive up to 20% of the pancreatic blood flow through a dense capillary network that perfuses into the islet [29]. As part of the isolation procedure, this dense vascular network is disrupted. In addition, the isolation process directly damages the islets, as evidenced by increased levels of unmethylated insulin DNA—a marker for dying beta cells—in the supernatant of the islet product before infusion [10, 30]. Upon islet infusion into the portal vasculature, an inflammatory reaction referred to as the instant blood-mediated inflammatory reaction is generated, with significant elevations of circulating cytokines and chemokines, most notably interleukin (IL)-8, IL-10, monocyte chemoattractant protein (MCP)-1, and IL-6 [30–32]. Ongoing islet death after infusion is suggested by elevations of the beta-cell–specific markers unmethylated insulin DNA and microRNA-375 [10, 33]. In sum, immediately after transplant, islets are in a hypoxic and damaged state, with some islets not surviving the transplant process.

In order to maximize the number of islets surviving the islet transplant process, we recommend aiming for normoglycemia or near-normoglycemia in the first few weeks to months after islet transplantation. It is well documented in animal models that beta-cell apoptosis is significantly higher in the setting of hyperglycemia than when insulin therapy is administered [34]. Under the conditions of hypoxia, islets are not fully functional initially after transplant and may be more vulnerable to hyperglycemic stress. Over a period of around 3 months, transplanted islets will elicit new vascularization, and vascular density will improve while relative hypoxia decreases [35–37].

All patients undergoing TPIAT start insulin therapy during the operative procedure. Insulin is initially given as a continuous intravenous infusion, which allows for rapid dose adjustments. This is particularly important over the first few days as nutrition is advanced, which, at our center, is done with continuous gastrojejunal feeds [38]. Around 5–7 days postoperatively, as clinically appropriate, patients are transitioned from the intravenous insulin drip to subcutaneous insulin therapy [39]. Subcutaneous insulin therapy is a basal-bolus regimen that can be delivered using multiple daily injections with a long-acting and rapid-acting insulin analog or by continuous subcutaneous insulin infusion using an insulin pump. Insulin pump use may be particularly appropriate for patients who require small and very precise doses of insulin [27, 40, 41]. At our center, all children are transitioned directly from intravenous insulin to an insulin pump. Insulin pump use does require special considerations: Individuals require additional diabetes education and training, must be comfortable with technology, and must either be alert and well enough to operate the pump system or have a family member or other caregiver who can do so. It is important that patients on insulin pump systems still receive basic education on subcutaneous injections and know how and when to administer an injection if the pump catheter or pump device fails.

Soon after TPIAT, target glucose is 80–125 mg/dl based on glucometer readings every 4 h if on enteral feeds and nothing by mouth, or on fasting, premeal, and bedtime readings if on an oral diet [4]. All patients are trained on a basic home glucometer, and insulin dosing in the hospital typically requires use of a hospital-calibrated glucometer for safety. In the current era, most patients are also started on continuous glucose monitoring (CGM) systems as either inpatients or outpatients [22, 24].

CGM is a particularly helpful tool for alerting to hypoglycemia and hyperglycemia, sometimes greatly reducing the need for fingerstick glucose measurements in the outpatient setting, and, in insulin pump users, integrating with pump systems for automated insulin delivery. However, it is important to also note the limitations of CGM. CGM reads interstitial glucose and can have inaccuracies, especially in the first 24 h after a new sensor start. Some pediatric TPIAT patients receive hydroxyurea for severe thrombocytosis resulting from splenectomy, and hydroxyurea will create false hyperglycemia on some CGM systems (at the time of this writing, on Dexcom G6 and G7); therefore, CGM should not be used for dosing insulin in these cases [23]. Patients need to be educated on how to process the sheer volume of data received by CGM—hundreds or even thousands of glucose readings per 24 h depending on the system (glucose values every 1–5 min). It is not feasible to maintain target range 24 h per day, and patients should be educated not to overreact to data. However, at our center, we will target as much time at 70–140 mg/dl as is safe to achieve in the first few weeks after TPIAT to protect the engrafting islets. Insulin dose adjustments are needed frequently during surgical recovery—sometimes even several days per week—as physiologic stress improves, activity increases, and dietary intake changes. Close communication with a physician or nurse after hospital discharge is critical.

8.4 Management of Diabetes in the Outpatient Setting Long-Term After TPIAT

At our center, we continue insulin therapy until at least 3 months after TPIAT. We target HbA1c ≤6.5%, fasting and premeal glucose 80–125 mg/d, and 2-h postmeal glucose <150 mg/d [3]. After the 3 months, if patients are near normoglycemia, are meeting glycemic goals based on home readings and HbA1c, and have relatively normal glucose and reassuring C-peptide response on mixed-meal testing, we may begin to slowly reduce insulin therapy. Up to 30% of patients will come off insulin, with this timing of insulin discontinuation most often occurring between 6 months and 2 years after TPIAT [3]. The odds of achieving insulin independence vary greatly by islet mass transplanted. Individuals who receive a low islet mass of <2500 islet equivalents per kilogram body weight (IEQ/kg) rarely discontinue insulin, while as many as two-thirds of individuals with >5000 IEQ/kg transplanted reach insulin independence (Fig. 8.1) [8, 9]. Those with a moderate islet mass between 2500 and 5000 IEQ/kg are more likely to come off insulin if they had a higher number of small islets (rather than large islets) transplanted, presumably because these small islets may survive better in the hypoxic conditions early after TPIAT [42]. Children have higher insulin independence rates than adults, and, in particular, young children come off insulin more often than adolescents (Fig. 8.2).

Using CGM data in post-TPIAT management, we have identified >75% time in the standard target range of 70–180 mg/dl and > 50% time in the tight target range of 70–140 mg/dl to be minimal goals, with high sensitivity and specificity for predicting an HbA1c ≤6.5% (*internal data, in submission*). However, these are

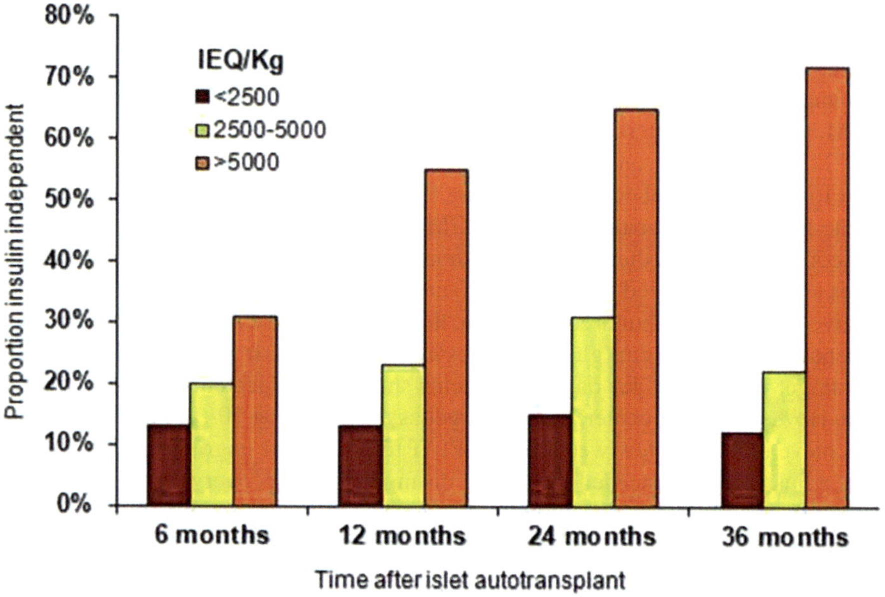

Fig. 8.1 Insulin independence based on transplanted islet mass at various time points after TPIAT, illustrating higher rates of insulin independence in patients with high islet mass. (Adapted from: Bellin et al. [4].)

Fig. 8.2 Time to discontinuation of insulin in children vs. adolescent patients undergoing TPIAT, showing the higher insulin independence rates in younger children. Data were collected from 134 pediatric patients (n = 52 children aged 3–11 years and n = 82 adolescents aged 12–18 years). (Adapted from: Gnikpingo et al. [18].)

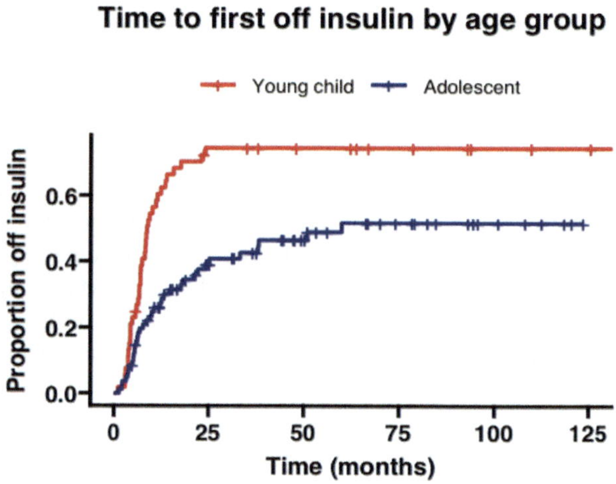

minimum goals, and achieving >75% time in the tight target of 70–140 mg/dL is likely optimal and predicts HbA1c ≤6.5% with greater specificity.

For laboratory monitoring in all patients, we recommend comprehensive post-TPIAT labs that include a mixed-meal tolerance test and HbA1c level at 3 months, 6 months, 1 year, and then yearly after TPIAT [18]. Individuals who are on insulin should additionally have HbA1c monitored every 3 months, consistent with current standards of care for insulin-treated diabetes. HbA1c between annual labs may also be considered on a case-by-case basis for individuals with increasing glucose or who are at the upper end of the goal HbA1c range.

There is an attrition of islet function over time, and patients who are insulin independent are expected to eventually need to resume insulin therapy. Duration of insulin independence is highly variable and, at our center, may range from only a year to >15 years, with the longest case that we are aware of at 22 years of insulin independence [43]. Young age and healthy body weight appear to be associated with greater chance of sustaining insulin independence and islet graft function long-term [8, 9]. We recommend all patients off insulin monitor glucose at home. This can be done by using a glucometer to test fasting and nonfasting glucose levels 3–4 days per week, or wearing a CGM. Glucose monitoring in insulin-independent patients has two benefits: (1) it allows for early intervention with low-dose insulin when mild hyperglycemia develops, to reduce ongoing metabolic stress on the beta cells that may exacerbate islet loss, and (2) it prevents acute presentations of hyperglycemia such as diabetic ketoacidosis. Close monitoring is also recommended during times of illness or subsequent surgeries, because temporary insulin use may be required.

Of note, we strongly recommend avoiding any systemic or injected (intramuscular or intra-articular) corticosteroids when possible because these do induce hyperglycemia and require either transient insulin coverage in insulin-independent patients or increased insulin doses. Failure to appropriately manage glycemia during corticosteroid administration has been associated with permanent declines in islet function, so patients are asked to contact their TPIAT team before receiving planned courses of corticosteroids or as soon as possible after administration in an emergency [44].

Non-insulin therapies are mostly unstudied in TPIAT. There was one randomized trial of the dipeptidyl peptidase-4 inhibitor sitagliptin started on the day of TPIAT and continued for 1 year to try to preserve beta cells during islet engraftment. However, there was no benefit in preserving islet mass, and even insulin doses and glycemic control were no different in sitagliptin users than in those who received placebo, suggesting little role for this medication in general in TPIAT [45]. Glucagon-like peptide-1 (GLP-1) receptor agonists cause delayed gastric emptying and, when tried in TPIAT anecdotally, are often poorly tolerated because these patients are already prone to gastrointestinal dysmotility. Interestingly, patients can have an exaggerated endogenous GLP-1 response after TPIAT, likely due to the change in intestinal anatomy with the surgery, while levels of glucose-dependent insulinotropic peptide (GIP)—which is produced in the duodenum that is mostly resected with surgery—are reduced 50% at 1 year after TPIAT from levels before surgery [46, 47]. Insulin sensitizers like metformin may have a role for individuals with a type 2 diabetes phenotype of insulin resistance but are not likely to provide any benefit for thin and insulin-sensitive patients whose diabetes primarily results from the insulin deficiency induced by surgery.

8.5 Challenges Around Hypoglycemia After TPIAT

A subset of patients report problematic hypoglycemia after TPIAT, even in the setting of insulin independence. This hypoglycemia most often occurs either after meals or with exercise [48–50]. The mechanisms for this hypoglycemia are not entirely clear. The exaggerated GLP-1 response in the setting of intestinal reconstruction may be contributing to an exaggerated postprandial insulin response [46]. There also appears to be a dysfunctional alpha-cell glucagon response to hypoglycemia, even in the setting of high islet mass, when all islets are transplanted into the liver (Fig. 8.3); this dysfunction may be particularly specific to islets transplanted in the standard hepatic site [50]. First-line management is small and frequent meals of low-carbohydrate and low-glycemic index foods and appropriate snacks for activity to avoid triggering a robust insulin response to high-carbohydrate meals [51]. For patients more severely affected by hypoglycemia, we have, in rare cases, used medication approaches, including acarbose, diazoxide, or mini-dose glucagon, tailored to the specific patient situation. The published literature on alpha-cell function and hypoglycemia is much sparser at the current time than on beta-cell function. Other causes of hypoglycemia including adrenal insufficiency should be ruled out. Insulinoma has never been reported in TPIAT and can be excluded, if needed, by prolonged inpatient fasting to document absence of hypoglycemia and to assess

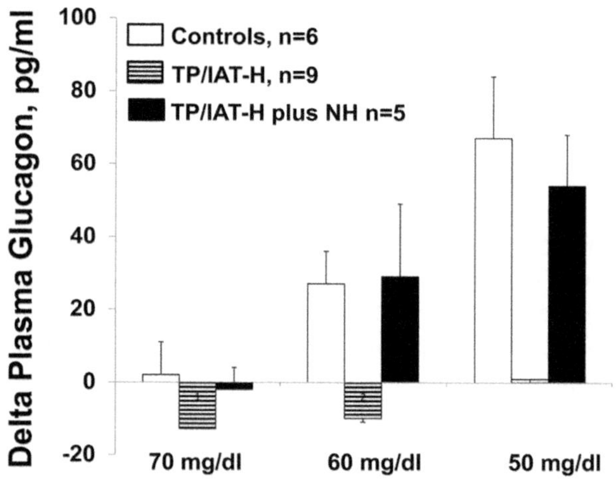

Fig. 8.3 Glucagon response to hypoglycemia in patients off insulin or on minimal basal insulin after TPIAT, all with high islet mass transplanted and documented alpha-cell function based on arginine stimulation testing. Hypoglycemia clamp tests suggested that individuals with all islets intrahepatic (TP/IAT-H, gray hatch) had a defective glucagon response to hypoglycemia compared with healthy volunteers (Controls, white), while those with some islets transplanted outside the liver (TP/IAT-H plus NH, black) had a glucagon response to hypoglycemia that was more similar to that of healthy volunteers. This was interpreted as potentially a result of hypoglycemia being masked in the liver environment due to glycogen flux within the liver (the major location of glycogen stores). (Adapted from: Bellin et al. [50].)

insulin and C-peptide levels if hypoglycemia does occur. For patients who are on insulin therapy, exogenous insulin should also be considered as a likely cause of hypoglycemia and adjustments should be made to insulin dosing as needed.

8.6 Other Endocrine Considerations in TPIAT

Individuals with chronic pancreatitis are at a two- to four-fold increased risk for osteoporosis and fractures, presumably due to malnutrition, vitamin D deficiency, reduced activity, and chronic inflammation [52, 53]. Patients after TPIAT are also at risk for vitamin D deficiency and have a period of reduced activity after operation. We have observed a decrease in bone mass in adults in the first year after TPIAT and recommend periodic bone health assessment by dual-energy X-ray absorptiometry (DEXA) post-TPIAT [53]. Vitamin D and calcium intake should be optimized in any patient with low bone density, and for those with osteoporosis or pathologic fracture, consideration of other pharmacologic agents may be warranted. Opioid users are at risk for opioid-induced central adrenal insufficiency [54]. While we do not routinely perform testing at our center, individuals with clinical concerns for adrenal insufficiency may warrant low-dose cosyntropin stimulation testing to evaluate for central adrenal insufficiency.

References

1. Abu-El-Haija M, Anazawa T, Beilman GJ, Besselink MG, Del Chiaro M, Demir IE, et al. The role of total pancreatectomy with islet autotransplantation in the treatment of chronic pancreatitis: a report from the International consensus guidelines in chronic pancreatitis. Pancreatology. 2020;20(4):762–71. https://doi.org/10.1016/j.pan.2020.04.005.
2. Bellin MD, Ramanathan K, Chinnakotla S. Total Pancreatectomy with islet auto-transplantation: surgical procedure, outcomes, and quality of life. Adv Surg. 2023;57(1):15–30. https://doi.org/10.1016/j.yasu.2023.03.002.
3. Sutherland DE, Radosevich DM, Bellin MD, Hering BJ, Beilman GJ, Dunn TB, et al. Total pancreatectomy and islet autotransplantation for chronic pancreatitis. J Am Coll Surg. 2012;214(4):409–24.; discussion 24–6. https://doi.org/10.1016/j.jamcollsurg.2011.12.040.
4. Bellin MD, Balamurugan AN, Pruett TL, Sutherland DE. No islets left behind: islet autotransplantation for surgery-induced diabetes. Curr Diab Rep. 2012;12(5):580–6. https://doi.org/10.1007/s11892-012-0296-1.
5. Kobayashi T, Manivel JC, Bellin MD, Carlson AM, Moran A, Freeman ML, et al. Correlation of pancreatic histopathologic findings and islet yield in children with chronic pancreatitis undergoing total pancreatectomy and islet autotransplantation. Pancreas. 2010;39(1):57–63. https://doi.org/10.1097/MPA.0b013e3181b8ff71.
6. Kobayashi T, Manivel JC, Carlson AM, Bellin MD, Moran A, Freeman ML, et al. Correlation of histopathology, islet yield, and islet graft function after islet autotransplantation in chronic pancreatitis. Pancreas. 2011;40(2):193–9. https://doi.org/10.1097/mpa.0b013e3181fa4916.
7. Mattke J, Eaton A, Wijkstrom M, Witkowski P, Trikudanathan G, Singh VK, et al. Islet isolation outcomes in patients undergoing Total Pancreatectomy with islet autotransplantation in the POST consortium. Transplantation. 2024; https://doi.org/10.1097/tp.0000000000005127.
8. Bellin MD, Eaton A, Ramanathan K, Beilman G, Downs E, Schwarzenberg SJ, et al. Long-term islet graft functional assessments in more than 500 patients undergoing Total Pancreatectomy

with Intraportal islet autotransplantation. J Am Coll Surg. 2025; https://doi.org/10.1097/xcs.0000000000001294.
9. Chinnakotla S, Beilman GJ, Dunn TB, Bellin MD, Freeman ML, Radosevich DM, et al. Factors predicting outcomes after a Total Pancreatectomy and islet autotransplantation lessons learned from over 500 cases. Ann Surg. 2015;262(4):610–22. https://doi.org/10.1097/sla.0000000000001453.
10. Bellin MD, Clark P, Usmani-Brown S, Dunn TB, Beilman GJ, Chinnakotla S, et al. Unmethylated insulin DNA is elevated after Total Pancreatectomy with islet autotransplantation: assessment of a novel Beta cell marker. Am J Transplant. 2017;17(4):1112–8. https://doi.org/10.1111/ajt.14054.
11. Parra Villasmil MG, Bellin MD. Risk factors and mechanisms for diabetes in pancreatitis. Gastroenterol Clin N Am. 2025;54(1):175–88. https://doi.org/10.1016/j.gtc.2024.08.002.
12. Schwarzenberg SJ, Uc A, Zimmerman B, Wilschanski M, Wilcox CM, Whitcomb DC, et al. Chronic pancreatitis: pediatric and adult cohorts show similarities in disease Progress despite different risk factors. J Pediatr Gastroenterol Nutr. 2019;68(4):566–73. https://doi.org/10.1097/mpg.0000000000002279.
13. Rickels MR, Bellin M, Toledo FG, Robertson RP, Andersen DK, Chari ST, et al. Detection, evaluation and treatment of diabetes mellitus in chronic pancreatitis: recommendations from PancreasFest 2012. Pancreatology. 2013;13(4):336–42. https://doi.org/10.1016/j.pan.2013.05.002.
14. Bellin MD. Pancreatogenic diabetes in children with recurrent acute and chronic pancreatitis: risks, screening, and treatment (mini-review). Front Pediatr. 2022;10:884668. https://doi.org/10.3389/fped.2022.884668.
15. Bellin MD, Lowe M, Zimmerman MB, Wilschanski M, Werlin S, Troendle DM, et al. Diabetes mellitus in children with acute recurrent and chronic pancreatitis: data from the INternational study Group of Pediatric Pancreatitis: in search for a CuRE cohort. J Pediatr Gastroenterol Nutr. 2019;69(5):599–606. https://doi.org/10.1097/mpg.0000000000002482.
16. Committee ADAPP. 2. Diagnosis and classification of diabetes: standards of Care in Diabetes—2025. Diabet Care. 2024;48(Supplement_1):S27–49. https://doi.org/10.2337/dc25-S002.
17. Nanno Y, Wastvedt S, Freeman ML, Trikudanathan G, Schwarzenberg SJ, Downs EM, et al. Metabolic measures before surgery and long-term diabetes outcomes in recipients of total pancreatectomy and islet autotransplantation. Am J Transplant. 2021;21(10):3411–20. https://doi.org/10.1111/ajt.16573.
18. Gnikpingo T, Benson S, Hodges JS, Downs E, Cook M, Schwarzenberg SJ, et al. Islet graft function by mixed meal tolerance testing is sustained over 4 years in young children undergoing total pancreatectomy with islet autotransplantation. Clin Transpl. 2023;37(12):e15106. https://doi.org/10.1111/ctr.15106.
19. Kizilgul M, Wilhelm JJ, Dunn TB, Beilman GJ, Pruett TL, Chinnakotla S, et al. The prognostic significance of glutamic acid decarboxylase antibodies in patients with chronic pancreatitis undergoing total pancreatectomy with islet autotransplantation. Diabetes Metab. 2019;45(3):301–5. https://doi.org/10.1016/j.diabet.2018.01.001.
20. Bellin MD, Moran A, Wilhelm JJ, O'Brien TD, Gottlieb PA, Yu L, et al. Development of autoimmune-mediated β cell failure after Total Pancreatectomy with autologous islet transplantation. Am J Transplant. 2015;15(7):1991–4. https://doi.org/10.1111/ajt.13216.
21. Kharoud HK, Mettler T, Freeman ML, Trikudanathan G, Beilman GJ, Chinnakotla S, et al. Type 1 diabetes mellitus in patients with recurrent acute and chronic pancreatitis: a case series. Pancreatology. 2021;21(1):95–7. https://doi.org/10.1016/j.pan.2020.12.006.
22. McEachron KR, Potlapalli N, Rayannavar A, Downs EM, Schwarzenberg SJ, Kirchner VA, et al. Early use of continuous glucose monitoring in children and adolescents after total pancreatectomy with islet autotransplantation. Pediatr Diabetes. 2021;22(3):434–8. https://doi.org/10.1111/pedi.13168.

23. Tellez SE, Hornung LN, Courter JD, Abu-El-Haija M, Nathan JD, Lawson SA, et al. Inaccurate glucose sensor values after Hydroxyurea administration. Diabetes Technol Ther. 2021;23(6):443–51. https://doi.org/10.1089/dia.2020.0490.
24. Segev N, Hornung LN, Tellez SE, Courter JD, Lawson SA, Nathan JD, et al. Continuous glucose monitoring in the intensive care unit following Total Pancreatectomy with islet autotransplantation in children: establishing accuracy of the Dexcom G6 model. J Clin Med. 2021;10(9) https://doi.org/10.3390/jcm10091893.
25. Bellin MD, Beilman GJ, Dunn TB, Pruett TL, Chinnakotla S, Wilhelm JJ, et al. Islet autotransplantation to preserve beta cell mass in selected patients with chronic pancreatitis and diabetes mellitus undergoing total pancreatectomy. Pancreas. 2013;42(2):317–21. https://doi.org/10.1097/MPA.0b013e3182681182.
26. Quartuccio M, Hall E, Singh V, Makary MA, Hirose K, Desai N, et al. Glycemic predictors of insulin Independence after Total Pancreatectomy with islet autotransplantation. J Clin Endocrinol Metab. 2017;102(3):801–9. https://doi.org/10.1210/jc.2016-2952.
27. Tellez SE, Hornung LN, Vitale DS, Lawson SA, Abu-El-Haija MA, Elder DA. Endocrine management and clinical outcomes in a cohort of pediatric patients undergoing Total Pancreatectomy with islet autotransplantation. Diabetes Technol Ther. 2023;25(11):800–7. https://doi.org/10.1089/dia.2023.0243.
28. Chinnakotla S, Bellin MD, Schwarzenberg SJ, Radosevich DM, Cook M, Dunn TB, et al. Total pancreatectomy and islet autotransplantation in children for chronic pancreatitis: indication, surgical techniques, postoperative management, and long-term outcomes. Ann Surg. 2014;260(1):56–64. https://doi.org/10.1097/sla.0000000000000569.
29. Jansson L, Barbu A, Bodin B, Drott CJ, Espes D, Gao X, et al. Pancreatic islet blood flow and its measurement. Ups J Med Sci. 2016;121(2):81–95. https://doi.org/10.3109/03009734.2016.1164769.
30. Abdel-Karim TR, Hodges JS, Herold KC, Pruett TL, Ramanathan KV, Hering BJ, et al. Peri-transplant inflammation and long-term diabetes outcomes were not impacted by either Etanercept or Alpha-1-antitrypsin treatment in islet autotransplant recipients. Transpl Int. 2024;37:12320. https://doi.org/10.3389/ti.2024.12320.
31. Bellin MD, Gelrud A, Arreaza-Rubin G, Dunn TB, Humar A, Morgan KA, et al. Total pancreatectomy with islet autotransplantation: summary of an NIDDK workshop. Ann Surg. 2015;261(1):21–9. https://doi.org/10.1097/sla.0000000000001059.
32. Itoh T, Iwahashi S, Kanak MA, Shimoda M, Takita M, Chujo D, et al. Elevation of high-mobility group box 1 after clinical autologous islet transplantation and its inverse correlation with outcomes. Cell Transplant. 2014;23(2):153–65. https://doi.org/10.3727/096368912x658980.
33. Kanak MA, Takita M, Shahbazov R, Lawrence MC, Chung WY, Dennison AR, et al. Evaluation of MicroRNA375 as a novel biomarker for graft damage in clinical islet transplantation. Transplantation. 2015;99(8):1568–73. https://doi.org/10.1097/tp.0000000000000625.
34. Biarnés M, Montolio M, Nacher V, Raurell M, Soler J, Montanya E. Beta-cell death and mass in syngeneically transplanted islets exposed to short- and long-term hyperglycemia. Diabetes. 2002;51(1):66–72. https://doi.org/10.2337/diabetes.51.1.66.
35. Lau J, Carlsson PO. Low revascularization of human islets when experimentally transplanted into the liver. Transplantation. 2009;87(3):322–5. https://doi.org/10.1097/TP.0b013e3181943b3d.
36. Carlsson PO. Influence of microenvironment on engraftment of transplanted β-cells. Ups J Med Sci. 2011;116(1):1–7. https://doi.org/10.3109/03009734.2010.548609.
37. Olsson R, Olerud J, Pettersson U, Carlsson PO. Increased numbers of low-oxygenated pancreatic islets after intraportal islet transplantation. Diabetes. 2011;60(9):2350–3. https://doi.org/10.2337/db09-0490.
38. Downs EM, Brun A, Bellin MD. Nutrition support in the pediatric total pancreatectomy with islet autotransplantation recipient. Nutr Clin Pract. 2024;39(1):100–8. https://doi.org/10.1002/ncp.11101.

39. Forlenza GP, Chinnakotla S, Schwarzenberg SJ, Cook M, Radosevich DM, Manchester C, et al. Near-euglycemia can be achieved safely in pediatric total pancreatectomy islet autotransplant recipients using an adapted intravenous insulin infusion protocol. Diabetes Technol Ther. 2014;16(11):706–13. https://doi.org/10.1089/dia.2014.0061.
40. Forlenza GP, Nathan BM, Moran AM, Dunn TB, Beilman GJ, Pruett TL, et al. Successful application of closed-loop artificial pancreas therapy after islet autotransplantation. Am J Transplant. 2016;16(2):527–34. https://doi.org/10.1111/ajt.13539.
41. Tellez S, Hornung L, Abu-El-Haija M, Elder D. Metabolic outcomes in pediatric patients one-year post-Total Pancreatectomy with islet autotransplantation after early pump initiation. J Clin Med. 2023;12(9) https://doi.org/10.3390/jcm12093319.
42. Suszynski TM, Wilhelm JJ, Radosevich DM, Balamurugan AN, Sutherland DE, Beilman GJ, et al. Islet size index as a predictor of outcomes in clinical islet autotransplantation. Transplantation. 2014;97(12):1286–91. https://doi.org/10.1097/01.TP.0000441873.35383.1e.
43. Bellin MD, Beilman GJ, Sutherland DE, Ali H, Petersen A, Mongin S, et al. How durable is Total Pancreatectomy and Intraportal islet cell transplantation for treatment of chronic pancreatitis? J Am Coll Surg. 2019;228(4):329–39. https://doi.org/10.1016/j.jamcollsurg.2018.12.019.
44. Ngo A, Sutherland DE, Beilman GJ, Bellin MD. Deterioration of glycemic control after corticosteroid administration in islet autotransplant recipients: a cautionary tale. Acta Diabetol. 2014;51(1):141–5. https://doi.org/10.1007/s00592-011-0315-8.
45. Bellin MD, Beilman GJ, Dunn TB, Pruett TL, Sutherland DE, Chinnakotla S, et al. Sitagliptin treatment after Total Pancreatectomy with islet autotransplantation: a randomized, Placebo-Controlled Study. Am J Transplant. 2017;17(2):443–50. https://doi.org/10.1111/ajt.13979.
46. McEachron KR, Yang Y, Hodges JS, Beilman GJ, Pruett TL, Kirchner VA, et al. Alterations in Enteroendocrine hormones after Total Pancreatectomy with islet autotransplantation. Pancreas. 2020;49(6):806–11. https://doi.org/10.1097/mpa.0000000000001582.
47. McEachron KR, Beilman GJ, Bellin MD. Sitagliptin treatment increases GLP-1 without improving diabetes outcomes after total pancreatectomy with islet autotransplantation. Am J Transplant. 2019;19(3):958–9. https://doi.org/10.1111/ajt.15119.
48. Bogachus LD, Bellin MD, Vella A, Robertson RP. Deficient glucagon response to hypoglycemia during a mixed meal in Total Pancreatectomy/islet autotransplantation recipients. J Clin Endocrinol Metab. 2018;103(4):1522–9. https://doi.org/10.1210/jc.2017-02182.
49. Bogachus LD, Oseid E, Bellin M, Vella A, Robertson RP. Deficient endogenous glucose production during exercise after Total Pancreatectomy/islet autotransplantation. J Clin Endocrinol Metab. 2017;102(9):3288–95. https://doi.org/10.1210/jc.2017-00923.
50. Bellin MD, Parazzoli S, Oseid E, Bogachus LD, Schuetz C, Patti ME, et al. Defective glucagon secretion during hypoglycemia after intrahepatic but not nonhepatic islet autotransplantation. Am J Transplant. 2014;14(8):1880–6. https://doi.org/10.1111/ajt.12776.
51. Lin YK, Faiman C, Johnston PC, Walsh RM, Stevens T, Bottino R, et al. Spontaneous hypoglycemia after islet autotransplantation for chronic pancreatitis. J Clin Endocrinol Metab. 2016;101(10):3669–75. https://doi.org/10.1210/jc.2016-2111.
52. Ramai D, Facciorusso A, Maida M, Capurso G, Chandan S, Spadaccini M, et al. Prevalence of osteopathy in chronic pancreatitis: a systematic review and meta-analysis. Clin Transl Gastroenterol. 2023;14(8):e00623. https://doi.org/10.14309/ctg.0000000000000623.
53. Wothe JK, Aidoo R, KR ME, Harindhanavudhi T, Trikudanathan G, Freeman ML, et al. Reduced bone mineral density in the first year after total pancreatectomy with islet autotransplantation (TPIAT). Pancreatology. 2021;21(8):1491–7. https://doi.org/10.1016/j.pan.2021.08.013.
54. Coluzzi F, LeQuang JAK, Sciacchitano S, Scerpa MS, Rocco M, Pergolizzi J. A closer look at opioid-induced adrenal insufficiency: a narrative review. Int J Mol Sci. 2023;24(5) https://doi.org/10.3390/ijms24054575.

Gastrointestinal and Nutritional Management After TPIAT

9

Elissa M. Downs, Rachel P. Jacobsen, and Sarah Jane Schwarzenberg

Abstract

Gastrointestinal management after total pancreatectomy with islet autotransplantation (TPIAT) requires support in the immediate postoperative period for the dysmotility that results from enteric reconstruction and postoperative ileus, among other factors, and may be further aggravated by opioid-induced constipation. Gastrojejunal feeding tubes can allow early introduction of enteral nutrition if gastroparesis limits oral intake, allowing proximal decompression and distal feeding. Due to iatrogenic complete exocrine pancreatic insufficiency, TPIAT recipients will need lifelong pancreatic enzyme replacement therapy, as well as fat-soluble vitamin (FSV) replacement. Deficiencies of FSV and essential fatty acids can be encountered and should be screened for at regular intervals. A low-oxalate diet is encouraged to prevent kidney stone formation. Growth improvements have been observed after TPIAT, especially in children. As with any major abdominal operation, gastrointestinal symptoms related to the procedure may occur later in life. Because splenectomy usually accompanies TPIAT, vaccines are administered preoperatively, and children are started on antibiotic prophylaxis, generally for 1 year postoperatively. All are advised to seek emergent eval-

E. M. Downs (✉)
Division of Pediatric Gastroenterology, Hepatology and Nutrition, University of Minnesota Medical School, Minneapolis, MN, USA
e-mail: down0015@umn.edu

R. P. Jacobsen
M Health Fairview Masonic Children's Hospital, Minneapolis, MN, USA

S. J. Schwarzenberg
Department of Pediatric Gastroenterology, Hepatology and Nutrition, University of Minnesota, Minneapolis, MN, USA

S. Chinnakotla et al. (eds.), *Total Pancreatectomy and Islet Auto Transplantation*,
https://doi.org/10.1007/978-981-92-0018-4_9

uation in the event of fevers due to the risk of overwhelming postsplenectomy infection.

Key Points

- Gastroparesis is common after TPIAT and frequently requires interventions such as enteral feeding tube placement; antiemetics, prokinetic agents, and other interventions for gastroparesis; and an aggressive bowel regimen to prevent constipation.
- Because most TPIAT operations will include splenectomy, prophylactic vaccination and antibiotics are needed; aspirin is used as prophylaxis due to increased risk of portal vein thrombosis.
- Postoperative nutrition protocols are not standardized.
    - Enteral feeding may be started first, usually with an extensively hydrolyzed peptide-based formula containing high medium-chain triglycerides.
      Oral intake can be advanced when gastroparesis and dysmotility improve.
- TPIAT causes complete exocrine pancreatic insufficiency (EPI). Pancreatic enzyme replacement therapy (PERT) and fat-soluble vitamin supplementation will be needed for life.
    - Several noninterchangeable oral PERT formulations have been approved for use in this setting, as well as an in-line immobilized lipase-only cartridge for enteral feeds.
      If EPI is not managed adequately, malabsorption will lead to poor weight gain, impaired growth, and nutrient deficiencies, among other complications.

9.1 Introduction

In this chapter, we will review our standard practices for gastrointestinal and nutritional management after total pancreatectomy with islet autotransplantation (TPIAT), although practices may vary from institution to institution. Despite the focus here on gastrointestinal and nutritional issues, post-TPIAT care does require a multidisciplinary, collaborative approach, with integrated management.

9.2 Postoperative Dysmotility

Although gastrointestinal tract reconstruction techniques during TPIAT may vary (see details in Chaps. 5 and 14), children may be more likely to undergo pylorus-preserving techniques and Roux-en-Y enteric reconstruction than adults [1, 2]. Early postoperative dysmotility is common among the various types of gastrointestinal reconstruction [3] but can be more common in pylorus-preserving operations, as seen in other pancreatic surgeries [4]. The dysmotility may be further compounded by potential ileus, vagal nerve injury, or other factors. In one adult cohort, delayed gastric emptying was reported in 36% in the post-TPIAT recovery period [5], but rates have not been investigated in children due to near-universal use of prokinetic agents postoperatively. Persistence of dysmotility in the longer term has not been as well described.

Several key features of postoperative management may be necessary because of this dysmotility: enteral feeding tube placement; antiemetics, prokinetic agents, and other interventions for gastroparesis; and an aggressive bowel regimen to prevent constipation.

In a large, multicenter study of recent surgical practices, children were more likely to have enteral (predominantly gastrojejunostomy) tubes placed during transplant than adults (93% vs. 63%, respectively, $p < 0.0001$) [2]. This allows enteral nutrition to be provided distally and gastric contents to be decompressed proximally. Dysmotility will slowly improve over a few weeks postoperatively, and improvement will be evident by decreased gastric output, improved nausea and vomiting, or improved pain. Dysmotility may take longer to resolve if preoperative dysmotility existed, surgical complications occurred, complex pain management requiring prolonged opioid use was needed, or opioid-induced constipation developed, among other factors. With resolution of gastroparesis and dysmotility, and when full nutritional and fluid needs are met orally, the gastrojejunostomy tube can be removed; this often occurs between 2 and 3 months postoperatively.

Antiemetics are scheduled per protocol early on and then transitioned to delivery as needed when improvement is noted. Prokinetic agents, including either amoxicillin–clavulanic acid or macrolides in the case of a penicillin allergy (as these will also cover splenectomy prophylaxis), are scheduled. If additional support is needed, metoclopramide can be added for short-term prokinetic support and antiemetic properties, although adverse effects may limit therapy [6]. Cyproheptadine, a serotonin and histamine antagonist, may also be considered for its effects on improving appetite and decreasing nausea and may help with any overlay of functional abdominal pain symptoms [7].

All patients are started on acid suppression due to the potential hypersecretory state, postoperative aspirin use, and longer-term risk for gastritis and anastomotic ulceration, leading to potential gastrointestinal bleeding [8].

An aggressive bowel regimen with scheduled osmotic and stimulant laxatives is started postoperatively, given the high incidence of constipation that can be seen in children in the intensive care unit after abdominal surgeries and due to opioid-induced constipation [9]. In the setting of severe opioid-induced constipation, methylnaltrexone, a peripherally acting mu-opioid receptor antagonist, can be added, which may counteract the side effects of opioids on the gut and has demonstrated safety and efficacy in children [10, 11]. A bowel regimen is continued as long as patients remain on opioids but may need to be continued longer based on a patient's prior history of constipation, dietary fiber and fluid intake, or other factors.

Supportive care for dysmotility may include early physical therapy, integrative medicine, and psychological support.

9.3 Splenectomy

Most current surgical techniques for TPIAT include splenectomy. A recent study of practices at 11 centers in the United States found that splenectomy was performed in 100% of 84 children and 91% of 195 adults ($p = 0.002$) [2], although some surgeons advocate for spleen-preserving procedures [12]. Because splenectomy leads to immunocompromise, it is recommended that patients receive vaccinations against encapsulated bacteria (including pneumococcal, meningococcal, and *Haemophilus influenzae* type b vaccinations) 14 days before or as soon as possible after splenectomy when stable per Centers for Disease Control and Prevention guidelines [13]. Children <18 years remain on prophylactic daily antibiotics through the first postoperative year or until 5 years old (if TPIAT was performed at younger than 4 years) because the risk for overwhelming postsplenectomy infection is higher in children [14]. This risk is lifelong, and patients are counseled to seek urgent evaluation for any febrile illnesses and to wear a medical alert bracelet.

Splenectomy also leads to a reactive thrombocytosis, although post-TPIAT peak platelet counts are uniquely extreme when compared with splenectomy for other indications [15]. The instant blood-mediated inflammatory response triggered by islets infused in the portal vein likely contributes [16]. All patients are started on aspirin to decrease the risk of thrombosis, particularly portal vein thrombosis. They are temporarily put on hydroxyurea if they develop thrombocytosis, even though this phenomenon is short-lived, to further minimize the risk of thromboembolic events.

9.4 Postoperative and Short-Term Nutrition

Postoperative nutrition protocols, developed in collaboration with a registered dietitian experienced in gastrointestinal and pancreatic disease, may include the oral, enteral, or (rarely) parenteral route but are not standardized across institutions performing TPIAT [17]. However, due to the dysmotility described previously, patients may have challenges advancing oral intake quickly. If a gastrojejunostomy or other feeding tube has been placed intraoperatively, enteral feeds will be started by postoperative day 2 and slowly advanced to promote gut integrity, wound healing, and euglycemia. While a standard formula may be used [18], more often a peptide-based (extensively hydrolyzed) formula with a higher medium-chain triglyceride content will be used to optimize fat and protein absorption in the setting of complete iatrogenic exocrine pancreatic insufficiency (EPI) [19]. An ultra-low-fat formula, along with intravenous (IV) lipid emulsion to prevent essential fatty acid deficiency (EFAD) [20], may be needed in the setting of operative traumatic lymphatic system injury leading to postoperative accumulation of chylous ascites [21, 22], which has been observed in both open and laparoscopic-assisted TPIAT in children [23]. Elimination of most long-chain fats will minimize lymphatic flow in the thoracic duct and assist with closure of most leaks [22].

Most patients will require additional free water added to the feeds to meet maintenance fluid needs as gastroparesis and nausea may limit oral hydration.

Pancreatic enzyme replacement therapy (PERT) is instituted with all enteral or oral nutritional intake due to EPI, with recommended dosing described in Sect. 9.5.

Parenteral nutrition may be used in rare circumstances of postoperative gut compromise, other complications, or severe feeding intolerance, but is generally avoided to minimize stress to the newly transplanted hepatic islets.

While no specific standardized protocol exists for advancement of enteral feeds once started postoperatively, it is our practice to advance enteral feeds to a continuous 24-h nutritional goal within 1–3 days. Tight glycemic control is achieved postoperatively with an insulin drip to minimize stress on the newly transplanted islets [24]. As enteral feeds are advanced to nutritional goal, the established insulin drip needs can then be transitioned to an insulin pump with a continuous glucose monitoring system [25, 26] while awaiting islet engraftment over the next several months [27]. Further posttransplant endocrine management is discussed in Chap. 8.

As gastroparesis and dysmotility improve, patients are encouraged to advance their oral intake with small, frequent meals to start. If needed based on the degree of ongoing gastroparesis, these meals should be low fat and low fiber [28]. They are instructed on carbohydrate counting, mealtime insulin coverage, and PERT. They are additionally instructed on a lower-oxalate diet to prevent kidney stones; see the discussion in Sect. 9.6.3. As intake improves, enteral support is first weaned to 12-h nocturnal feeds to allow for more convenient insulin pump programming. As intake steadily improves, the 12-h nocturnal feeds are then discontinued. This stepwise reduction allows further assessment of the patient's ability to advance to a fully oral diet to prevent weight loss, dehydration, or other complications. Only then do we transition liquid medications that have been administered enterally to tablet or capsule formulations by mouth. The gastrojejunostomy tube is subsequently removed after a period of observation without use; for most, this is around 2–3 months after TPIAT, but, again, only when full nutritional and fluid needs are met and oral medications are tolerated.

9.5 Pancreatic Enzyme Replacement Therapy

Because the exocrine pancreas is lost during TPIAT, patients now have complete iatrogenic EPI and require lifelong PERT and lifelong fat-soluble vitamin (FSV) supplementation. Strict adherence to PERT with every meal and snack beyond simple carbohydrates is critical to prevent complications of malabsorption. Skipping enzymes with intake in the short term may lead to bloating, flatulence, malodorous stools, and steatorrhea; skipping enzymes chronically will lead to vitamin deficiencies, essential fatty acid deficiencies, and malnutrition [19].

Multiple Food and Drug Administration (FDA)-approved PERT formulations are currently available in the United States, but these are not considered interchangeable and are not bioequivalent due to varying capsule amounts of lipase, amylase, and protease. Nonproprietary enzymes from health food stores or other companies are unregulated and not recommended. Approved formulations include a nonenteric-coated enzyme tablet (*Viokace*, Nestlé Health Science), capsules of enzyme microbeads/microtablets with an enteric coating protecting them from stomach acid degradation and designed to be released at duodenal pH (*CREON*, AbbVie, Inc.; *Zenpep*, Nestlé Health Science; *PERTZYE*, Digestive Care, Inc.; *PANCREAZE*, Ortho-McNeil-Janssen Pharmaceuticals, Inc.), and an immobilized lipase-only cartridge used in-line for continuous or bolus enteral feeds (*RELiZORB*, Alcresta Therapeutics, Inc.)..

PERT is immediately started with continuous enteral feeds postoperatively, preferably with an in-line cartridge containing only immobilized lipase, RELiZORB [29]. This cartridge is now approved in children down to 6 months of age (as of November 2025) [30]. In another condition associated with EPI (cystic fibrosis), it reduced gastrointestinal symptoms of malabsorption [29] and improved anthropometrics [31]. The current version of the one-time use cartridge can accomplish fat hydrolysis for up to 500 mL of formula, with maximum use of 6 per day. It is connected in-line with the enteral feeding set (Fig. 9.1) and hydrolyzes fats in the formula prior to entering the body. The lipase units are immobilized in the cartridge and are not counted toward daily dosing if also using oral PERT. Formula compatibility, fat hydrolysis percentages, and infusion rates can be checked on the manufacturer's website for the most up-to-date information (https://www.relizorb.com).

Only one enteric-coated enzyme capsule, PERTZYE, is FDA-approved for enzyme coverage of formula through a gastrostomy tube. The capsule, which contains 4000 lipase units, can be opened, mixed with a small amount of juice, nectar-thick liquid, or applesauce, and administered through a gastrostomy tube size 14

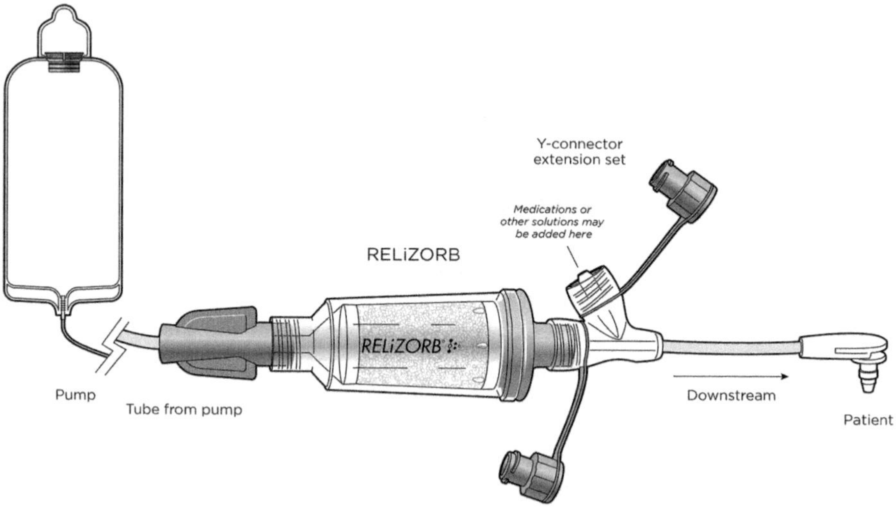

Fig. 9.1 Connection of RELiZORB (immobilized lipase-only enzyme cartridge) in-line with an enteral feeding set for bolus (G-tube) or continuous (G-tube or J-tube) enteral feeds. (Used with permission from Alcresta, Inc.)

French or larger [32], at a suggested dosing range of 2000 (range 500–4000) lipase units per gram of fat in the enteral feed bolus volume [33]. With these formulations available, other approaches (e.g., crushed nonenteric-coated enzymes added to feeds, enteric-coated enzyme capsules given orally throughout the duration of a tube feeding, or activating an enteric-coated enzyme with sodium bicarbonate and mixing in a feed) are not preferred.

When advancing oral intake in children, PERT dosing is most often based on body weight but can also be based on the number of fat grams consumed at a meal. This approximates pancreatic lipase output at an amount that corrects steatorrhea and prevents malabsorption [34]. For children unable to swallow the capsules whole, these can be opened, the contents sprinkled on a small amount of acidic soft food, and the beads swallowed without being crushed or chewed.

For weight-based dosing, we follow consensus recommendations outlined for management of EPI in cystic fibrosis [35], with a dosing range of 500–2500 lipase units/kg/meal, with a half dose for snacks. Children less than 4 years may require a starting dose at or above 1000 lipase units/kg/meal. If following fat gram–based dosing, this may range from 500 to 4000 lipase units/g fat. Adults may be given a standard 75,000–100,000 lipase unit dose/meal, similar in range to severe EPI dosing, up to a maximum of 2500 lipase units/kg/meal. This is concordant with a large European multicenter study demonstrating that those undergoing pancreaticoduodenectomy require higher PERT for nutrient status and to relieve malabsorption than those with their pancreas intact (such as in acute or chronic pancreatitis), as well as twice-daily antacid dosing [34].

The dose should be adjusted based on response (poor weight gain, cramping, gassiness, bloating, diarrhea, and/or steatorrhea), taking into account that not all patients will endorse significant symptoms or even steatorrhea when they are not adherent to enzymes, and steatorrhea may occur even with good adherence [36]. Threshold doses of 2500 lipase units/kg/meal and 10,000 lipase units/kg/day are recommended due to complications of fibrosing colonopathy in patients with cystic fibrosis with high-dose enzyme capsules and at much higher enzyme intake amounts, such as >6000 lipase units/kg/meal [37, 38]. With implementation of these recommendations and reformulation of available PERT, the incidence of fibrosing colonopathy is now very low [39].

During long-term follow-up, PERT dosing adequacy should be reassessed at every visit, taking into account weight gain, symptoms, and other proxy signs of absorption (see summary in Table 9.1). Adherence to the PERT regimen should be elicited with motivational interviewing techniques to improve adherence if lacking. When adherence to PERT was assessed in children with EPI due to cystic fibrosis, 61% had only moderate adherence [40], which included taking insufficient doses for snacks and dosing enzymes after meals. When this was specifically assessed in children after TPIAT, adherence was more consistent at 80% at a 2-year follow-up [36]. Even with self-reported consistent adherence, steatorrhea was noted in 62% of one cohort at 1-year follow-up, with gastrointestinal symptoms impacting daily life in about 50% [36].

Table 9.1 Suggested monitoring after TPIAT for growth and issues related to exocrine pancreatic insufficiency

Category and components to review		Timeline for review
Anthropometrics	Height, weight, consider functional assessments and body composition (as available)	Baseline Post-op: 3, 6, 12 months, yearly As needed
PERT	Timing with intake, enzyme storage, adherence, doses per meal and snack	Baseline Post-op: 3, 6, 12 months, yearly As needed
Fat-soluble vitamins	Intake, doses, other supplementation, levels of individual vitamins	Baseline (if EPI) Post-op: 3, 6, 12 months, yearly Follow-up of correction of deficiencies
Essential fatty acids	Dosing, dietary intake, current fish oil supplementation, essential fatty acid panel	Baseline (if EPI) Post-op: 3, 6, 12 months, yearly Follow-up of correction of deficiencies

EPI exocrine pancreatic insufficiency, *PERT* pancreatic enzyme replacement therapy, *TPIAT* total pancreatectomy with islet autotransplantation

Antacid therapy could be considered if improved responsiveness to PERT is needed and may allow lower dosing that is equally effective [41]. If PERT seems like it is failing despite being taken correctly and after dose optimization, a different formulation could be trialed. Each brand has differences in the size or uniformity of their microbeads (CREON, PERTZYE) or microtablets (Zenpep, PANCREAZE). In addition, PERTZYE is unique among enteric-coated capsules in that it contains a bicarbonate buffer, which may aid in earlier duodenal release if stomach acid is not sufficiently neutralized.

If signs and symptoms of malabsorption persist after these methods are tried, other etiologies such as celiac disease, small intestinal bacterial overgrowth (SIBO) [42], chronic inflammatory or infectious enteritis, or others should be investigated and addressed [43].

9.6 Nutritional and Related Complications Due to EPI and/or TPIAT

In the recovery period after TPIAT, patients experience a mixed anemia from surgical blood loss, a pro-inflammatory state altering iron homeostasis, and partial duodenal resection limiting iron absorption. While the anemia improves over time, rates of iron deficiency increase [44], and some may require IV iron replacement if oral iron is insufficient [45].

If EPI is inadequately managed, resultant malabsorption will lead to poor weight gain, impaired growth, macro- and micronutrient deficiencies, and, in children, potentially developmental delay [19].

9.6.1 Fat-Soluble Vitamins and Vitamin Deficiencies

Because of EPI, it is recommended that TPIAT recipients remain on FSV supplementation for life. FSV supplementation is started with specific formulations where the vitamins have been altered to be water soluble to enhance absorption. These are available by prescription only. FSV dosing is based on recommendations developed for EPI in children [46, 47] and adults [47, 48] with cystic fibrosis. Monitoring intervals are suggested in Table 9.1, with biochemical assays and FSV dosing by age in Table 9.2.

FSV deficiencies are not uncommon in both adults and children with chronic pancreatitis and at follow-up assessments after TPIAT [49, 50]. Ongoing FSV deficiencies can occur despite PERT in adequate dosing ranges because not all providers prescribe FSV supplementation in the specific water-soluble preparation. However, use of these specialty FSV formulations may be inadequate because of decreased knowledge of their importance or lack of insurance coverage. Pediatric providers may be more likely to prescribe these formulations than adult providers [49].

A small potential risk of overdoing vitamin supplementation remains. The specialty FSV preparations are not complete multivitamins, so it is possible that when using these in combination with other complete multivitamin and mineral supplements, oral or enteral nutritional supplementation, and dietary intake, patients could be receiving well over the recommended dietary intake of certain vitamins.

9.6.2 Essential Fatty Acid Deficiencies

Essential fatty acids cannot be synthesized directly in the human body. These fatty acids include linoleic acid, the omega-6 precursor to arachidonic acid, and alpha-linolenic acid, the omega-3 precursor to eicosapentaenoic acid and docosahexaenoic acid [51]. EFAD can be diagnosed by an elevated triene-to-tetraene ratio (T:T), which adjusts in the setting of decreased intake of linoleic acid and arachidonic acid. Our institution uses the established T:T of ≥ 0.05 if <18 years old or ≥ 0.038 if ≥ 18 years old [52], with suggested monitoring shown in Table 9.1.

At our institution, we found that risk for EFAD was increased after TPIAT in a large study including children and adults. Overall, the prevalence of EFAD was 33% at 1-year follow-up, but adults were more affected than children (46% vs. 6%, respectively, $p = 0.0024$) [20]. A suggested protocol for optimization of intake and replacement of deficiencies is in Box 9.1.

Table 9.2 Vitamin monitoring and daily dosing recommendations after TPIAT

Vitamin	1st tier monitoring	Recommendations for daily dosing by age		
A	Retinol Retinol-binding protein	1–3 y: 1500 mcg	4–8 y: 1500–3000 mcg	>8 y: 3000 mcg
E	α-Tocopherol α-Tocopherol:Serum lipids	1–3 y: 80–150 mg	4–8 y: 100–200 mg	>8 y: 200–400 mg
D	25-hydroxy vitamin D	1–10 y: 20–25 mcg	>10 y: 20–50 mcg	
K	PIVKA-II* Prothrombin time	All ages: 0.3–0.5 mg		

PIVKA-II protein induced by vitamin K absence II (*as available), *TPIAT* total pancreatectomy with islet autotransplantation

9.6.3 Nephrolithiasis

At our institution, we found a 30% incidence of kidney stones by 15 years after TPIAT, with 44% having more than one episode [53]. The underlying pathophysiology is thought to be due to fat malabsorption (if enzymes are not taken, if enzyme dosing is inadequate, or if there is a mismatch of food and enzyme arrival times in the intestines), leading to the presence of luminal free fatty acids. Calcium will then preferentially bind to these unabsorbed free fatty acids instead of ingested dietary oxalate. Greater intestinal oxalate absorption will now be renally excreted, increasing risk for kidney stones [54]. We discuss limiting high-oxalate foods (with highest content found in foods such as leafy greens, rhubarb, and soy, but also almonds, white potatoes, chocolate, and raspberries, among others) and pairing oxalate intake with calcium or calcium-rich foods [55].

9.7 Growth and Nutrition Outcomes

Optimization of nutrition in the pre- and postoperative period is important to minimize complications of TPIAT. As discussed, FSV deficiencies are not uncommon in both children and adults before TPIAT [49, 50] and should be corrected prior to surgery. Although almost half of adults are normal weight prior to TPIAT, the other half are split between overweight and obese individuals, with a small number underweight [49]. Among children, approximately one-third are overweight and obese prior to TPIAT, with only a small number underweight [49]. Sarcopenia, or skeletal muscle loss, may not be obvious by these standard anthropometrics, requiring functional testing or body composition analysis [17]. Sarcopenia was present in one-third of adults undergoing TPIAT and led to low islet yield and increased likelihood of discharge to a rehabilitation facility [56]. Sarcopenia has not been extensively studied in children with pancreatitis. In an assessment of those with chronic pancreatitis prior to TPIAT, low bone mineral density (with z-scores greater than −2) was seen in 12% of adults [57]. To improve outcomes, nutritional rehabilitation should be undertaken prior to TPIAT if feasible.

Children and adults who are carrying excess weight before TPIAT are encouraged to reach a nonobese body mass index (BMI) to improve liver health (i.e., $<30\ kg/m^2$ in adults or < 85th percentile for children). Values above this threshold in adults were associated with greater mortality [1], although BMI elevations may lose significance when adjusted for age in other models [58]..

The smallest children are generally deferred as surgical candidates until their liver reaches a size of 400 cubic centimeters to hold an adequate volume of infused islets, but children as young as 3 years have been successfully transplanted [59].

Growth is carefully monitored after TPIAT. At a minimum, height and weight should be followed. Other measures could also be considered, such as body composition and calculation of lean body mass, if noninvasive, easy to obtain, low cost, and clinically available over time. Suggested intervals for monitoring are included in Table 9.1, with closer follow-up with a gastroenterologist and a specialized registered dietitian if faltering is observed.

Children have demonstrated gains in height, weight, and BMI z-scores through 1 and 2 years postoperatively [59], with the fraction with normal BMI rising from 62% to 73% at 1-year follow-up in a large multicenter series, compared with 54% of adults having normal BMI at follow-up ($P < 0.001$) [49]. Bone mineral density declines of approximately 4% have been seen in adults at 12 months after TPIAT, although other markers at this time point suggest bone remodeling, followed by stability in density through 18 months postoperatively [57].

In children and adults with growth declines after TPIAT, we review adherence to PERT, optimize dosing, and evaluate for malabsorption. In conjunction with specialized registered dietitians, we discuss high-energy-density intake and nutritional supplementation. More rarely, ongoing use of a feeding tube, or even replacement of a feeding tube for reinitiation of enteral nutrition support, may be required.

9.8 Other Management of Gastrointestinal Issues

Patients may experience gastrointestinal symptoms associated with acute, recurrent, or chronic pancreatitis, or unrelated to the pancreas. The latter may not resolve after TPIAT. Additionally, the surgical procedure and recovery can be associated with gastrointestinal complications. Evaluating a post-TPIAT patient with gastrointestinal symptoms requires an understanding of their preoperative gastrointestinal history as well as an understanding of TPIAT.

9.8.1 Gastrointestinal Symptoms

There is limited published information on post-TPIAT gastrointestinal complications and management. Crosby et al. reviewed gastrointestinal questionnaires from 184 individuals aged 5–66 years [36]. The most common symptom 12 months after TPIAT was diarrhea, endorsed by 80% of patients, and another 62% complained of steatorrhea. At the 12-month follow-up, post-TPIAT patients complained of constipation (41%) and weight loss or difficulty maintaining weight (31%). Among adult patients, 51% felt their symptoms interfered with their life. Children reported fewer symptoms and less symptom impact on their lives.

John et al. provided patient-reported outcome measures related to gastrointestinal symptoms in 33 post-TPIAT adults (mean age 42 years) [3]. Symptoms of dysmotility were present in 45% of these patients. Patients reported decreased quality of life and impaired daily function related to dysmotility. There was no association in this study between reports of abdominal symptoms and dysmotility.

The high frequency of steatorrhea and difficulty gaining or maintaining weight suggests that the initial evaluation of gastrointestinal symptoms should include a review of pancreatic enzyme dose and use. Of course, the differential of any gastrointestinal symptom in a post-TPIAT patient must include conditions common to any patient in the same age group. There are three issues to be aware of that affect TPIAT patients more frequently than the general population: SIBO, dysmotility, and partial bowel obstruction.

9.8.2 Small Intestinal Bacterial Overgrowth

Gastrointestinal symptoms associated with excessive numbers of bacteria in the small intestine include abdominal pain, nausea, bloating, flatulence, and diarrhea [60]. If left untreated, this can lead to deficiencies in vitamins B12 and D, as well as iron deficiency.

SIBO can often be seen in patients with chronic pancreatitis prior to TPIAT, with diabetes and opioid use as potential covariables [60]. Risk factors for post-TPIAT SIBO include postoperative gastroparesis [3], opioid-induced dysmotility, and Roux-en-Y reconstruction [61]. Testing for SIBO is controversial. Jejunal aspirate with quantitative bacterial cultures is the "gold standard," but it is a difficult test for many reasons. Breath testing is simple and recommended by the American College of Gastroenterology [60] but requires that patients stop many medications, including laxatives, promotility agents, and antibiotics, before testing [62]. In addition, correlation between jejunal aspirates and breath testing is poor [62]. In many cases, clinicians diagnose SIBO based on symptoms.

Treatment for SIBO includes antibiotic therapy. First-line treatment is rifaximin, an antibiotic that is not systemically absorbed [62]. The dose and time course of therapy have not been standardized. Other antibiotics, for example, amoxicillin–clavulanic acid, metronidazole, and tetracycline, have been used [62]. Studies of probiotics have not demonstrated statistically significant improvement [62, 63]. Improvement in risk factors for SIBO, including reduction of opioids and, possibly, promotility agents, may be helpful to prevent a relapse after treatment [62].

9.8.3 Dysmotility

Gastroparesis and dysmotility immediately postoperatively were discussed above. Utilizing the Gastroparesis Cardinal Symptom Index, John et al. demonstrated that 45% of TPIAT patients studied had dysmotility at some point after the procedure, with some having dysmotility more than 2 years after the procedure [3]. Ongoing severe dysmotility led to lower physical health scores on quality-of-life assessment. Few of these patients were being treated long-term for their dysmotility, suggesting an opportunity for improving gastrointestinal symptoms after TPIAT.

9.8.4 Partial Small Bowel Obstruction

As with any abdominal surgery, TPIAT may result in intra-abdominal adhesions [64]. These can be a source of chronic abdominal pain or can present as acute abdominal pain with partial small bowel obstruction. Conservative management, such as nasogastric suction for 2–3 days with intravenous fluid support, may allow the obstruction to resolve, preventing the need for adhesiolysis. Reoperation is undertaken with care, as adhesions are likely to reform.

9.9 Conclusions

With the challenges of altered intestinal anatomy after TPIAT and the loss of the exocrine pancreas, children and adults are at increased risk for gastrointestinal and nutritional complications, requiring a multidisciplinary team and a standardized approach to curtail these risks. Whenever possible, TPIAT candidates should undergo nutritional rehabilitation prior to TPIAT to minimize postoperative risks and improve outcomes.

Postoperative dysmotility is common, potentially requiring gastric decompression and distal intestinal feeds, antiemetics, prokinetic agents, and an aggressive bowel regimen. However, long-term dysmotility is not uncommon, even once off opioids, causing more chronic constipation and abdominal pain. Other issues such as SIBO, partial bowel obstructions due to adhesions, malabsorption, and more should be considered as potential causes of acute or chronic gastrointestinal symptoms.

With complete EPI, lifelong PERT and specialty FSV preparations are required. Detailed nutritional assessments at multiple follow-up visits are recommended in the first year after TPIAT and annually thereafter at a minimum, but at any time sooner if concerns arise. Adherence to PERT should be continually reassessed, and patients should be queried for gastrointestinal and other symptoms affecting their quality of life but also suggestive of developing complications, such as vitamin deficiencies, essential fatty acid deficiencies, nephrolithiasis, and others.

With close follow-up and monitoring, improvements in growth, with normalization of BMI status, can be seen post-TPIAT.

Box 9.1: Suggested Protocol to Treat Essential Fatty Acid Deficiency in Teens and Adults

1. *Dietary modifications:*
   (a) Increase intake of low-mercury fish at least twice weekly (such as salmon, whitefish, herring, canned white tuna).
   (b) Increase intake of ground flax seeds or flaxseed oil, chia seeds, pumpkin seeds, walnuts, or soybeans.
   (c) Consume 30–40% calories as fat. Specifically, limit saturated fats, eliminate trans fats, increase mono- and polyunsaturated fats.

(continued)

Box 9.1 (continued)

2. *Supplementation:*

(a) Start with 1 gram of fish oil daily and increase up to 3 grams daily as tolerated.
(b) Look for products with certifications from United States Pharmacopeia (USP), Labdoor, or International Fish Oil Standards (IFOS)..
(c) Consider use at bedtime or use of "burpless" products to decrease fish taste.
(d) Consider vegan/vegetarian algal, flaxseed, or other oil-based supplements.

3. *Follow-up:*

(a) Retest fatty acid panel 6–12 weeks after initiation of modifications and therapy.

Adapted from reference [20]

References

1. Bellin MD, Beilman GJ, Sutherland DER, Ali H, Petersen A, Mongin S, et al. How durable is Total Pancreatectomy and Intraportal islet cell transplantation for treatment of chronic pancreatitis? J Am Coll Surg. 2019;228:329–39.
2. Nathan JD, Yang Y, Eaton A, Witkowski P, Wijkstrom M, Walsh M, et al. Surgical approach and short-term outcomes in adults and children undergoing total pancreatectomy with islet autotransplantation: a report from the prospective observational study of TPIAT. Pancreatol Off J Int Assoc Pancreatol IAP Al 2022;22:1–8.
3. John GK, Singh VK, Moran RA, Warren D, Sun Z, Desai N, et al. Chronic gastrointestinal Dysmotility and pain following Total Pancreatectomy with islet autotransplantation for chronic pancreatitis. J Gastrointest Surg Off J Soc Surg Aliment Tract. 2017;21:622–7.
4. Wu W, Hong X, Fu L, Liu S, You L, Zhou L, et al. The effect of pylorus removal on delayed gastric emptying after Pancreaticoduodenectomy: a meta-analysis of 2,599 patients. PLoS One. 2014;9:e108380.
5. John GK, Singh VK, Pasricha PJ, Sinha A, Afghani E, Warren D, et al. Delayed gastric emptying (DGE) following Total Pancreatectomy with islet auto transplantation in patients with chronic pancreatitis. J Gastrointest Surg Off J Soc Surg Aliment Tract. 2015;19:1256–61.
6. Rodriguez L, Irani K, Jiang H, Goldstein AM. Clinical presentation, response to therapy, and outcome of gastroparesis in children. J Pediatr Gastroenterol Nutr. 2012;55:185–90.
7. Madani S, Cortes O, Thomas R. Cyproheptadine use in children with functional gastrointestinal disorders. J Pediatr Gastroenterol Nutr. 2016;62:409–13.
8. Robbins AJ, Lusczek E, Bellin MD, Alwan FS, Hodges JS, Chapman SA, et al. Gastrointestinal bleed after Total Pancreatectomy with islet autotransplant. Pancreas. 2021;50:841–6.
9. Roller MD, Panchal A, Duesing L, Mikhailov TA. Incidence of opioid-induced constipation in the pediatric intensive care unit: a descriptive cohort study. JPEN J Parenter Enteral Nutr. 2024;48:354–9.
10. Smith CJ, Sierra CM, Robbins J, Chang NY, Mirza F. Methylnaltrexone for opioid-induced Dysmotility in critically ill infants and children: a pilot study. J Pediatr Pharmacol Ther JPPT Off J PPAG. 2023;28:136–42.

11. Mills KP, McPherson CC, Said AS, Lahart MA. Successful use of intravenous Methylnaltrexone for opioid-induced constipation in critically ill pediatric patients. J Pediatr Intensive Care. 2024;13:25–31.
12. Coluzzi M, Naziruddin B, Kumano K, Saracino G, Testa G, Beecherl E, et al. Spleen-preserving total pancreatectomy and islet autotransplantation with complete preservation of the splenic arterial and venous supply does not impact islet yield and function. Am J Surg. 2022;224:1295–300.
13. CDC. Vaccines & Immunizations [Internet]. Vaccines Immun. 2024 [cited 23 Jan 2025]. Available from: https://www.cdc.gov/vaccines/index.html.
14. Davidson RN, Wall RA. Prevention and management of infections in patients without a spleen. Clin Microbiol Infect Off Publ Eur Soc Clin Microbiol Infect Dis. 2001;7:657–60.
15. Boucher AA, Luchtman-Jones L, Palumbo JS, Cancelas JA, Abu-El-Haija M, Jenkins TM, et al. Extreme thrombocytosis after pediatric Pancreatectomy with islet autotransplantation is unique compared to other Postsplenectomy states. J Pediatr Surg. 2020;55:1645–50.
16. Naziruddin B, Iwahashi S, Kanak MA, Takita M, Itoh T, Levy MF. Evidence for instant blood-mediated inflammatory reaction in clinical autologous islet transplantation. Am J Transplant. 2014;14:428–37.
17. Hasse JM, Meng S, Silpe S, Naziruddin B. Nutrition challenges following total pancreatectomy with islet autotransplantation. Nutr Clin Pract Off Publ Am Soc Parenter Enter Nutr. 2024;39:86–99.
18. Chinnakotla S, Bellin MD, Schwarzenberg SJ, Radosevich DM, Cook M, Dunn TB, et al. Total pancreatectomy and islet auto-transplantation in children for chronic pancreatitis. Indication, surgical techniques, post operative management and Long-term outcomes. Ann Surg 2014;260:56–64.
19. Sankararaman S, Schindler T, Sferra TJ. Management of Exocrine Pancreatic Insufficiency in children. Nutr Clin Pract Off Publ Am Soc Parenter Enter Nutr. 2019;34(Suppl 1):S27–42.
20. Downs EM, Hodges JS, Trikudanathan G, Freeman ML, Chinnakotla S, Kirchner V, et al. Essential fatty acid deficiency is common after Total Pancreatectomy and islet autotransplantation. Pancreas. 2024;53:e689–93.
21. Singh H, Pandit N, Krishnamurthy G, Gupta R, Verma GR, Singh R. Management of chylous ascites following pancreaticobiliary surgery. JGH Open Access J Gastroenterol Hepatol. 2019;3:425–8.
22. Leibovitch I, Mor Y, Golomb J, Ramon J. The diagnosis and management of postoperative chylous ascites. J Urol. 2002;167:449–57.
23. Berger M, Bellin MD, Kirchner V, Schwarzenberg SJ, Chinnakotla S. Laparoscopic-assisted versus open total pancreatectomy and islet autotransplantation: a case-matched study of pediatric patients. J Pediatr Surg. 2020;55:558–63.
24. Forlenza GP, Chinnakotla S, Schwarzenberg SJ, Cook M, Radosevich DM, Manchester C, et al. Near-euglycemia can be achieved safely in pediatric total pancreatectomy islet autotransplant recipients using an adapted intravenous insulin infusion protocol. Diabetes Technol Ther. 2014;16:706–13.
25. McEachron KR, Potlapalli N, Rayannavar A, Downs EM, Schwarzenberg SJ, Kirchner VA, et al. Early use of continuous glucose monitoring in children and adolescents after total pancreatectomy with islet autotransplantation. Pediatr Diabetes. 2021 May;22(3):434-438.
26. Tellez SE, Hornung LN, Courter JD, Abu-El-Haija M, Nathan JD, Lawson SA, et al. Improved glycemic outcomes with early initiation of insulin pump therapy in pediatric postoperative Total Pancreatectomy with islet autotransplantation. J Clin Med. 2021;10:2242.
27. Olsson R, Olerud J, Pettersson U, Carlsson P-O. Increased numbers of low-oxygenated pancreatic islets after intraportal islet transplantation. Diabetes. 2011;60:2350–3.
28. Saliakellis E, Fotoulaki M. Gastroparesis in children. Ann Gastroenterol. 2013;26:204–11.
29. Stevens J, Wyatt C, Brown P, Patel D, Grujic D, Freedman SD. Absorption and safety with sustained use of RELiZORB evaluation (ASSURE) study in patients with cystic fibrosis receiving enteral feeding. J Pediatr Gastroenterol Nutr. 2018;67:527–32.

30. Alcresta Therapeutics Announces FDA Clearance for Expanded Use of RELiZORB® (iMMOBILIZED LIPASE) Cartridge for Neonates and Infants [internet]. Alcresta 2025. [cited 14 May 2026]. Available from: https://www.alcresta.com/news/alcresta-therapeutics-announces-fda-clearance-for-expanded-use-of-relizorb-immobilized-lipase-cartridge-for-neonates-and-infants/
31. Hendrix SJ, Flume PA, First ER, Stone AA, Van Buskirk M. Improvements in anthropometric measures and gastrointestinal tolerance in patients with cystic fibrosis by using a digestive enzyme cartridge with overnight enteral nutrition. Nutr Clin Pract. 2022;37:344–50.
32. GlobalNewswire. Digestive Care, Inc. Announces FDA labeling revision approval for PERTZYE(R) (pancrelipase) [Internet] GlobeNewswire News Room 2017 [cited 24 Oct 2023]. Available from: https://www.globenewswire.com/news-release/2017/07/12/1180176/0/en/Digestive-Care-Inc-Announces-FDA-Labeling-Revision-Approval-for-PERTZYE-R-pancrelipase.html.
33. Freswick PN, Reid EK, Mascarenhas MR. Pancreatic enzyme replacement therapy in cystic fibrosis. Nutrients. 2022;14:1341.
34. Domínguez-Muñoz JE, Martínez-Seara X, Hegyi P, Rollet S, Phillips M, Bolado F, et al. Optimal dose of pancreatic enzyme replacement therapy (PERT) for pancreatic exocrine insufficiency (PEI) in different pancreatic diseases: results of the European PEI registry. Pancreatology. 2024;24:e18.
35. Singh VK, Schwarzenberg SJ. Pancreatic insufficiency in cystic fibrosis. J Cyst Fibros. 2017;16:S70–8.
36. Crosby J, Bellin MD, Radosevich DM, Chinnakotla S, Dunn TB, Pruett TL, et al. Gastrointestinal symptoms before and after Total Pancreatectomy with islet autotransplantation: the role of pancreatic enzyme dosing and adherence. Pancreas. 2015;44:453–8.
37. FitzSimmons SC, Burkhart GA, Borowitz D, Grand RJ, Hammerstrom T, Durie PR, et al. High-dose pancreatic-enzyme supplements and fibrosing colonopathy in children with cystic fibrosis. N Engl J Med. 1997;336:1283–9.
38. Reichard KW, Vinocur CD, Franco M, Crisci KL, Flick JA, Billmire DF, et al. Fibrosing colonopathy in children with cystic fibrosis. J Pediatr Surg. 1997;32:237–41. discussion 241–242
39. Chiuve SE, Fife D, Leitz G, Peterson C, Campbell NM, Rennig A, et al. Incidence of fibrosing colonopathy with pancreatic enzyme replacement therapy in patients with cystic fibrosis. J Cyst Fibros Off J Eur Cyst Fibros Soc. 2023;22:1017–23.
40. Schall JI, Bentley T, Stallings VA. Meal patterns, dietary fat intake and pancreatic enzyme use in preadolescent children with cystic fibrosis. J Pediatr Gastroenterol Nutr. 2006;43:651–9.
41. Vecht J, Symersky T, Lamers CBHW, Masclee AAM. Efficacy of lower than standard doses of pancreatic enzyme supplementation therapy during acid inhibition in patients with pancreatic exocrine insufficiency. J Clin Gastroenterol. 2006;40:721–5.
42. Avelar Rodriguez D, Ryan PM, Toro Monjaraz EM, Ramirez Mayans JA, Quigley EM. Small intestinal bacterial overgrowth in children: a state-of-the-art review. Front Pediatr. 2019;7:363.
43. Whitcomb DC, Buchner AM, Forsmark CE. AGA clinical practice update on the epidemiology, evaluation, and Management of Exocrine Pancreatic Insufficiency: expert review. Gastroenterology. 2023;165:1292–301.
44. Downs EM. Iron status and total pancreatectomy with islet autotransplantation [abstract]. NASPGHAN. Hollywood, Florida; 2018.
45. DeLoughery TG, Jackson CS, Ko CW, Rockey DC. AGA clinical practice update on Management of Iron Deficiency Anemia: expert review. Clin Gastroenterol Hepatol Off Clin Pract J Am Gastroenterol Assoc. 2024;22:1575–83.
46. Borowitz D, Baker RD, Stallings V. Consensus report on nutrition for pediatric patients with cystic fibrosis. J Pediatr Gastroenterol Nutr. 2002;35:246–59.
47. Tangpricha V, Kelly A, Stephenson A, Maguiness K, Enders J, Robinson KA, et al. An update on the screening, diagnosis, management, and treatment of vitamin D deficiency in individuals

with cystic fibrosis: evidence-based recommendations from the Cystic Fibrosis Foundation. J Clin Endocrinol Metab. 2012;97:1082–93.
48. Yankaskas JR, Marshall BC, Sufian B, Simon RH, Rodman D. Cystic fibrosis adult care: consensus conference report. Chest. 2004;125:1S–39S.
49. Downs EM, Eaton A, Witkowski P, Wijkstrom M, Walsh M, Trikudanathan G, et al. Nutritional risks in patients undergoing Total Pancreatectomy islet AutoTransplantation in the POST consortium. J Gastrointest Surg. 2023;27(9):1893–902.
50. McEachron KR, Downs EM, Schwarzenberg SJ, Chinnakotla S, Bellin MD. Fat-soluble vitamin deficiency is common in children with chronic pancreatitis undergoing Total Pancreatectomy with islet autotransplantation. J Pediatr Gastroenterol Nutr. 2021;72:123–6.
51. Mogensen KM. Essential fatty acid deficiency. Pract Gastroenterol. 2017;41(6):37–44.
52. Lagerstedt SA, Hinrichs DR, Batt SM, Magera MJ, Rinaldo P, McConnell JP. Quantitative determination of plasma c8-c26 total fatty acids for the biochemical diagnosis of nutritional and metabolic disorders. Mol Genet Metab. 2001;73:38–45.
53. Avula N, Hodges JS, Beilman G, Chinnakotla S, Freeman ML, Ramanathan K, et al. Increased kidney stone risk following total pancreatectomy with islet autotransplantation. Pancreatol Off J Int Assoc Pancreatol IAP Al. 2024;24:1167–73.
54. Vujasinovic M, Dugic A, Thiel T, Kjellman A, Yang C, Löhr J-M. Pancreatic exocrine insufficiency is a risk factor for kidney stones in patients with chronic pancreatitis. Pancreatology. 2023;23:294–8.
55. Mitchell T, Kumar P, Reddy T, Wood KD, Knight J, Assimos DG, et al. Dietary oxalate and kidney stone formation. Am J Physiol-Ren Physiol. 2019;316:F409–13.
56. Trikudanathan G, Feussom G, Teigen L, Munigala S, Price K, Dirweesh A, et al. Pre-operative sarcopenia predicts low islet cell yield following Total Pancreatectomy with islet autotransplantation for chronic pancreatitis. J Gastrointest Surg Off J Soc Surg Aliment Tract. 2020;24:2423–30.
57. Wothe JK, Aidoo R, KR ME, Harindhanavudhi T, Trikudanathan G, Freeman ML, et al. Reduced bone mineral density in the first year after total pancreatectomy with islet autotransplantation (TPIAT). Pancreatol Off J Int Assoc Pancreatol IAP Al. 2021;21:1491–7.
58. Hooks G, Lu H, Eaton A, Trikudanathan G, Downs E, Freeman ML, et al. Addressing long-term mortality risk in patients undergoing total pancreatectomy with islet autotransplant (TPIAT): causes of death and risk factors. HPB. 2024;26:664–73.
59. Bellin MD, Forlenza G, Majumder K, Berger M, Freeman ML, Beilman GJ, et al. Total pancreatectomy with islet autotransplantation resolves pain in young children with severe chronic pancreatitis. J Pediatr Gastroenterol Nutr. 2017;64:440–5.
60. Pimentel M, Saad RJ, Long MD, Rao SSC. ACG clinical guideline: small intestinal bacterial overgrowth. Off J Am Coll Gastroenterol ACG. 2020;115:165.
61. Kitaghenda FK, Hong J, Shao Y, Yao L, Zhu X. The prevalence of small intestinal bacterial overgrowth after roux-en-Y gastric bypass (RYGB): a systematic review and meta-analysis. Obes Surg. 2024;34:250–7.
62. Zafar H, Jimenez B, Schneider A. Small intestinal bacterial overgrowth: current update. Curr Opin Gastroenterol. 2023;39:522–8.
63. Zhong C, Qu C, Wang B, Liang S, Zeng B. Probiotics for preventing and treating small intestinal bacterial overgrowth: a meta-analysis and systematic review of current evidence. J Clin Gastroenterol. 2017;51:300–11.
64. Liakakos T, Thomakos N, Fine PM, Dervenis C, Young RL. Peritoneal adhesions: etiology, pathophysiology, and clinical significance. Recent advances in prevention and management. Dig Surg. 2001;18:260–73.

Surgical Complications After Total Pancreatectomy with Islet Autotransplantation (TPIAT)

10

Varvara A. Kirchner

Abstract

Total pancreatectomy with islet autotransplantation (TPIAT) is a complex surgical procedure aimed at alleviating symptoms in patients with chronic and acute recurrent pancreatitis while minimizing postoperative diabetic complications. This surgery presents significant challenges, particularly during pancreatectomy. The inherent operative risks arise from the retroperitoneal location of the gland and its proximity to vital structures; the inflammatory etiology of the disease process, resulting in destruction of normal anatomic planes; and prior pancreatic interventions, leading to a significant burden of adhesions, difficult dissection, and increased risk of intraoperative complications.

Meticulous reconstruction techniques with a focus on well-vascularized anastomoses are critical to avoid postoperative complications. The choice of intestinal reconstruction, e.g., Roux-en-Y, modified Billroth II, or pylorus preservation, may affect the specifics of the postoperative challenges. Irrespective of islet infusion technique, large tissue volume and portal pressure greater than 25 cm H_2O are associated with risks of portal vein thrombosis and bleeding. Careful hemostasis of the operative field, monitoring of intraportal pressures, and heparinization during islet infusion are critical to avoid these complications. Postoperative bleeding, infection, and small-bowel obstruction are the most common causes for reoperation following TPIAT; gastrointestinal and infectious complications are the most frequent reasons for early readmissions.

A minimally invasive approach to TPIAT is feasible with comparable surgical outcomes, but complications during port placement, effects of CO_2 pneumoperitoneum on the cardiovascular and respiratory systems, and injuries associated with introduction and manipulation of surgical instruments should be considered.

V. A. Kirchner (✉)
Division of Abdominal Transplantation, Stanford University, Palo Alto, CA, USA
e-mail: kirc0079@stanford.edu

S. Chinnakotla et al. (eds.), *Total Pancreatectomy and Islet Auto Transplantation*,
https://doi.org/10.1007/978-981-92-0018-4_10

Comprehensive preoperative evaluation, technical expertise, careful patient selection, and effective postoperative care are essential to mitigate risks and improve overall outcomes in this complex surgical procedure.

Key Points

- Total pancreatectomy for chronic and acute recurrent pancreatitis is a complex procedure with the potential for life-threatening complications.
- Severe inflammation and adhesions that are associated with pancreatitis and prior endoscopic and surgical interventions contribute to the complexity of pancreatectomy, increasing the risk of bleeding and injury to intra-abdominal organs and vasculature.
- During islet infusion, large tissue volume and a rise in intraportal pressures are associated with an increased risk of portal vein thrombosis and bleeding due to transient portal hypertension.
- Bleeding, infection, and bowel obstruction are the most common complications necessitating return to the operating room postoperatively.
- In the presence of technical expertise, a minimally invasive approach is an acceptable option for TPIAT but is associated with significant rate of conversion to open operation.

10.1 Introduction

Surgical complications associated with total pancreatectomy with islet autotransplantation (TPIAT) can be divided into four major temporal categories: pancreatectomy, bowel and biliary reconstruction, islet infusion, and postoperative short- and long-term surgical complications.

Pancreatectomy is an inherently complex procedure and is associated with potentially life-threatening complications due to the retroperitoneal location of the pancreas and its proximity to the major blood vessels and associated vital organs such as the liver, spleen, kidneys, and intestine. Chronic inflammation, preexisting pancreatic pseudocysts, abscesses, pancreatic duct disruption, and fistulas lead to inflammation of anatomical planes around the organ, making the dissection more treacherous (Fig. 10.1a, b).

Two additional factors exacerbate the complexity of the procedure: preexisting interventions and the goal of minimizing ischemia to the pancreas during the dissection. Frequently, patients presenting for TPIAT have already undergone procedures to manage their symptoms, ranging from celiac plexus nerve block, endoscopic cyst gastrostomy, and cholecystectomy to complex pancreatic drainage and partial resection procedures. These interventions may compromise the dissection planes, increasing the risk of damage to surrounding tissue and blood vessels. In addition, the unique goal of TPIAT is to minimize future diabetic complications by

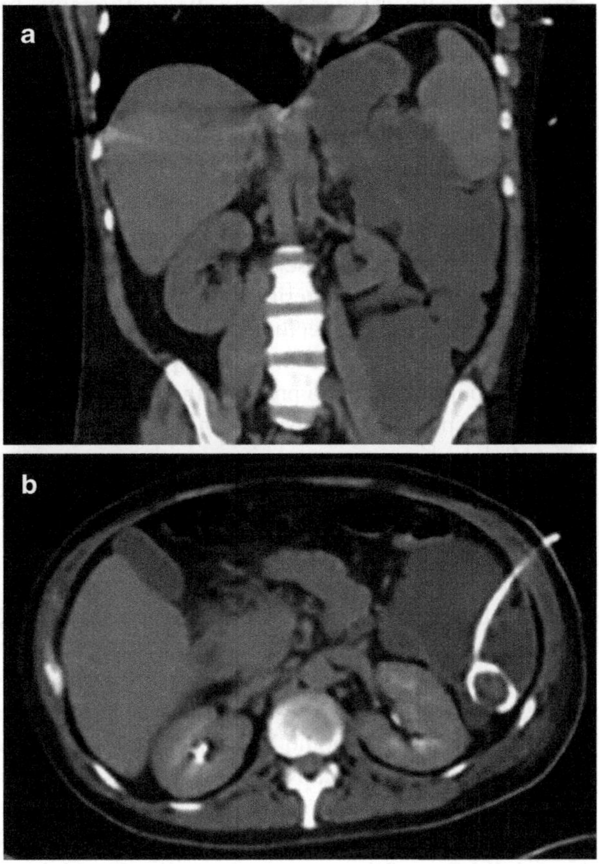

Fig. 10.1 (**a**, **b**) Patient presented 6 m prior to TPIAT with severe acute-on-chronic pancreatitis, multisystem organ failure, and pancreatic duct leak requiring percutaneous drainage

preserving and transplanting the islets. Therefore, maintenance of pancreatic blood flow throughout the dissection with the goal of minimizing warm ischemia to the gland and avoiding damage to the islets is critical for the islet quality and the success of autotransplantation; however, this maneuver increases the risk of bleeding during pancreatectomy.

The current chapter will discuss intraoperative and intraprocedural surgical complications during pancreatectomy, reconstruction, and islet infusion, as well as postoperative complications, referencing both open and minimally invasive techniques.

10.2 Intraoperative and Periprocedural Complications

10.2.1 Pancreatectomy

Injury to adjacent structures or intraoperative bleeding can occur at any point during total pancreatectomy. At the initial entry into the abdomen, significant scarring and adhesions may be observed, especially in the areas of the hepatic hilum and lesser sac, where the stomach can be adherent to the pancreas, and at the root of the mesentery, which is frequently shortened and sucked in toward the pancreatic bed due to chronic inflammation. During initial exposure of the anterior surface of the pancreatic body, injuries can occur to the stomach, especially in the setting of prior pseudocyst drainage.

Again, given the degree of inflammation, care must be taken around the vessels to prevent major hemorrhage. As the pancreatic tail and body are exposed, the path of the splenic artery is observed at the superior border of the pancreas, with the splenic vein traveling posterior to the body. Although historically the majority of surgeons performed splenectomy at the time of TPIAT [1], spleen preservation techniques are being adopted with advances in surgical techniques [2]. In this setting, an attempt should be made to preserve the short gastric and left gastroepiploic vasculature to the spleen with division of the splenic artery and vein away from the splenic hilum. Spleen-preserving techniques with preservation of splenic vessels should be discouraged because they increase ischemic injury to the pancreas during ligation of vascular perforators to the splenic body. In contrast, spleen-preserving techniques with ligation of the splenic vasculature preserve perfusion of the gland throughout the operation but are associated with an increased risk of splenic infarcts that may result in abscesses or development of gastric varices [3] or may necessitate delayed splenectomy.

During the mobilization of splenic flexure to expose the splenic hilum, sigmoid injuries may result in the setting of significant omental fat and adhesions. If splenectomy is planned, care should be taken during hilar dissection as well as around the spleen to avoid splenic capsular damage and hemorrhage. As the pancreas is dissected from the retroperitoneum, adhesions and distorted planes may result in the violation of Gerota's fascia and injury to the left adrenal gland and left kidney. With the mobilization of the pancreas medially, the origin of the splenic artery from the celiac trunk is exposed. Prior celiac plexus block for pain relief may be associated with additional scarring in this area (Fig. 10.2a–d); therefore, if TPIAT is planned, it is recommended to avoid celiac plexus block within 2–3 months prior to the procedure.

During the exposure of the pancreatic head, after the division of the gastrocolic ligament, ligation of the right gastroepiploic artery and mobilization of the transverse colon is performed. The transverse colon mesentery should be carefully mobilized to preserve the middle colic artery, which may be scarred due to the shortened mesentery and can be easily injured while exposing the infrapancreatic superior mesenteric vein (SMV). At the time of the Kocher maneuver, care should be taken to avoid injury to retroperitoneal structures such as the inferior vena cava and the right gonadal vein, which can be avulsed off the inferior vena cava during mobilization of the duodenum. Following the Kocher maneuver, the hilar dissection is performed with careful attention to hepatic arterial anatomy. Preoperative imaging (e.g., computed tomography [CT] or magnetic resonance imaging) is critical for detailed evaluation of vascular variations in order to avoid injuries such as replaced or accessory right hepatic arteries that usually originate from the superior

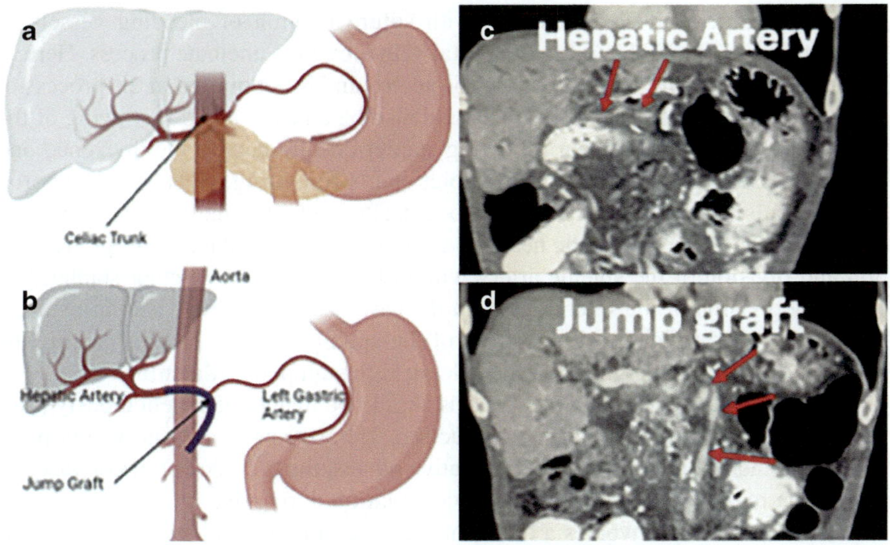

Fig. 10.2 Patient with chronic pancreatitis and extensive inflammatory involvement of the celiac trunk with subsequent erosion of the celiac trunk during dissection (**a**), which necessitated a jump graft to the hepatic artery and left gastric artery (**b**–**d**) to maintain perfusion to the liver and stomach

mesenteric artery (SMA) and travel behind or through the head of the pancreas, although a course anterior to the pancreatic head has also been reported [4]. If the head of the pancreas is involved in the inflammatory process, the planes between the common bile duct (CBD), portal vein, hepatic artery, and gastroduodenal artery (GDA) may be distorted. Intraoperative vascular ultrasound or aspiration of bile using a 25-gauge needle from the CBD prior to the division of the structure may be helpful. Although historically it has been recommended to avoid division of the GDA until the end of the pancreatic dissection, in the setting of extensive inflammation it is often not possible, and the GDA has to be sacrificed during exploration of the hepatic hilum. To avoid potential intraluminal dissection during ligation of the GDA with propagation into the hepatic artery, individual division of the anterior and posterior superior pancreatoduodenal arteries can be attempted.

A pylorus-preserving technique is recommended in order to avoid dumping syndrome postoperatively. The division of the first portion of the duodenum can be performed at any point when the surgeon is committed to the resectability of the pancreas. Following division of the ligament of Treitz, the fourth portion of the duodenum is divided and pulled through behind the superior mesenteric vasculature to facilitate completion of the pancreatectomy. Meticulous technique is necessary while creating a dissection plane between the pancreatic neck and the SMV/splenic vein confluence and portal vein to avoid injury to the trunk of Henle, which can have variable anatomy and can contribute to significant bleeding complications [5]. Lastly, the uncinate process is dissected away from the portal vein. Several techniques can be utilized for division of the uncinate process, including use of a harmonic scalpel and electrocautery with suture ligation of bleeding vessels or application of a stapler lateral to the portal vein along the uncinate process. Here, it is critical to make sure that the SMA is protected and is not injured in the process of transection. If a stapler is used, care should also be taken to avoid narrowing of the portal vein, which can happen following stapler closure next to the thickened and inflamed tissue. After closure of the stapler and before firing, patency of the portal vein and pulse of the SMA, as well as good perfusion to the small bowel, should be confirmed. Once the pancreatic head, body, and tail are free, the final steps are ligation and division of the splenic artery with either suture or a vascular stapler, followed by division of the splenic vein. In the case of intraoperative islet infusion, it is recommended to leave a long stump of the splenic vein for ease of placing the infusion catheter, with ligation of the splenic vein stump after the infusion.

Following pancreatectomy, hemostasis should be maintained meticulously prior to biliary and gastrointestinal reconstruction. Hemostasis is critical at this point because, in addition to challenging operative planes, the presence of major vasculature in the region, and the need for anticoagulation during and after islet infusion, the TPIAT procedure involves a transient increase in portal and mesenteric venous pressure following infusion of islets into the portal system, which increases backpressure on venous branches ligated during pancreatectomy, thus increasing the risk of intra- and postoperative bleeding.

10.2.2 Reconstruction

During the reconstruction phase, there are different variations of biliary and intestinal reconstruction. The Prospective Observational Study of TPIAT (POST) on surgical approach and outcomes reported Roux-en-Y duodenojejunostomy or gastrojejunostomy as the most common methods of intestinal reconstruction for adults (65%) and children (98%) [1]. Based on a meta-analysis, pylorus preservation during pancreatic resection increases the risk of delayed gastric emptying [6] but also reduces the risk of postoperative dumping syndrome [7]. Other variations of biliary reconstruction include modified Billroth II with in-line retrocolic end-to-side hepaticojejunostomy and antecolic side-to-side duodenojejunostomy [8]. Historically, Billroth II has been associated with an increased bile reflux incidence of 42%, versus 10% with Roux-en-Y [9]; the addition of a pylorus-preserving technique to Billroth II is meant to decrease the risk of this complication.

10.2.3 Islet Infusion

Following biliary and intestinal reconstruction, islets can be infused into the stump of the splenic vein prior to closure of the abdomen. If islet infusion is delayed, the patient can be closed, with islet infusion happening subsequently in interventional radiology suite (IR), either through the more commonly adopted transhepatic approach or through an externalized catheter left in the mesenteric vasculature during the index operation [10].

Independent of the method, the complication profile during islet infusion includes bleeding due to the increased intraportal pressure and portal vein thrombosis (PVT). In a study of 233 patients undergoing TPIAT, rates of bleeding and PVT were 7.73% and 3.43%, respectively [11]. The total tissue volume per kilogram of body weight was the best predictor of change in portal pressure during islet infusion. Both tissue volume >0.25 cc/kg and a change in portal pressure with δ pressure exceeding 25 cm H_2O were associated with increased complication rates [11]. Therefore, in the setting when portal venous pressure exceeds 25 cm H_2O, islet infusion should be stopped temporarily and portal pressures should be reassessed prior to reinitiation of infusion; if the pressures do not decline, islet infusion may need to be stopped entirely. Administration of heparin at 70 units/kg dose during islet infusion is routine to decrease the risk of thrombosis and prevent islet destruction due to the instant blood-mediated inflammatory reaction [12]. Some providers perform routine postinfusion liver biopsy to document liver health and the presence of transplanted islets, although increased portal pressures may lead to an increased risk of bleeding from biopsy sites. Thus, meticulous hemostasis is critical in this setting.

To avoid a missed diagnosis of PVT, all patients undergoing TPIAT should be monitored with postinfusion liver function test panel and liver Doppler ultrasound. In the majority of cases, PVT resolves with anticoagulation therapy over the course of several months, although this depends on the original extent of the thrombosis; in rare critical cases, IR and surgical thrombectomy can be used.

In the setting of IR infusion, additional complications should be considered, including risk of intraperitoneal or liver subcapsular bleeding, which has an incidence of up to 13% [13]. Therefore, effective hepatic tract ablation, reduction in the number of passes through the liver during cannulation, and minimization of the rise in portal pressures are recommended. When an externalized mesenteric venous catheter is used for infusion, dysfunction or bleeding at the site of a dislodged catheter can occur.

10.3 Postoperative Complications

10.3.1 Bleeding

Hemorrhage following pancreatectomy can be divided into early (e.g., within 24 h after the operation) and late events. Early bleeding complications are frequently due to inadequate hemostasis and coagulopathy. Late complications may be associated with arterial stump erosions, although this occurs less frequently in the setting of total pancreatectomy because the majority of the gland is removed and the risk of activated amylase leak is rare compared with that during partial pancreatectomy procedures [14]. Intraluminal hemorrhage due to staple line bleeding or ulcers may present as early or late events.

According to the report from the POST study, postoperative hemorrhage, although rare, was one of the two primary indications for reoperation in adults, with an incidence of 27%, and the primary indication in children following TPIAT [1].

In the non-TPIAT pancreatectomy population, mortality has been reported following major hemorrhagic episodes from postoperative stump erosion of the splenic and left gastric arteries [15]. The diagnostic modality for hemorrhage will depend on the initial presentation and will include CT with intravenous contrast, angiography, and endoscopy. The management will depend on the extent and location of the bleed and may include observation with correction of coagulopathy, IR techniques, or open or endoscopic surgical techniques. Based on non-TPIAT outcomes, open surgical exploration following postoperative bleeding is associated with the highest mortality, at 37%, compared with interventional angiography at 17% [14].

10.3.2 Infection

The infectious complications after TPIAT may range from wound infections and intra-abdominal abscesses in the setting of clean-contaminated or contaminated operation to infections associated with biliary or intestinal anastomotic leaks.

Infection is the other of the two most common causes for reoperation in adults following TPIAT, with an estimated frequency of over 20% [1]. It was also diagnosed in 63% of TPIAT patients who were readmitted to the hospital within the first year after the procedure [16].

In a retrospective analysis of complications within the first year after TPIAT, 21% of patients (38/179) presented with wound infection, 17% (31/179) with intra-abdominal infection, 9% (17/179) with urinary tract infection, 8% (14/179) with bacteremia, 8% (14/179) with *Clostridioides difficile* colitis, and 2% (4/179) with sepsis [16]. Depending on the presentation, management ranged from antimicrobial therapy to drainage of the infected area or surgical anastomotic revision and abdominal washout.

Surveillance cultures of isolated islets often demonstrate polymicrobial contamination, with reported estimates between 53% and 61%. This contamination is mostly attributed to the prevalence of biliary interventions and drainage procedures, as well as to the duration of pancreatitis prior to TPIAT in this patient population [16–18]. The incidence of infection in individuals with positive surveillance cultures has been reported to be between 22% and 57%; however, only 5% of patients had an infectious complication caused by the same organism as the surveillance cultures from their pancreas or islet cell preparation [17, 18]. Despite the liver being the most common site for islet infusion, hepatic abscesses are extremely infrequent in this patient population. The recommendation for post-TPIAT antimicrobial management includes prophylactic perioperative antibiotics, followed by an additional 5–7 days of tailored antimicrobial therapy in the case of positive pancreas or islet cell surveillance cultures [17].

10.3.3 Gastrointestinal Complications

Post-TPIAT gastrointestinal complications include intestinal and biliary leaks, strictures, small-bowel obstruction, chyle leak, marginal anastomotic ulcers, delayed gastric emptying, constipation, and dumping syndrome. They significantly increase early and late morbidity and contribute to a high rate of readmissions (between 50% and 70%) in the early postoperative period [16, 19].

Nathan et al. reported that small-bowel obstruction necessitated reoperation in 14% of patients [1]. Late presentations of bowel obstruction are likely secondary to adhesions or progressive weight loss and thinning of the mesentery with an increased risk of internal hernias given the presence of mesenteric defects due to prior intestinal reconstruction. Biliary leaks and strictures occur at the low frequency of 1–2% and are managed either endoscopically or by reoperation [1, 16].

Chyle leak in pancreatic surgery has been reported in 1.3–22.1% of patients, with the main risk factors being the extent of the surgery and early enteral feeding [20]. In the multivariable analysis of intra- and postoperative events following TPIAT, chyle leak was associated with higher rates of readmission within the first year; 17% of readmitted patients (21/125) and 4% of non-readmitted patients (2/54) were diagnosed with chyle leak [16]. The majority of leaks resolve spontaneously with conservative management, including a switch to a nonfat diet or elemental enteric formula, with occasional need for cessation of oral intake and transition to total parenteral nutrition. Somatostatin analogs and drainage of collected intra-abdominal fluid may be needed. Diagnosis is based on the presence of triglycerides in the analyzed fluid. If conservative management fails, further investigation with lymphoscintigraphy and sclerotic embolization may be performed [20].

In the modern era, marginal ulcers have been reported in 2.5–10% of cases following pancreaticoduodenectomy [21]. The presentation of marginal ulcers may include discomfort during or after meals but may also evolve into persistent pain and gastrointestinal bleeding. Intraoperatively, it is critical to ensure robust vascularization of the intestinal anastomosis to avoid future risk of ulcers and anastomotic strictures [22]. Postoperatively, risk factors include advanced age, alcohol and tobacco consumption, chronic use of nonsteroidal anti-inflammatory drugs (NSAIDs), and failure to take antacid therapy [21, 23]. Although some of these risk factors cannot be modified, it is strongly recommended for patients following TPIAT to avoid excessive alcohol consumption, cease tobacco use, avoid NSAIDs, and continue scheduled antacid therapy [23, 24].

Delayed gastric emptying may be a preexisting condition in patients prior to TPIAT due to the chronic use of narcotics to address severe pain, but it can also be a new symptom due to variations in surgical technique such as pylorus-preserving duodenectomy or disruption of the autonomic neural network during pancreatectomy, as well as changes in hormone production [6, 25, 26]. Delayed gastric emptying often presents with prolonged nausea, vomiting, feeling of fullness, early satiety, and food intolerance. After ruling out mechanical obstruction, multiple invasive and noninvasive diagnostic modalities may aid diagnosis, including gastric-emptying scintigraphy, capsule motility studies, manometry, and CO_2 breath test [26]. To minimize patient symptoms after TPIAT, some programs routinely place intraoperative gastrojejunostomy tubes following surgery to provide gastric decompression and recovery through the gastric port and, at the same time, to ensure timely initiation of enteric nutrition via a jejunostomy port [1]. Scheduled prokinetic medications such as metoclopramide or erythromycin may be employed to expedite gastrointestinal motility [24, 26].

Although post-TPIAT constipation is not directly related to surgical complications, it is a prevalent symptom in the given patient population that can be exacerbated by opioids pre- and postoperatively, as well as by dehydration due to poor oral intake and insufficient use of pancreatic enzyme replacement therapy (PERT). Management usually focuses on weaning off opioids, introducing mu-opioid antagonists to selectively target the wall of the gut, adjusting PERT doses, and scheduling a robust bowel regimen to avoid recurrent constipation episodes [24, 27]. In certain instances, patients with chronic constipation may develop severe colonic dysfunction that, in rare cases, may necessitate colectomy to relieve symptoms [28, 29].

In TPIAT, dumping syndrome may present after pylorectomy or greater gastric resection followed by gastrojejunostomy. Although the prevalence of dumping syndrome after bariatric surgery may be near 50%, the incidence after pancreatic surgery is closer to 10% and is primarily associated with resection of the pylorus [30, 31]. Early symptoms occur within the first hour after a meal and include abdominal pain, bloating, nausea, diarrhea, flushing, palpitations, tachycardia, hypotension, and syncope; the underlying mechanism involves osmotic effect, hormone release, and autonomic neural response [32]. Late symptoms begin 1–3 h following a meal and primarily manifest as hypoglycemia, which has been well described in bariatric surgery [32]. Management of the syndrome is most often with dietary modifications, including smaller, more frequent meals; separation of liquids and solid meals; minimizing intake of simple sugars and milk; and encouraging fiber-rich foods. Pharmaceutical options include somatostatin analogs and inhibitors of oligosaccharide metabolism. Surgical revisions are reserved for cases in which dietary and medical management are not successful [33].

10.4 Consideration of a Minimally Invasive Approach

Minimally invasive surgery (MIS) is well established as a less painful approach for the patient and frequently has faster recovery, shorter length of stay, and improved cosmetic outcomes [34]. In the case of TPIAT for chronic or acute recurrent pancreatitis, MIS is slowly gaining popularity, with several centers reporting laparoscopic and robotic techniques with comparable surgical outcomes to the open approach [35–37]. However, adoption is slow because the complexity of the operation requires advanced MIS skills, and the operative field is frequently treacherous as a result of chronic inflammation, adhesions, and prior interventions. Conversion to open surgery has been reported to occur in 10–16% of cases [35, 37]. The need for preservation of the vascular supply to the pancreas until the end of the explant in order to ensure islet viability makes pancreatectomy for TPIAT more challenging and may present an additional challenge in the setting of MIS. The potential additional complications in the setting of an MIS approach include rare but potentially severe injuries to structures during port placement (incidence of 0.38%), respiratory acidosis due to the use of carbon dioxide for insufflation, decreased cardiac output by up to 30%, increased systemic vascular resistance secondary to pneumoperitoneum, and gas embolism necessitating cardiorespiratory recovery maneuvers, pneumothorax, pneumomediastinum, and injuries related to the introduction and manipulation of laparoscopic surgical instruments that may result in unrecognized organ lacerations, perforations, and burns [38, 39].

References

1. Nathan JD, Yang Y, Eaton A, Witkowski P, Wijkstrom M, Walsh M, et al. Surgical approach and short-term outcomes in adults and children undergoing total pancreatectomy with islet autotransplantation: a report from the prospective observational study of TPIAT. Pancreatology. 2022;22(1):1–8.
2. Granieri S, Bonomi A, Frassini S, Gjoni E, Germini A, Kersik A, et al. Kimura's vs Warshaw's technique for spleen preserving distal pancreatectomy: a systematic review and meta-analysis of high-quality studies. HPB. 2023;25(6):614–24.
3. Wang L, Wu D, Cheng Y-g, Xu J-w, Chu H-b, Zhang G-y, et al. Warshaw technique in laparoscopic spleen-preserving distal pancreatectomy: surgical strategy and late outcomes of splenic preservation. Biomed Res Int. 2019;2019:1–10.
4. Raghavendra D, Balachandar TG, Prabhakaran R, Swain SK, Nirmal J, Sunil N, et al. Replaced right hepatic artery passing anterior to pancreas: a rare and challenging anatomical variant during pancreaticoduodenectomy. Egypt J Radiol Nucl Med. 2022;53(1):1–2.
5. Gao Y, Lu Y. Variations of Gastrocolic trunk of Henle and its significance in Gastrocolic surgery. Gastroenterol Res Pract. 2018;2018:1–8.
6. Zhou Y, Lin L, Wu L, Xu D, Li B. A case-matched comparison and meta-analysis comparing pylorus-resecting pancreaticoduodenectomy with pylorus-preserving pancreaticoduodenectomy for the incidence of postoperative delayed gastric emptying. HPB. 2015;17(4):337–43.
7. Tran KTC, Smeenk HG, van Eijck CHJ, Kazemier G, Hop WC, Greve JWG, et al. Pylorus preserving Pancreaticoduodenectomy versus standard Whipple procedure. Ann Surg. 2004;240(5):738–45.
8. Park JY, Kwon OK, Jeon J-H, Choi Y-K, Park KB. Impact of the different biliopancreatic limb length on diabetes and incretin hormone secretion following distal gastrectomy in gastric cancer patients. Sci Rep. 2021;11(1):22451.
9. Thong DQ, Le Minh QH, Dat TQ, Hai NV, Nguyen DT, Tuan Anh NV, et al. Billroth-II modified with hinged anti-peristaltic afferent loop versus Roux-en-Y reconstruction after distal gastrectomy for gastric cancer: a propensity-score match analysis. Surgery. 2024;175(6):1524–32.
10. Gaba RC, Garcia-Roca R, Oberholzer J. Pancreatic islet cell transplantation: an update for interventional radiologists. J Vasc Interv Radiol. 2012;23(5):583–94.
11. Wilhelm JJ, Bellin MD, Dunn TB, Balamurugan AN, Pruett TL, Radosevich DM, et al. Proposed thresholds for pancreatic tissue volume for safe intraportal islet autotransplantation after total pancreatectomy. Am J Transplant. 2013;13(12):3183–91.
12. Abdel-Karim TR, Hodges JS, Herold KC, Pruett TL, Ramanathan KV, Hering BJ, et al. Peri-transplant inflammation and long-term diabetes outcomes were not impacted by either Etanercept or Alpha-1-antitrypsin treatment in islet autotransplant recipients. Transpl Int. 2024;37:1–2.

13. Villiger P, Ryan EA, Owen R, O'Kelly K, Oberholzer J, Saif FA, et al. Prevention of bleeding after islet transplantation: lessons learned from a multivariate analysis of 132 cases at a single institution. Am J Transplant. 2005;5(12):2992–8.
14. Floortje van Oosten A, Smits FJ, van den Heuvel DAF, van Santvoort HC, Molenaar IQ. Diagnosis and management of postpancreatectomy hemorrhage: a systematic review and meta-analysis. HPB. 2019;21(8):953–61.
15. Janot MS, Belyaev O, Kersting S, Chromik AM, Seelig MH, Sülberg D, et al. Indications and early outcomes for total pancreatectomy at a high-volume pancreas center. HPB Surg. 2010;2010:1–8.
16. Kirchner V, Bagdiwala A, Vock D, Bellin M, Beilman G, Berry L, et al. Patterns and associated risk factors for early readmissions post total pancreatectomy and islet auto-transplantation (TP-IAT). Am J Transplant. 2017;17(3).
17. Colling KP, Blondet JJ, Balamurugan AN, Wilhelm JJ, Dunn T, Pruett TL, et al. Positive sterility cultures of transplant solutions during pancreatic islet autotransplantation are associated infrequently with clinical infection. Surg Infect. 2015;16(2):115–23.
18. Gołębiewska JE, Bachul PJ, Fillman N, Kijek MR, Basto L, Para M, et al. Early infectious complications after total pancreatectomy with islet autotransplantation: a single center experience. J Gastrointest Surg. 2019;23(11):2201–10.
19. Shahbazov R, Naziruddin B, Yadav K, Saracino G, Yoshimatsu G, Kanak MA, et al. Risk factors for early readmission after total pancreatectomy and islet auto transplantation. HPB. 2018;20(2):166–74.
20. Muzzolini M, Araujo RLC, Kingham TP, Peschaud F, Paye F, Lupinacci RM. Incidence and risk factors for Chyle leak after pancreatic surgery for cancer: a comprehensive systematic review. Eur J Surg Oncol. 2022;48(4):707–17.
21. Fan S, Chen G, Zhang K, Zhao L, Yuan H, Wu J, et al. The incidence and risk factors of marginal ulcers in the short and medium term in symptomatic post-pancreaticoduodenectomy patients—single-center experience. Am J Surg. 2024;233:94–9.
22. Morgan KA, Fontenot BB, Harvey NR, Adams DB. Revision of anastomotic stenosis after pancreatic head resection for chronic pancreatitis: is it futile? HPB. 2010;12(3):211–6.
23. Gross A, Gentle C, Wehrle CJ, Nimylowycz K, Said Al-deen S, Aminian A, et al. Nonsteroidal anti-inflammatory drug (NSAID) prescribing after gastrojejunostomy: a preventable cause of morbidity. Surgery. 2025;179:108806.
24. Reid TD, Madduri SS, Agala CB, Weng C, McEwan S, Desai CS. Perioperative management of patients undergoing total pancreatectomy with/without islet cell autotransplantation: a single center experience. J Clin Med. 2023;12(12):3993.
25. Jehangir A, Parkman HP. Chronic opioids in gastroparesis: relationship with gastrointestinal symptoms, healthcare utilization and employment. World J Gastroenterol. 2017;23(40):7310–20.
26. Kim YH. Management and prevention of delayed gastric emptying after pancreaticoduodenectomy. Korean J Hepato-Biliary-Pancreat Surg. 2012;16(1):1.
27. Brown B, Price ST. Mu-opioid antagonists for the treatment of opioid-induced bowel dysfunction. Am Fam Physician. 2023;107(2):131–2.
28. Chaichanavichkij P, Vollebregt PF, Tee SZY, Scott SM, Knowles CH. Slow-transit constipation and criteria for colectomy: a cross-sectional study of 1568 patients. BJS Open. 2021;5(3):1–2.
29. Thaler K, Dinnewitzer A, Oberwalder M, Weiss EG, Nogueras JJ, Efron J, et al. Quality of life after colectomy for colonic inertia. Tech Coloproctol. 2005;9(2):133–7.
30. Linehan IP, Russell RC, Hobsley M. The dumping syndrome after pancreatoduodenectomy. Surg Gynecol Obstet. 1988;167(2):114–8.
31. Vavricka SR, Greuter T. Gastroparesis and dumping syndrome: current concepts and management. J Clin Med. 2019;8(8):1127.
32. Scarpellini E, Arts J, Karamanolis G, Laurenius A, Siquini W, Suzuki H, et al. International consensus on the diagnosis and management of dumping syndrome. Nat Rev Endocrinol. 2020;16(8):448–66.

33. Hui C, Bauza G. Dumping Syndrome. StatPearls [Internet]. 2023; Available from: https://www.ncbi.nlm.nih.gov/books/NBK470542/
34. Singh SS, Shinde RK. Minimally invasive gastrointestinal surgery: a review. Cureus. 2023;15:e48864.
35. Fan CJ, Hirose K, Walsh CM, Quartuccio M, Desai NM, Singh VK, et al. Laparoscopic Total pancreatectomy with islet autotransplantation and intraoperative islet separation as a treatment for patients with chronic pancreatitis. JAMA Surg. 2017;152(6):550.
36. Galvani CA, Rilo HR, Samamé J, Porubsky M, Rana A, Gruessner RWG. Fully robotic-assisted technique for Total pancreatectomy with an autologous islet transplant in chronic pancreatitis patients: results of a first series. J Am Coll Surg. 2014;218(3):e73–e8.
37. Kinny-Köster B, Walsh CM, Sun Z, Faghih M, Desai NM, Warren DS, et al. Minimally invasive total pancreatectomy with islet autotransplantation for chronic pancreatitis: the robotic approach. Surg Endosc. 2024;38(7):3948–56.
38. Maskal S, Ellis R, Prabhu A, Miller B, Beffa L, Krpata D, et al. Injuries incurred from minimally invasive access for abdominal surgery. Surg Endosc. 2023;37(7):5368–73.
39. Morales AA, Echevarría YL, Mursulí AL, Rodriguez P. General complication of laparoscopic surgery, necessary review. Clin Surg. 2024;9:3705.

Medical Complications and Management After Total Pancreatectomy with Islet Autotransplantation

11

Petr Vanek, Justin Howard, and Guru Trikudanathan

Abstract

Total pancreatectomy with islet autotransplantation (TPIAT) offers unique advantages over standard total pancreatectomy, retaining some endogenous insulin production to improve quality of life. However, TPIAT also carries a risk of postoperative complications. Beyond endocrine and exocrine insufficiency, patients may be prone to gastrointestinal dysmotility syndromes (e.g., obstipation, gastroparesis). Furthermore, susceptibility to infections, both intra-abdominal and systemic, can increase due to anatomic alterations and changes in immune regulation, especially after splenectomy. Late postoperative issues include nutritional deficiencies, bone density loss, and psychological challenges, emphasizing the value of a comprehensive, multidisciplinary care model with close endocrine follow-up, thorough nutritional support, and regular screening for treatable complications. Moreover, recognizing risk factors, implementing preventive strategies, and standardizing treatment protocols remain priorities for centers offering TPIAT. In this chapter, we provide an overview of the most significant medical complications that can arise after TPIAT and outline evidence-based management approaches based on the latest research and our own clinical experience.

P. Vanek
Department of Gastroenterology, Masaryk Memorial Cancer Institute, Brno, Czech Republic

J. Howard · G. Trikudanathan (✉)
Division of Gastroenterology, Hepatology and Nutrition, Department of Medicine, University of Minnesota Medical School, Minneapolis, MN, USA
e-mail: triku001@umn.edu

S. Chinnakotla et al. (eds.), *Total Pancreatectomy and Islet Auto Transplantation*, https://doi.org/10.1007/978-981-92-0018-4_11

Key Points

1. TPIAT improves quality of life, yet it introduces complex postoperative challenges that demand a robust, multidisciplinary approach for optimal long-term outcomes.
2. Many patients remain partially or fully insulin-dependent, necessitating close glycemic surveillance; exocrine insufficiency is universal, requiring lifelong pancreatic enzyme replacement therapy.
3. Gastroparesis, obstipation, and dysmotility frequently occur after TPIAT, often exacerbated by opioids and altered anatomy. Malabsorption and nutrient deficiencies require dietary modifications, vitamin supplementation, and DEXA screening for osteoporosis.
4. Risk of postsplenectomy infections and portal vein thrombosis necessitate appropriate vaccinations, antibiotic prophylaxis, and anticoagulation protocols. Gut microbiota alterations can aggravate GI symptoms and infection risks, highlighting the importance of microbiota-focused research.
5. Because opioid dependence is common before TPIAT, structured tapering and multimodal pain management are crucial to minimizing long-term reliance postoperatively.

11.1 Introduction

Total pancreatectomy with islet autotransplantation (TPIAT) is increasingly utilized as a management option for chronic and recurrent acute pancreatitis refractory to other intervention modalities [1, 2]. Although TPIAT confers significant improvements in quality of life (QoL) in carefully selected patients, it also involves risks, demands a prolonged recovery, and requires commitment from the patient, their caregivers, and the healthcare team.

Patients with chronic pancreatitis (CP) inherently face risks of multiple complications, and TPIAT adds certain technical and postoperative challenges [3]. Nevertheless, compared to TP alone, TPIAT confers key advantages that lead to improved QoL, even when full pain relief is not achieved [4]. Although the overall mortality rate after TPIAT remains incompletely characterized, timely and proactive management of potential complications has been shown to reduce life-threatening events [5]. Importantly, while postoperative complications may increase hospital stay and readmissions, they generally do not adversely impact islet graft function [6–8].

This chapter explores the medical complications and management after TPIAT, including nutritional deficiencies, gastrointestinal (GI) dysmotility, infection risks, and other significant issues such as thrombotic events, psychological challenges, opioid dependence, increased cholangitis risk, microbiome alterations, nephrolithiasis, and pancreatic cancer (Fig. 11.1). Endocrine and exocrine insufficiencies are only briefly discussed here, as they are covered in detail in Chaps. 8 and 9, respectively. Notably, most complications following TPIAT arise from the surgical aspects

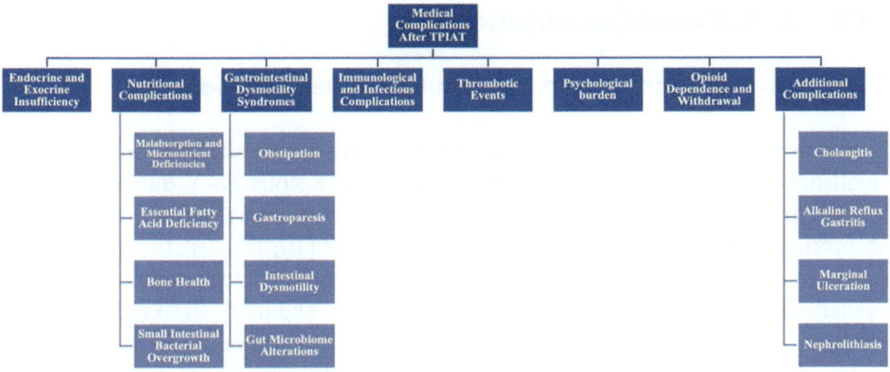

Fig. 11.1 Overview of medical complications after TPIAT, categorized into key areas discussed in detail throughout the chapter

of the procedure, whereas issues directly related to IAT are relatively uncommon [7, 9].

Patients typically undergo regular follow-up during the first postoperative year (at 3, 6, and 12 months) and annually thereafter. These visits commonly involve fasting and stimulated glucose measurements, C-peptide levels, HbA1c, nutritional assessments, liver function tests, and complete blood counts, facilitating early detection of complications and the maintenance of long-term graft function [10]. Recent data from the Prospective Observational Study in TPIAT (POST) show a median initial hospital stay of 11 days for adults and 15 days for children, with pediatric patients less likely to require readmission [11]. In-hospital mortality rates range from 0% to 2% [12–17], but as surgical expertise evolves, the risk has declined. For instance, the University of Minnesota (UMN) has reported no immediate postoperative deaths in the past 15 years [11, 18].

11.2 Endocrine and Exocrine Insufficiency

IAT preserves varying degrees of insulin-producing capacity, though many patients remain partially or fully insulin-dependent [15, 19–21]. Nonetheless, residual islet function often mitigates the severity of diabetes, providing notable benefit over TP without IAT. Hypoglycemic episodes may still arise, likely due to altered anatomy and insufficient glucagon responses, highlighting the need for close glycemic surveillance and patient education [22–24]. Yet, even with these complexities, partial islet function frequently translates into better overall metabolic control and increased QoL than would be expected in the absence of an islet graft [4, 25]. Concurrently, inevitable exocrine pancreatic insufficiency (EPI) necessitates lifelong pancreatic enzyme replacement therapy (PERT) to prevent malabsorption and associated complications (e.g., fat-soluble vitamin [FSV] deficiencies) [26–28].

11.3 Nutritional Complications

11.3.1 Malabsorption and Micronutrient Deficiencies

In addition to EPI, TPIAT introduces further nutritional risks by altering normal small-bowel continuity (often maintained through a Roux-en-Y duodenojejunostomy with partial duodenectomy and biliary reconstruction) which can affect the absorption of iron, calcium, and other micronutrients [10, 18, 29]. To mitigate these risks, clinicians should conduct annual or biannual nutritional assessments [1]. Such evaluations include iron studies, FSVs, vitamin B12, and markers of nutrition (e.g., albumin, prealbumin), as well as monitoring for steatorrhea, stool patterns, and abdominal symptoms. Serial weight measurements are crucial for quantifying PERT effectiveness [1]. For pediatric patients, height and weight should be recorded at every visit, with growth parameters reviewed every 3 months [1].

A recent multicenter POST analysis of 348 TPIAT recipients revealed increased FSV deficiencies by 1 year, despite adequate enzyme replacement [30]. Adults were especially prone to vitamin A deficiency, and underweight patients faced higher risks for vitamin A and E deficiencies. Only one-third of adults and two-thirds of children used pancreatic-specific multivitamins, suggesting that standard multivitamins may be inadequate [30]. Identifying those who are underweight or who exhibit evidence of insufficient nutrient absorption may help target higher-risk groups, warranting aggressive supplementation and closer follow-up. Furthermore, supplementation with specialized pancreatic multivitamins, which deliver water-soluble FSV formulations, improves absorption [10].

At our institution, once patients are on a normal oral diet, we aim for 1000 lipase units/kg/meal (range 500–2000 IU) and introduce a pancreatic multivitamin [26]. We then adjust the multivitamin regimen and add 25(OH)D supplementation as needed based on FSV levels checked at 3, 6, and 12 months after TPIAT.

11.3.2 Essential Fatty Acid Deficiency

Essential fatty acid deficiency (EFAD) may also occur after TPIAT due to EPI and anatomic alterations. A recent study of 197 TPIAT recipients found that the prevalence of EFAD was 33% at 1 year posttransplant, increasing to 49% at 2 years and 53.5% at 3 or more years [31]. Significant predictors at 1 year included older age at transplant, being an adult, and having an obstructive etiology. Notably, only 6% of children had EFAD 1 year after TPIAT, compared with 46% of adults.

EFAD may be diagnosed clinically, presenting as dry, scaly skin, hair loss, poor wound healing, increased susceptibility to infections, and, in severe cases, growth retardation and impaired neurological function [32]. Laboratory assays for essential fatty acids levels, available at large research centers, can confirm the diagnosis. Treatment involves dietary supplementation to restore normal levels.

11.3.3 Bone Health

Patients with CP already have increased risks of osteopenia and osteoporosis [1, 3, 33]. After TPIAT, factors such as malabsorption, changes in inflammatory compounds, altered GI hormones, and reduced mobility can further exacerbate bone loss [29, 34–37]. Conversely, removing the source of the pancreatitis may reduce chronic inflammation and improve overall health and activity with positive impacts on bone mineral density (BMD) [15]. A recent study from the UMN group reported declines in lumbar spine, hip, and overall BMD during the first year after TPIAT, with possible stabilization between 12 and 18 months [29]. This suggests that negative impacts on bone health may be limited to the early postoperative period. However, further studies are required to determine the long-term effects of TPIAT on bone health.

Dual-energy X-ray absorptiometry (DEXA) is recommended to screen for osteopenia and osteoporosis in CP [33, 38]. However, the optimal timing and target screening population remain unclear [33]. According to the American Gastroenterological Association, patients with at least one additional osteoporosis risk factor should undergo DEXA screening [39]. Similarly, the HaPanEU guidelines advise DEXA for CP patients with added risk factors, including postmenopausal status, previous low-trauma fractures, men over 50 years old, and those with malabsorption [38]. They also suggest baseline screening for all CP patients, with follow-up scans every 2 years if initial results detect bone pathology [38].

Vitamin D status significantly contributes to overall bone health. In cases of vitamin D deficiency, current guidelines recommend high-dose cholecalciferol (vitamin D_3) to rapidly replenish stores, typically 50,000 IU (1250 mcg) once weekly or 6000 IU (150 mcg) daily for 8–12 weeks in adults [40]. After reassessment of 25(OH)D levels, a maintenance dose of 1000–2000 IU/day (25–50 mcg) is often employed to maintain serum concentrations above 30 ng/ml. Pediatric dosing varies by body weight and deficiency severity but generally follows similar principles. Notably, post-TPIAT vitamin D recommendations extrapolated from cystic fibrosis guidelines suggest 800–1000 IU (20–25 mcg) daily for children 1–10 years old and 800–2000 IU (20–50 mcg) daily for children over 10 years [41]. Monitoring 25(OH) D levels at 8–12 weeks and periodically thereafter ensures adequate correction, particularly in TPIAT patients with persistent malabsorption.

Early detection of bone density loss facilitates interventions such as high-dose vitamin D or bone-protective therapies (e.g., bisphosphonates) in selected cases. Coupling an aggressive rehabilitation program with adequate calcium and protein intake may help limit postoperative bone loss.

11.3.4 Additional Factors Affecting Nutrition

Postoperatively, GI symptoms may shift. Constipation may diminish, though steatorrhea and diarrhea may increase due to altered enzyme output and surgical changes in anatomy [26]. These issues usually respond to optimal enzyme supplementation but can recur if dosing is inadequate or if other GI disturbances arise. For example, persistent steatorrhea despite escalating PERT doses should prompt suspicion of small intestinal bacterial overgrowth (SIBO) [42].

The development of SIBO after TPIAT is multifactorial, involving disruptions in small-bowel motility, reduced gastric acid secretion (patients on proton pump inhibitors), and anatomical changes, altogether disrupting the homeostatic mechanisms surrounding the intestinal microbiome [43]. Those with Roux-en-Y reconstruction may face an elevated risk due to stasis in the afferent limb. SIBO presents with a range of symptoms, including abdominal pain, bloating, nausea, vomiting, flatulence, diarrhea, constipation, or soft stools [44]. Importantly, it may contribute to persistent malabsorption and micronutrient depletion [45, 46].

Diagnosis is often clinical, and treatment is frequently initiated empirically based on symptoms, though hydrogen breath testing can be used for confirmation. Antibiotic therapy typically leads to rapid symptom relief, which further supports the diagnosis. However, recurrence of SIBO is common, often requiring repeated courses of treatment.

11.4 Gastrointestinal Dysmotility Syndromes

CP can precipitate dysmotility preoperatively, and these issues often persist or worsen after TPIAT. Contributing factors include mechanical causes, altered hormonal regulation, neurologic changes, medications such as opioid analgesics, and postoperative complications such as adhesive disease [47–50]. Patients develop a range of issues, including obstipation, gastroparesis, or intestinal dysmotility. Importantly, multiple problems often overlap. Up to 69% of patients experience GI symptoms in the months after surgery that significantly impact their daily lives [26]. Additionally, as many as 45% of TPIAT recipients report persistent dysmotility symptoms [51].

11.4.1 Obstipation

Postoperative obstipation is a frequent cause of abdominal pain in TPIAT patients, particularly in the context of long-term opioid therapy. Symptoms vary: some report reduced stool output, straining, or hard stools, while others may have overflow diarrhea. Imaging (e.g., abdominal X-rays or computed tomography [CT]) often reveals a significant stool burden, though radiologists may not always comment on it directly. Management centers around weaning or stopping opioids.

A standard bowel cleanout protocol is employed when obstipation occurs, followed by daily maintenance with osmotic laxatives such as polyethylene glycol (MiraLAX). Osmotic laxatives are generally preferred over stool softeners like docusate and stimulant laxatives such as bisacodyl and senna. Long-term management includes hydration, fiber intake, and routine pharmacologic measures (e.g., laxatives or motility agents). Because many TPIAT patients remain on opioids, prokinetic agents such as linaclotide, lubiprostone, and plecanatide can be beneficial for recurrent obstipation. Pelvic floor evaluation should be considered if this standard management fails.

11.4.2 Gastroparesis

Delayed gastric emptying (DGE) is a well-recognized complication after TPIAT, ranging from mild to severe [51, 52]. Symptoms typically include nausea, vomiting, early satiety, and abdominal pain, and the condition is strongly associated with opioid use [53, 54]. Notably, up to 35% of TPIAT recipients experience persistent DGE symptoms [55], often correlating with lower QoL and underscoring the importance of proactive management [51]. Post-TPIAT patients with DGE have readmission rates three times higher than those without the condition, further highlighting its clinical significance [8].

Diagnosis of gastroparesis should be confirmed with objective testing rather than relying on symptoms alone. The American College of Gastroenterology (ACG) recommends gastric emptying scintigraphy as the gold standard, with alternatives including breath testing or wireless motility capsule assessment [56]. The United European Gastroenterology and European Society for Neurogastroenterology and Motility (UEG/ESNM) guidelines emphasize differentiating gastroparesis from functional dyspepsia because the two conditions share overlapping symptoms [57].

Because postoperative GI function is frequently delayed, DGE is anticipated early on and managed by gastric decompression via a gastrojejunal tube placed at surgery to maintain adequate nutrition until motility recovers [11]. Patients are also counseled preoperatively about the potential for DGE following TPIAT. Interestingly, early DGE may be less pronounced in laparoscopic TPIAT [58]. If gastroparesis persists after resuming oral intake, dietary therapy is critical and should be done in conjunction with a GI dietitian. The ACG recommends a small-particle, low-fat, low-fiber diet to optimize gastric emptying [56]. Similarly, the UEG/ESNM advise a nutritional approach tailored to symptom severity, which can include enteral nutrition for refractory cases [57].

Pharmacologic therapy primarily involves prokinetic agents, though options remain limited. Metoclopramide is the only Food and Drug Administration (FDA)-approved prokinetic agent, but it should be used at the lowest effective dose for the shortest duration possible due to the risk of extrapyramidal effects and tardive dyskinesia [56]. Erythromycin is another prokinetic option, but tachyphylaxis limits its long-term efficacy. Domperidone, widely used internationally, remains unavailable in the United States [56, 59]. Newer agents such as prucalopride (5-HT4 receptor agonist) and ghrelin receptor agonists are promising but need further validation [56].

For patients with refractory gastroparesis, minimally invasive or surgical options may be required. Gastric peroral endoscopic pyloromyotomy (G-POEM) has emerged as a potential third-line therapy for gastroparesis, and ACG guidelines suggest pyloromyotomy over no treatment for symptom control (conditional recommendation, low quality of evidence) when medical therapy fails [56]. However,

UEG/ESNM did not endorse the statement that pyloromyotomy is effective, citing a lack of controlled validation in observational studies [57]. Gastric electrical stimulation is generally an option for diabetic gastroparesis, though its use is limited and evidence remains mixed [56]. In selected severe cases, a percutaneous gastrostomy tube with jejunal extension may be necessary for gastric venting and enteral nutrition.

11.4.3 Intestinal Dysmotility

Beyond the stomach, dysmotility can affect the small intestine and colon. Ileus is the most extreme form in the immediate postoperative period, but longer-term motility disorders may result from innervation changes or altered GI hormones following TPIAT [60]. Mechanical factors (e.g., adhesions) also contribute [61]. Increasing evidence suggests the gut microbiome influences motility, and surgical reconfiguration of the GI tract likely alters microbial composition in ways that can exacerbate or perpetuate dysmotility [62, 63].

It is crucial to exclude other causes (e.g., mechanical obstruction) before attributing symptoms to dysmotility alone. Most patients adapt over time to achieve a new baseline, but some develop severe, persistent issues. Dietary modifications and prokinetic drugs (e.g., metoclopramide, linaclotide, lubiprostone) may provide relief, while optimizing PERT can prevent undigested nutrients from aggravating symptoms [64]. Lastly, minimizing opioid use whenever feasible or employing multimodal pain management may improve GI function.

11.4.4 Gut Microbiome Alterations

CP has been associated with altered gut microbial profiles, including lower alpha diversity (i.e., reduced richness and evenness) and diminished levels of beneficial genera, such as *Faecalibacterium* [65, 66]. A recent study by the UMN group correlated lower alpha diversity with worse functional GI symptoms among CP patients undergoing evaluation for TPIAT, with sex differences and opioid use potentially influencing these relationships [67]. Additionally, the study found that TPIAT patients exhibited significant postoperative microbiome shifts, including an increase in *Bacteroides*, a genus associated with nutrient synthesis and reduced inflammatory peptides [68, 69]. However, alpha diversity did not change significantly from pre- to post-TPIAT, and the microbial structure remained statistically different from that of healthy controls [67]. While the clinical implications remain unclear, these findings open the door for targeted microbiota-based interventions to enhance postoperative outcomes.

Support for this approach comes from a recent UMN case report, where microbiota transplant therapy (MTT) successfully treated nonobstructive recurrent cholangitis in a post-TPIAT patient [70]. In this case, dysbiosis and bacterial overgrowth in the surgically modified biliary limb were implicated as drivers of infection.

Factors such as GI tract disruption, periodic antibiotic use, enteral feeding, and opioid fluctuations were thought to contribute to dysbiosis by promoting bacterial overgrowth and translocation [67, 71–73].

Although antibiotics remain the standard medical therapy for cholangitis, repeated treatment failures in this patient prompted the use of MTT to restore a healthy microbial balance. By transplanting a complete microbial community, MTT can potentially reduce the burden of resistant or virulent strains [73–75]. While not yet standard practice in this context, microbiota restructuring with MTT may merit further evaluation as an adjunctive therapy in selected cases.

11.5 Immunological and Infectious Complications

Common complications following TPIAT include surgical site infections, pneumonia, urinary tract infections, and sepsis [76, 77]. While infection profiles are generally similar between pediatric and adult cohorts, late-onset issues in children, such as overwhelming postsplenectomy infection, require further study [78]. Although spleen-sparing procedures are an option, they carry higher risks of reoperation for ischemia or bleeding (1–10%), exceeding the risks typically associated with standard splenectomy and vaccination [15, 79].

Bacterial contamination of the islet autograft represents a significant infection risk, often stemming from chronic bacterial colonization of the pancreatic duct, especially in patients with prior endoscopic or surgical interventions [76, 80]. Earlier studies found that 22–50% of islet preparations were culture-positive, yet postoperative infection rates did not rise if adequate perioperative antibiotics were administered [76, 80–82]. While most studies find no adverse effect on insulin independence, a small 27-patient study linked contaminated grafts to poorer metabolic outcomes [82].

A recent single-center study of 28 TPIAT recipients also found no direct correlation between pathogens in islet preparations and clinical infections, but the authors found islet contamination might be a surrogate marker for greater infection susceptibility, particularly in patients with advanced or long-standing CP[83]. Colonization of the pancreatic ductal system (e.g., via stenting or ductal obstruction) is believed to predispose grafts to contamination [80, 82].

Antimicrobial prophylaxis guidelines for surgery do not specifically address IAT, and the standard 24-hour broad-spectrum antibiotic course [83] may be inadequate for culture-positive islet preparations [84]. Extended regimens (up to 7 days) have been proposed, but universal guidelines are lacking [76, 80, 84]. The extent of prophylaxis and type of agent(s) typically depend on institutional protocols. Empiric regimens typically cover gram-positive, gram-negative, and anaerobic bacteria, such as piperacillin/tazobactam or a combination of metronidazole, ciprofloxacin, and cefazolin [85].

Postoperative infections are often better predicted by patient-related factors, such as poor nutrition, long-standing CP, or altered immunity, than by bacterial contamination alone. Nevertheless, detecting islet-product contamination is clinically relevant, and further research is needed to evaluate extended antibiotic prophylaxis and other strategies for preventing infections after TPIAT.

Furthermore, postsplenectomy patients require specialized precautions, including prompt medical evaluation for fever, appropriate antibiotic prophylaxis, and adherence to Centers for Disease Control and Prevention (CDC)-recommended vaccines for asplenic individuals [1, 78]. These patients face an increased risk of infections from encapsulated bacteria, including *Streptococcus pneumoniae*, *Haemophilus influenzae* type b, and *Neisseria meningitidis* [86]. Wearing medical alert bracelets is also advised for asplenic individuals.

11.6 Thrombotic Events

Thrombotic events are a notable concern after TPIAT, especially portal vein thrombosis (PVT). Potential contributors include the persistent inflammatory state in CP, prolonged surgery, and the instant blood-mediated inflammatory response (IBMIR) when tissue factor–expressing islet cells contact large volumes of portal blood [6, 11]. Such processes are usually localized rather than systemic, with IBMIR limited to presinusoidal and sinusoidal hepatic circulation [6, 87, 88]. Reported incidences vary, but partial PVT occurs in up to 10% of adult recipients and 2% of pediatric patients [11, 89], indicating children may be somewhat protected, although their overall complication profile is otherwise similar to adults [11].

Anticoagulants play a dual role in reducing thrombotic risk and supporting islet engraftment; however, balancing bleeding and thrombosis is critical. Practices vary widely among centers in terms of agent selection, monitoring, and duration [6, 90, 91]. Immediate postoperative prophylaxis with unfractionated or low-molecular-weight heparin is standard to reduce PVT risk [6, 85], and Doppler ultrasound surveillance is recommended for early detection [10]. If thrombosis is detected, patients often receive a 3-month anticoagulation course (warfarin or a direct oral anticoagulant), followed by imaging to confirm resolution [92]. Elevated risk occurs with larger islet volumes or higher portal pressures [93].

Reactive thrombocytosis is another consideration after TPIAT. It commonly occurs following splenectomy, and its timing after TPIAT mirrors that seen in other postsplenectomy states but tends to be more pronounced [94]. Reactive thrombocytosis is typically self-limiting and generally does not require treatment [95]. However, given the need for anticoagulation post-TPIAT and the risk of thrombosis, particularly PVT, aspirin is often used to reduce platelet activation and aggregation [91]. A survey found that 5 of 15 TPIAT centers initiate aspirin in adult patients between postoperative days 1 and 7 [91]. The optimal duration of antiplatelet therapy remains unclear, but discontinuing aspirin is reasonable once thrombocytosis resolves, unless otherwise indicated.

11.7 Psychological Burden

The PancreaFest Recommendations emphasize identifying clear psychological contraindications to TPIAT and distinguishing when psychiatric illnesses are modifiable [1]. Studies show TPIAT often significantly improves pain and QoL [2]. However, psychological factors extend beyond immediate surgical outcomes.

Despite the potential QoL gains, TPIAT recipients frequently have preexisting psychiatric comorbidities or chronic pain that heighten vulnerability to mental health challenges. A large retrospective review found that 38% of TPIAT patients had documented psychiatric diagnoses, typically depression and substance misuse [96]. Although perioperative mortality is low, several deaths from nonaccidental self-harm or overdose noted in an analysis from the UMN group [97] highlight the need for robust psychological assessment and support. High-risk features, such as prior suicide attempts or long-standing opioid dependence, demand careful consideration. More data are needed to determine which psychiatric conditions most strongly predict poor outcomes and how psychosocial screening can best be implemented. Ultimately, a coordinated multidisciplinary approach is critical to help patients not only survive but also achieve lasting QoL improvements.

11.8 Opioid Dependence and Withdrawal

Essentially all patients undergoing TPIAT are opioid-dependent prior to surgery [15, 90]. Postoperatively, pain management typically combines their baseline opioid requirements with adjunctive analgesia for major abdominal surgery. Multimodal strategies such as perioperative paravertebral catheters, dexmedetomidine, and ketamine are emphasized to limit overall opioid burden [85, 98].

Despite these measures, opioid withdrawal can still contribute to persistent abdominal pain after TPIAT. Weaning is often deferred until acute postoperative pain subsides, which usually occurs several weeks after surgery in the outpatient setting [90]. Standard regimens include both long- and short-acting opioids, tapering the short-acting agents first, followed by gradual reductions of long-acting formulations every 2–4 weeks. Patients and families should be counseled about potential withdrawal symptoms (e.g., nausea, vomiting, abdominal pain, anxiety) and reassured that these are generally self-limiting. In addition, involving pain specialists can help guide a safe taper and ensure optimal symptom control [1].

Recent unpublished data from the POST study provide further insight into postoperative opioid use in a large, multicenter cohort. Among 384 patients, 61% required opioids pre-TPIAT, but only 24% remained on any opioids at 1 year, underscoring the substantial decrease in opioid dependency following surgery. Notably, older age and preoperative opioid use were the strongest predictors of continued opioid requirements at 12 months. This highlights the importance of comprehensive preoperative counseling and individualized pain management plans, particularly for patients at higher risk for persistent opioid dependence.

Overall, these findings demonstrate that, although opioid therapy is nearly universal prior to TPIAT, the procedure can facilitate significant reductions in opioid burden for many patients. Achieving optimal outcomes requires proactive weaning protocols, multidisciplinary engagement, and cautious follow-up to address the complexities of pain management in the postoperative setting.

11.9 Additional Complication Considerations

11.9.1 Cholangitis

Cholangitis is a recognized complication of biliary reconstructive procedures [99, 100]. Several factors contribute to its development: removal of the sphincter of Oddi eliminates its protective role in blocking bacterial entry into the biliary tract, transient biliary stasis during the immediate postoperative period can trigger cholangitis, and anastomotic strictures from surgical technical errors may cause cholangitis months or even years later [99].

Cholangitis should be suspected in patients with abdominal pain, fever, and abnormal liver function tests. Initial evaluation includes right upper quadrant ultrasound to identify dilated bile ducts, often followed by CT or magnetic resonance cholangiopancreatography for further assessment. Recurrent cholangitis warrants investigation for anatomical causes, with endoscopic retrograde cholangiopancreatography frequently used to diagnose and treat biliary strictures. Most cases are managed endoscopically or through interventional radiology [101, 102]. Surgical reintervention may be required in rare, persistent strictures.

Importantly, recurrent cholangitis can occur after hepatobiliary tract diversions even without biliary obstruction [100, 103]. For example, 4.4% of patients with a nonstenotic hepaticojejunostomy have been reported to experience recurrent cholangitis [104]. Additionally, a recent systematic review found that small common bile duct diameter was a significant risk factor in only one of four studies analyzed [103].

Our unpublished data indicate that 22 patients with hepaticojejunostomy for benign indications experienced a total of 144 episodes of nonobstructive recurrent cholangitis over a median follow-up of 154 months, averaging 6.6 episodes per patient. These findings highlight a substantial disease burden in this population, frequently requiring recurrent hospitalizations. Moreover, this underreported condition leads to prolonged antibiotic use, reduced QoL, and increased health care costs.

Periodic antibiotic exposure may further exacerbate disease progression by increasing the pathogenic potential of commensal microbiota. This occurs through favoring the selection of antibiotic-resistant bacterial strains, suppressing nonpathogenic flora, and activating the bacterial SOS response that enhances virulence factor expression [70]. In addition, emerging evidence suggests that an altered gut microbiome may contribute to postoperative nonobstructive cholangitis, with backflow of dysbiotic microbiota into the biliary tract possibly playing a key role [70].

11.9.2 Alkaline Reflux Gastritis

TPIAT patients are prone to alkaline reflux gastritis due to disruptions in pyloric function caused by resection or altered innervation, resulting in bile backflow that damages the gastric mucosa [105]. Symptoms typically include epigastric pain, nausea, and bilious vomiting, often exacerbated by eating. This condition is more common in surgical reconstructions without a Roux limb [90]. Diagnosis is confirmed endoscopically and managed medically with proton pump inhibitors, sucralfate, and dietary adjustments. In severe or refractory cases, surgical revision to create a Roux limb may be required.

11.9.3 Marginal Ulceration

Marginal ulcers are a potential risk in all post-TPIAT patients, though their exact pathogenesis remains unclear. These ulcers often present with symptoms such as epigastric pain, nausea, vomiting, or, in some cases, GI bleeding. The UMN group reported that 35% of TPIAT patients presenting with GI bleeding were diagnosed with a marginal ulcer or an anastomotic bleed, with a median onset of 17 months after surgery [106]. In response, they implemented a protocol recommending proton pump inhibitor therapy for at least 1 year after surgery, or indefinitely if no contraindications exist. Patients with symptoms suggestive of gastritis or marginal ulcers (e.g., epigastric pain, food-related discomfort, nausea, early satiety, or burning sensation) should undergo evaluation with upper endoscopy.

11.9.4 Nephrolithiasis

Nephrolithiasis is increasingly recognized as a cause of abdominal or flank pain in post-TPIAT patients. Known complications include renal colic, recurrent urinary tract infections, and obstructive nephropathy, which can occasionally culminate in end-stage renal disease [107]. A retrospective analysis of 629 pediatric and adult TPIAT recipients found that nearly 30% developed calcium-oxalate kidney stones within 15 years after surgery [107]. This risk exceeds that of patients with CP or the general population. The rate of recurrence was high (44%), with roughly one in four episodes requiring stone removal. Older age and current or former smoker status were associated with greater risk for kidney stones [107].

Pathophysiology centers on long-standing EPI, which leads to binding of dietary calcium by unabsorbed fat and bile acids in the small intestine, reducing the availability of calcium for oxalate binding. Other explanations include altered calcium absorption, because vitamin D depends on pancreatic enzymes for absorption and its deficiency reduces intestinal calcium uptake [108]. Removal of the duodenum, a key site of calcium absorption, further impairs calcium metabolism [109]. These factors can lead to hypercalciuria and subsequent stone formation [107]. While management generally adheres to standard nephrolithiasis protocols, kidney stone risk mitigation strategies such as low-oxalate diet, adequate PERT dosage, increased fluid hydration, and calcium supplementation may be useful in those at high risk [107].

11.9.5 Pancreatic Cancer

The risk of pancreatic ductal adenocarcinoma (PDAC) poses a serious concern for CP patients, particularly those with inherited disease, although individual risk factors and optimal timing of TPIAT for high-risk cases remain unclear [1, 110]. Patients with hereditary pancreatitis and current or former smoker status have a two-fold increased likelihood of PDAC, developing cancer on average 20 years earlier than nonsmokers [111]. Although TPIAT is presumed to reduce cancer risk by removing pancreatic tissue, at least one post-TPIAT metastatic PDAC case has been reported [112].

This particular case demonstrates that neoplastic cells can potentially survive enzymatic digestion and embolize to the liver during autotransplantation into the portal venous system, resulting in metastatic disease. The patient, whose tumor markers (CEA and CA 19-9) were normal preoperatively but had pancreatic intraepithelial neoplasia found at surgery, later developed metastatic PDAC [112]. A retrospective analysis of stored preoperative serum identified three distinct microRNAs (miRNA-10b, −30c, and -106b) that were elevated. These small, noncoding RNAs are involved in biological processes such as cell proliferation, differentiation, migration, invasion, and survival. They have been implicated in PDAC pathogenesis, but not in CP [113]. Incorporating miRNA-10b, −30c, and −106b testing at this stage of care may provide a unique tool for detecting early preclinical PDAC not identified by conventional tumor markers. However, validation in larger prospective studies is needed.

11.10 Summary

TPIAT serves as a definitive solution for selected patients with chronic or recurrent acute pancreatitis, particularly when standard treatments fail. While universal exocrine insufficiency requires lifelong enzyme replacement and variable endocrine function necessitates close glycemic monitoring, the procedure distinctly improves QoL. Nevertheless, GI dysmotility (e.g., obstipation, gastroparesis), nutrition-related issues (e.g., vitamin deficiencies, bone density loss), and infection risks continue to pose challenges in postoperative care. Other concerns include thrombotic events, opioid dependence, nephrolithiasis, cholangitis, and dysbiosis.

A coordinated, multidisciplinary model—encompassing endocrinology, gastroenterology, surgery, nutrition, pain management, and mental health—is essential for long-term success. Ongoing research, especially through multicenter registries, will help refine preventive measures, monitoring protocols, and therapeutic strategies to further enhance patient outcomes after TPIAT.

References

1. Bellin MD, Freeman ML, Gelrud A, et al. Total pancreatectomy and islet autotransplantation in chronic pancreatitis: recommendations from PancreasFest. Pancreatology. 2014;14(1):27–35. https://doi.org/10.1016/j.pan.2013.10.009.
2. Abu-El-Haija M, Anazawa T, Beilman GJ, et al. The role of total pancreatectomy with islet autotransplantation in the treatment of chronic pancreatitis: a report from the international consensus guidelines in chronic pancreatitis. Pancreatology. 2020;20(4):762–71. https://doi.org/10.1016/j.pan.2020.04.005.
3. Vanek P, Freeman ML. Updates in the management of chronic pancreatitis. Gastroenterol. Clin. N. Am. 2024:S0889855324000499. https://doi.org/10.1016/j.gtc.2024.08.008.
4. Chinnakotla S, Beilman GJ, Vock D, et al. Intraportal islet autotransplantation independently improves quality of life after Total Pancreatectomy in patients with chronic refractory pancreatitis. Ann Surg. 2022;276(3):441–9. https://doi.org/10.1097/SLA.0000000000005553.
5. Hooks G, Lu H, Eaton A, et al. Addressing long-term mortality risk in patients undergoing total pancreatectomy with islet autotransplant (TPIAT): causes of death and risk factors. HPB. 2024;26(5):664–73. https://doi.org/10.1016/j.hpb.2024.02.002.
6. Robbins AJ, Skube ME, Bellin MD, et al. Portal vein thrombosis after Total Pancreatectomy and islet autotransplant: prophylaxis and graft impact. Pancreas. 2019;48(10):1329–33. https://doi.org/10.1097/MPA.0000000000001421.
7. Shahbazov R, Naziruddin B, Salam O, et al. The impact of surgical complications on the outcome of total pancreatectomy with islet autotransplantation. Am J Surg. 2020;219(1):99–105. https://doi.org/10.1016/j.amjsurg.2019.04.007.
8. Shahbazov R, Naziruddin B, Yadav K, et al. Risk factors for early readmission after total pancreatectomy and islet auto transplantation. HPB. 2018;20(2):166–74. https://doi.org/10.1016/j.hpb.2017.08.033.
9. Yamane K, Anazawa T, Nagai K, Ito T, Hatano E. Current status of total pancreatectomy with islet autotransplantation for chronic and recurrent acute pancreatitis. Annals of Gastroent Surgery. 2024;8(3):401–12. https://doi.org/10.1002/ags3.12767.
10. Bellin MD, Ramanathan K, Chinnakotla S. Total Pancreatectomy with islet auto-transplantation. Adv Surg. 2023;57(1):15–30. https://doi.org/10.1016/j.yasu.2023.03.002.
11. Nathan JD, Yang Y, Eaton A, et al. Surgical approach and short-term outcomes in adults and children undergoing total pancreatectomy with islet autotransplantation: a report from the prospective observational study of TPIAT. Pancreatology. 2022;22(1):1–8. https://doi.org/10.1016/j.pan.2021.09.011.
12. Dunderdale J, McAuliffe JC, McNeal SF, et al. Should Pancreatectomy with islet cell autotransplantation in patients with chronic alcoholic pancreatitis be abandoned? J Am Coll Surg. 2013;216(4):591–6. https://doi.org/10.1016/j.jamcollsurg.2012.12.043.
13. Garcea G, Weaver J, Phillips J, et al. Total Pancreatectomy with and without islet cell transplantation for chronic pancreatitis: a series of 85 consecutive patients. Pancreas. 2009;38(1):1–7. https://doi.org/10.1097/MPA.0b013e3181825c00.
14. Gruessner RWG, Cercone R, Galvani C, et al. Results of open and robot-assisted Pancreatectomies with autologous islet transplantations: treating chronic pancreatitis and preventing surgically induced diabetes. Transplant Proc. 2014;46(6):1978–9. https://doi.org/10.1016/j.transproceed.2014.06.005.
15. Sutherland DER, Radosevich DM, Bellin MD, et al. Total Pancreatectomy and islet autotransplantation for chronic pancreatitis. J Am Coll Surg. 2012;214(4):409–24. https://doi.org/10.1016/j.jamcollsurg.2011.12.040.
16. Wilson GC, Sutton JM, Abbott DE, et al. Long-term outcomes after Total Pancreatectomy and islet cell autotransplantation: is it a durable operation? Ann Surg. 2014;260(4):659–67. https://doi.org/10.1097/SLA.0000000000000920.

17. Wilson GC, Ahmad SA, Schauer DP, Eckman MH, Abbott DE. Cost-effectiveness of Total Pancreatectomy and islet cell autotransplantation for the treatment of minimal change chronic pancreatitis. J Gastrointest Surg. 2015;19(1):46–55. https://doi.org/10.1007/s11605-014-2612-3.
18. Kirchner VA, Dunn TB, Beilman GJ, et al. Total Pancreatectomy with islet autotransplantation for acute recurrent and chronic pancreatitis. Curr Treat Options Gastro. 2017;15(4):548–61. https://doi.org/10.1007/s11938-017-0148-9.
19. Webb MA, Illouz SC, Pollard CA, et al. Islet auto transplantation following Total Pancreatectomy: a long-term assessment of graft function. Pancreas. 2008;37(3):282–7. https://doi.org/10.1097/mpa.0b013e31816fd7b6.
20. Chinnakotla S, Radosevich DM, Dunn TB, et al. Long-term outcomes of Total Pancreatectomy and islet auto transplantation for hereditary/genetic pancreatitis. J Am Coll Surg. 2014;218(4):530–43. https://doi.org/10.1016/j.jamcollsurg.2013.12.037.
21. Chinnakotla S, Beilman GJ, Dunn TB, et al. Factors predicting outcomes after a Total Pancreatectomy and islet autotransplantation lessons learned from over 500 cases. Ann Surg. 2015;262(4):610–22. https://doi.org/10.1097/SLA.0000000000001453.
22. Bogachus LD, Oseid E, Bellin M, Vella A, Robertson RP. Deficient endogenous glucose production during exercise after Total Pancreatectomy/islet autotransplantation. J Clin Endocrinol Metab. 2017;102(9):3288–95. https://doi.org/10.1210/jc.2017-00923.
23. Bogachus LD, Bellin MD, Vella A, Robertson RP. Deficient glucagon response to hypoglycemia during a mixed meal in Total Pancreatectomy/islet autotransplantation recipients. J Clin Endocrinol Metabol. 2018;103(4):1522–9. https://doi.org/10.1210/jc.2017-02182.
24. Bellin MD, Parazzoli S, Oseid E, et al. Defective glucagon secretion during hypoglycemia after intrahepatic but not nonhepatic islet autotransplantation. Am J Transplant. 2014;14(8):1880–6. https://doi.org/10.1111/ajt.12776.
25. Bellin MD, Beilman GJ, Sutherland DER, et al. How durable is Total Pancreatectomy and Intraportal islet cell transplantation for treatment of chronic pancreatitis? J Am Coll Surg. 2019;228(4):329–39. https://doi.org/10.1016/j.jamcollsurg.2018.12.019.
26. Crosby J, Bellin MD, Radosevich DM, et al. Gastrointestinal symptoms before and after Total Pancreatectomy with islet autotransplantation: the role of pancreatic enzyme dosing and adherence. Pancreas. 2015;44(3):453–8. https://doi.org/10.1097/MPA.0000000000000266.
27. Keim V, Klar E, Poll M, Schoenberg MH. Postoperative care following pancreatic surgery. Deutsches Ärzteblatt international Published online November. 2009;27 https://doi.org/10.3238/arztebl.2009.0789.
28. McEachron KR, Downs EM, Schwarzenberg SJ, Chinnakotla S, Bellin MD. Fat-soluble vitamin deficiency is common in children with chronic pancreatitis undergoing Total Pancreatectomy with islet autotransplantation. J Pediatr Gastroenterol Nutr. 2021;72(1):123–6. https://doi.org/10.1097/MPG.0000000000002950.
29. Wothe JK, Aidoo R, McEachron KR, et al. Reduced bone mineral density in the first year after total pancreatectomy with islet autotransplantation (TPIAT). Pancreatology. 2021;21(8):1491–7. https://doi.org/10.1016/j.pan.2021.08.013.
30. Downs EM, Eaton A, Witkowski P, et al. Nutritional risks in patients undergoing Total Pancreatectomy islet AutoTransplantation in the POST consortium. J Gastrointest Surg. 2023;27(9):1893–902. https://doi.org/10.1007/s11605-023-05770-1.
31. Downs EM, Hodges JS, Trikudanathan G, et al. Essential fatty acid deficiency is common after Total Pancreatectomy and islet autotransplantation. Pancreas. 2024;53(8):e689–93. https://doi.org/10.1097/MPA.0000000000002365.
32. Mogensen KM. Essential fatty acid deficiency. Pract Gastroenterol. 2017;41(6):37–44.
33. Arvanitakis M, Ockenga J, Bezmarevic M, et al. ESPEN practical guideline on clinical nutrition in acute and chronic pancreatitis. Clin Nutr. 2024;43(2):395–412. https://doi.org/10.1016/j.clnu.2023.12.019.
34. Coates PS, Fernstrom JD, Fernstrom MH, Schauer PR, Greenspan SL. Gastric bypass surgery for morbid obesity leads to an increase in bone turnover and a decrease in bone mass. J Clin Endocrinol Metab. 2004;89(3):1061–5. https://doi.org/10.1210/jc.2003-031756.

35. Brzozowska MM, Tran T, Bliuc D, et al. Roux-en-Y gastric bypass and gastric sleeve surgery result in long term bone loss. Int J Obes. 2021;45(1):235–46. https://doi.org/10.1038/s41366-020-00660-x.
36. Hage MP, El-Hajj FG. Bone and mineral metabolism in patients undergoing roux-en-Y gastric bypass. Osteoporos Int. 2014;25(2):423–39. https://doi.org/10.1007/s00198-013-2480-9.
37. Orford NR, Lane SE, Bailey M, et al. Changes in bone mineral density in the year after critical illness. Am J Respir Crit Care Med. 2016;193(7):736–44. https://doi.org/10.1164/rccm.201508-1514OC.
38. Löhr JM, Dominguez-Munoz E, Rosendahl J, et al. United European gastroenterology evidence-based guidelines for the diagnosis and therapy of chronic pancreatitis (HaPanEU). UEG Journal. 2017;5(2):153–99. https://doi.org/10.1177/2050640616684695.
39. American Gastroenterological Association medical position statement: guidelines on osteoporosis in gastrointestinal diseases. This document presents the official recommendations of the American Gastroenterological Association (AGA) Committee on Osteoporosis in Gastrointestinal Disease. It was approved by the Clinical Practice Committee on September 21, 2002, and by the AGA Governing Board on November 1, 2002. *Gastroenterology*. 2003;124(3):791–794. doi:10.1053/gast.2003.50107.
40. Holick MF, Binkley NC, Bischoff-Ferrari HA, et al. Evaluation, treatment, and prevention of vitamin D deficiency: an Endocrine Society clinical practice guideline. J Clin Endocrinol Metabol. 2011;96(7):1911–30. https://doi.org/10.1210/jc.2011-0385.
41. Downs EM, Brun A, Bellin MD. Nutrition support in the pediatric total pancreatectomy with islet autotransplantation recipient. Nut in Clin Prac. 2024;39(1):100–8. https://doi.org/10.1002/ncp.11101.
42. Bures J, Cyrany J, Kohoutova D, et al. Small intestinal bacterial overgrowth syndrome. World J Gastroenterol. 2010;16(24):2978–90. https://doi.org/10.3748/wjg.v16.i24.2978.
43. Bushyhead D, Quigley EM. Small intestinal bacterial overgrowth. Gastroenterol Clin N Am. 2021;50(2):463–74. https://doi.org/10.1016/j.gtc.2021.02.008.
44. Kitaghenda FK, Hong J, Shao Y, Yao L, Zhu X. The prevalence of small intestinal bacterial overgrowth after roux-en-Y gastric bypass (RYGB): a systematic review and meta-analysis. Obes Surg. 2024;34(1):250–7. https://doi.org/10.1007/s11695-023-06974-9.
45. Adike A, DiBaise JK. Small intestinal bacterial overgrowth. Gastroenterol Clin N Am. 2018;47(1):193–208. https://doi.org/10.1016/j.gtc.2017.09.008.
46. Avelar Rodriguez D, Ryan PM, Toro Monjaraz EM, Ramirez Mayans JA, Quigley EM. Small intestinal bacterial overgrowth in children: a state-of-the-art review. Front Pediatr. 2019;7:363. https://doi.org/10.3389/fped.2019.00363.
47. Paraskevas KI, Avgerinos C, Manes C, Lytras D, Dervenis C. Delayed gastric emptying is associated with pylorus-preserving but not classical Whipple pancreaticoduodenectomy: a review of the literature and critical reappraisal of the implicated pathomechanism. World J Gastroenterol. 2006;12(37):5951–8. https://doi.org/10.3748/wjg.v12.i37.5951.
48. Hölzer HH, Turkelson CM, Solomon TE, Raybould HE. Intestinal lipid inhibits gastric emptying via CCK and a vagal capsaicin-sensitive afferent pathway in rats. Am J Phys. 1994;267(4 Pt 1):G625–9. https://doi.org/10.1152/ajpgi.1994.267.4.G625.
49. Yeo CJ, Barry MK, Sauter PK, et al. Erythromycin accelerates gastric emptying after Pancreaticoduodenectomy: a prospective, randomized. Placebo-Controlled Trial Annals of Surgery. 1993;218(3):229–38. https://doi.org/10.1097/00000658-199309000-00002.
50. Suzuki H, Mochiki E, Haga N, Shimura T, Itoh Z, Kuwano H. Effect of duodenectomy on gastric motility and gastric hormones in dogs. Ann Surg. 2001;233(3):353–9. https://doi.org/10.1097/00000658-200103000-00008.
51. John GK, Singh VK, Moran RA, et al. Chronic gastrointestinal Dysmotility and pain following Total Pancreatectomy with islet autotransplantation for chronic pancreatitis. J Gastrointest Surg. 2017;21(4):622–7. https://doi.org/10.1007/s11605-016-3348-z.
52. Robinson JR, Marincola P, Shelton J, Merchant NB, Idrees K, Parikh AA. Perioperative risk factors for delayed gastric emptying after a pancreaticoduodenectomy. HPB. 2015;17(6):495–501. https://doi.org/10.1111/hpb.12385.

53. Navas CM, Wadas ED, Zbib NH, Crowell MD, Lacy BE. Gastroparesis and severity of delayed gastric emptying: comparison of patient characteristics, treatments and medication adverse events. Dig Dis Sci. 2021;66(2):526–34. https://doi.org/10.1007/s10620-020-06258-7.
54. Jehangir A, Parkman HP. Chronic opioids in gastroparesis: relationship with gastrointestinal symptoms, healthcare utilization and employment. WJG. 2017;23(40):7310–20. https://doi.org/10.3748/wjg.v23.i40.7310.
55. McEachron KR, Bellin MD. Total pancreatectomy and islet autotransplantation for chronic and recurrent acute pancreatitis. Curr Opin Gastroenterol. 2018;34(5):367–73. https://doi.org/10.1097/MOG.0000000000000458.
56. Camilleri M, Kuo B, Nguyen L, et al. ACG Clinical Guideline: Gastroparesis. Am J Gastroenterol. 2022;117(8):1197–220. https://doi.org/10.14309/ajg.0000000000001874.
57. Schol J, Wauters L, Dickman R, et al. United European gastroenterology (UEG) and European Society for Neurogastroenterology and Motility (ESNM) consensus on gastroparesis. UEG J. 2021;9(3):287–306. https://doi.org/10.1002/ueg2.12060.
58. John GK, Singh VK, Pasricha PJ, et al. Delayed gastric emptying (DGE) following Total Pancreatectomy with islet auto transplantation in patients with chronic pancreatitis. J Gastrointest Surg. 2015;19(7):1256–61. https://doi.org/10.1007/s11605-015-2848-6.
59. Camilleri M, Parkman HP, Shafi MA, Abell TL, Gerson L. Clinical guideline: Management of Gastroparesis. Am J Gastroenterol. 2013;108(1):18–37. https://doi.org/10.1038/ajg.2012.373.
60. Browning KN, Travagli RA. Central nervous system control of gastrointestinal motility and secretion and modulation of gastrointestinal functions. In: Terjung R, editor Comprehensive physiology. 1st ed. Wiley; 2014:1339–1368. doi:https://doi.org/10.1002/cphy.c130055.
61. Tabibian N, Swehli E, Boyd A, Umbreen A, Tabibian JH. Abdominal adhesions: a practical review of an often overlooked entity. Ann. Med. Surg. 2017;15:9–13. https://doi.org/10.1016/j.amsu.2017.01.021.
62. Zheng Z, Tang J, Hu Y, Zhang W. Role of gut microbiota-derived signals in the regulation of gastrointestinal motility. Front Med. 2022;9:961703. https://doi.org/10.3389/fmed.2022.961703.
63. Zheng Z, Hu Y, Tang J, Xu W, Zhu W, Zhang W. The implication of gut microbiota in recovery from gastrointestinal surgery. Front Cell Infect Microbiol. 2023;13:1110787. https://doi.org/10.3389/fcimb.2023.1110787.
64. Dominguez-Muñoz JE, Vujasinovic M, De La Iglesia D, et al. European guidelines for the diagnosis and treatment of pancreatic exocrine insufficiency: UEG, EPC, EDS, ESPEN, ESPGHAN, ESDO, and ESPCG evidence-based recommendations. UEG J. Published online December 5, 2024:ueg2.12674. 2025; https://doi.org/10.1002/ueg2.12674.
65. Jandhyala SM, Madhulika A, Deepika G, et al. Altered intestinal microbiota in patients with chronic pancreatitis: implications in diabetes and metabolic abnormalities. Sci Rep. 2017;7:43640. https://doi.org/10.1038/srep43640.
66. Wang W, Xiao Y, Wang X, et al. Disordered gut microbiota in children who have chronic pancreatitis and different functional gene mutations. Clin Transl Gastroenterol. 2020;11(3):e00150. https://doi.org/10.14309/ctg.0000000000000150.
67. McEachron KR, Nalluri H, Beilman GJ, et al. Decreased intestinal microbiota diversity is associated with increased gastrointestinal symptoms in patients with chronic pancreatitis. Pancreas. 2022;51(6):649–56. https://doi.org/10.1097/MPA.0000000000002096.
68. Kelly CR, Khoruts A, Staley C, et al. Effect of fecal microbiota transplantation on recurrence in multiply recurrent Clostridium difficile infection: a randomized trial. Ann Intern Med. 2016;165(9):609–16. https://doi.org/10.7326/M16-0271.
69. Linares DM, Ross P, Stanton C. Beneficial microbes: the pharmacy in the gut. Bioengineered. 2016;7(1):11–20. https://doi.org/10.1080/21655979.2015.1126015.
70. Scott A, Khoruts A, Freeman ML, et al. Successful use of fecal microbiota transplantation in Management of Nonobstructive Recurrent Cholangitis Following Total Pancreatectomy and Islet Autotransplant. ACG Case Rep J. 2024;11(10):e01527. https://doi.org/10.14309/crj.0000000000001527.

71. Alverdy JC, Krezalek MA. Collapse of the microbiome, emergence of the Pathobiome, and the immunopathology of sepsis. Crit Care Med. 2017;45(2):337–47. https://doi.org/10.1097/CCM.0000000000002172.
72. Hasan N, Yang H. Factors affecting the composition of the gut microbiota, and its modulation. PeerJ. 2019;7:e7502. https://doi.org/10.7717/peerj.7502.
73. Bajaj JS, Shamsaddini A, Acharya C, et al. Multiple bacterial virulence factors focused on adherence and biofilm formation associate with outcomes in cirrhosis. Gut Microbes. 2021;13(1):1993584. https://doi.org/10.1080/19490976.2021.1993584.
74. Millan B, Park H, Hotte N, et al. Fecal microbial transplants reduce antibiotic-resistant genes in patients with recurrent *Clostridium difficile* infection. Clin Infect Dis. 2016;62(12):1479–86. https://doi.org/10.1093/cid/ciw185.
75. Bajaj JS, Shamsaddini A, Fagan A, et al. Fecal microbiota transplant in cirrhosis reduces gut microbial antibiotic resistance genes: analysis of two trials. Hepatol Commun. 2021;5(2):258–71. https://doi.org/10.1002/hep4.1639.
76. Berger MG, Majumder K, Hodges JS, et al. Microbial contamination of transplant solutions during pancreatic islet autotransplants is not associated with clinical infection in a pediatric population. Pancreatology. 2016;16(4):555–62. https://doi.org/10.1016/j.pan.2016.03.019.
77. Butterfield JT, Vakayil VR, Joppru K, Bellin MD, Beilman GJ, Harmon JV. Factors associated with morbidity following Total Pancreatectomy and islet autotransplantation: a NSQIP analysis. Transplant Proc. 2021;53(2):705–11. https://doi.org/10.1016/j.transproceed.2020.11.013.
78. Di Sabatino A, Carsetti R, Corazza GR. Post-splenectomy and hyposplenic states. Lancet. 2011;378(9785):86–97. https://doi.org/10.1016/S0140-6736(10)61493-6.
79. Kirchner VA, Finger EB, Bellin MD, et al. Long-term outcomes for living pancreas donors in the modern era. Transplantation. 2016;100(6):1322–8. https://doi.org/10.1097/TP.0000000000001250.
80. Colling KP, Blondet JJ, Balamurugan AN, et al. Positive sterility cultures of transplant solutions during pancreatic islet autotransplantation are associated infrequently with clinical infection. Surg Infect. 2015;16(2):115–23. https://doi.org/10.1089/sur.2013.224.
81. Johnson CN, Morgan KA, Owczarski SM, Wang H, Fried J, Adams DB. Autotransplantation of culture-positive islet product: is dirty always bad? HPB. 2014;16(7):665–9. https://doi.org/10.1111/hpb.12198.
82. Jolissaint JS, Langman LW, DeBolt CL, et al. The impact of bacterial colonization on graft success after total pancreatectomy with autologous islet transplantation: considerations for early definitive surgical intervention. Clin Transpl. 2016;30(11):1473–9. https://doi.org/10.1111/ctr.12842.
83. Bratzler DW, Dellinger EP, Olsen KM, et al. Clinical practice guidelines for antimicrobial prophylaxis in surgery. Am J Health Syst Pharm. 2013;70(3):195–283. https://doi.org/10.2146/ajhp120568.
84. Gołębiewska JE, Bachul PJ, Fillman N, et al. Early infectious complications after Total Pancreatectomy with islet autotransplantation: a single center experience. J Gastrointest Surg. 2019;23(11):2201–10. https://doi.org/10.1007/s11605-019-04118-y.
85. Szempruch KR, Walter K, Ebert N, Bridgens K, Desai CS. Pharmacological management of patients undergoing total pancreatectomy with auto-islet transplantation. Pancreatology. 2022;22(5):656–64. https://doi.org/10.1016/j.pan.2022.04.009.
86. Bonanni P, Grazzini M, Niccolai G, et al. Recommended vaccinations for asplenic and hyposplenic adult patients. Hum Vaccin Immunother. 2017;13(2):359–68. https://doi.org/10.1080/21645515.2017.1264797.
87. Boucher AA, Wastvedt S, Hodges JS, et al. Portal vein thrombosis may be more strongly associated with islet infusion than extreme thrombocytosis after Total Pancreatectomy with islet autotransplantation. Transplantation. 2021;105(11):2499–506. https://doi.org/10.1097/TP.0000000000003624.
88. Bergman ZR, Robbins AJ, Alwan FS, et al. Perioperative coagulation changes in Total Pancreatectomy and islet autotransplantation. Pancreas. 2022;51(6):671–7. https://doi.org/10.1097/MPA.0000000000002085.

89. Kawahara T, Kin T, Kashkoush S, et al. Portal vein thrombosis is a potentially preventable complication in clinical islet transplantation. Am J Transplant. 2011;11(12):2700–7. https://doi.org/10.1111/j.1600-6143.2011.03717.x.
90. Chinnakotla S, Bellin MD, Schwarzenberg SJ, et al. Total pancreatectomy and islet autotransplantation in children for chronic pancreatitis: indication, surgical techniques, postoperative management, and long-term outcomes. Ann Surg. 2014;260(1):56–64. https://doi.org/10.1097/SLA.0000000000000569.
91. Desai CS, Szempruch KR, Vonderau JS, et al. Anticoagulation practices in total pancreatectomy with autologous islet cell transplant patients: an international survey of clinical programs. Transpl Int. 2021;34(3):593–5. https://doi.org/10.1111/tri.13821.
92. Sheen CL. Clinical features, diagnosis and outcome of acute portal vein thrombosis. QJM. 2000;93(8):531–4. https://doi.org/10.1093/qjmed/93.8.531.
93. Wilhelm JJ, Bellin MD, Dunn TB, et al. Proposed thresholds for pancreatic tissue volume for safe Intraportal islet autotransplantation after Total Pancreatectomy. Am J Transplant. 2013;13(12):3183–91. https://doi.org/10.1111/ajt.12482.
94. Boucher AA, Luchtman-Jones L, Palumbo JS, et al. Extreme thrombocytosis after pediatric Pancreatectomy with islet autotransplantation is unique compared to other Postsplenectomy states. J Pediatr Surg. 2020;55(8):1645–50. https://doi.org/10.1016/j.jpedsurg.2019.09.019.
95. Bleeker JS, Hogan WJ. Thrombocytosis: diagnostic evaluation, thrombotic risk stratification, and risk-based management strategies. Thrombosis. 2011;2011:1–16. https://doi.org/10.1155/2011/536062.
96. Phillips AE, Steel JL, Amin A, et al. Psychosocial outcomes 1-year post total pancreatectomy and autologous islet cell transplant. Pediatr Transplant. 2022;26(2):e14167. https://doi.org/10.1111/petr.14167.
97. McEachron KR, Melton M, Beilman GJ, Bellin MD. Psychiatric comorbidities in patients undergoing Total Pancreatectomy with islet cell autotransplantation and associated mortality. Pancreas. 2018;47(4):e16–8. https://doi.org/10.1097/MPA.0000000000001010.
98. Hutchins J, Castro C, Wang Q, Chinnakotla S. Postoperative pain control with paravertebral catheters after pediatric total pancreatectomy and islet autotransplantation: a retrospective cohort study. Bosenberg a, ed. Pediatr Anesth. 2016;26(3):315–20. https://doi.org/10.1111/pan.12840.
99. Birgin E, Téoule P, Galata C, Rahbari NN, Reissfelder C. Cholangitis following biliary-enteric anastomosis: a systematic review and meta-analysis. Pancreatology. 2020;20(4):736–45. https://doi.org/10.1016/j.pan.2020.04.017.
100. Hata T, Sakata N, Aoki T, et al. Postoperative cholestasis and cholangitis after Total Pancreatectomy with biliary reconstruction impair the function of autotransplanted islets. Transplantation. 2013;96(5):e40–3. https://doi.org/10.1097/TP.0b013e3182a049bb.
101. Mohammad Alizadeh AH. Cholangitis: diagnosis, treatment and prognosis. J Clin Transl Hepatol. 2017;5(4):1–10. https://doi.org/10.14218/JCTH.2017.00028.
102. Miura F, Okamoto K, Takada T, et al. Tokyo guidelines 2018: initial management of acute biliary infection and flowchart for acute cholangitis. J Hepato Biliary Pancreat. 2018;25(1):31–40. https://doi.org/10.1002/jhbp.509.
103. Salaheddine Y, Henry AC, Daamen LA, et al. Risk factors for cholangitis after Pancreatoduodenectomy: a systematic review. Dig Dis Sci. 2023;68(7):3158–66. https://doi.org/10.1007/s10620-023-07929-x.
104. Overdevest AG, Fritzsche JA, Smit MAD, et al. Recurrent cholangitis in patients with a non-stenotic hepaticojejunostomy: incidence and risk factors. HPB. 2024;26(4):558–64. https://doi.org/10.1016/j.hpb.2024.01.003.
105. Burden WR, Hodges RP, Hsu M, O'Leary JP. Alkaline Reflux Gastritis. Surg Clin N Am. 1991;71(1):33–44. https://doi.org/10.1016/S0039-6109(16)45331-4.
106. Robbins AJ, Lusczek E, Bellin MD, et al. Gastrointestinal bleed after Total Pancreatectomy with islet autotransplant. Pancreas. 2021;50(6):841–6. https://doi.org/10.1097/MPA.0000000000001842.

107. Avula N, Hodges JS, Beilman G, et al. Increased kidney stone risk following total pancreatectomy with islet autotransplantation. Pancreatology. 2024;24(7):1167–73. https://doi.org/10.1016/j.pan.2024.09.004.
108. Christakos S, Dhawan P, Porta A, Mady LJ, Seth T. Vitamin D and intestinal calcium absorption. Mol Cell Endocrinol. 2011;347(1–2):25–9. https://doi.org/10.1016/j.mce.2011.05.038.
109. Bronner F. Mechanisms of intestinal calcium absorption. J Cell Biochem. 2003;88(2):387–93. https://doi.org/10.1002/jcb.10330.
110. Vanek P, Urban O, Zoundjiekpon V, Falt P. Current screening strategies for pancreatic cancer. Biomedicine. 2022;10(9):2056. https://doi.org/10.3390/biomedicines10092056.
111. Lowenfels AB, Maisonneuve P, Whitcomb DC, Lerch MM, DiMagno EP. Cigarette smoking as a risk factor for pancreatic cancer in patients with hereditary pancreatitis. JAMA. 2001;286(2):169–70. https://doi.org/10.1001/jama.286.2.169.
112. Muratore S, Zeng X, Korc M, et al. Metastatic pancreatic adenocarcinoma after Total Pancreatectomy islet autotransplantation for chronic pancreatitis. Am J Transplant. 2016;16(9):2747–52. https://doi.org/10.1111/ajt.13851.
113. Croce CM. Causes and consequences of microRNA dysregulation in cancer. Nat Rev Genet. 2009;10(10):704–14. https://doi.org/10.1038/nrg2634.

12 Total Pancreatectomy with Islet Autotransplantation (TPIAT) for Alcoholic Pancreatitis

Luis F. Lara and Gregory C. Wilson

Abstract

Alcohol use disorder (AUD) affects 7% of the world population and has a high health burden, including a high risk of acute and chronic pancreatitis. Over 80% of individuals with AUD also smoke, which is itself a risk factor for pancreatitis. Most centers require 6 months of sobriety before performing total pancreatectomy with islet autotransplantation (TPIAT), so patients require active counseling on remaining sober and abstinent from smoking. Studies of TPIAT rarely evaluate outcomes by etiology, but heavy alcohol consumption and smoking are both associated with an increased risk of postoperative complications. However, it is not clear whether light or moderate alcohol use is problematic or whether complete abstinence is needed for a successful TPIAT. Chronic pancreatitis is associated with an increased burden of psychological diseases, which are exacerbated by AUD; even those who achieve sobriety may be more prone to anxiety and depression after TPIAT and will need psychological support. Thus, the need to treat ongoing pain and distress from chronic pancreatitis with TPIAT or other procedures must be weighed against the risks inherent in treating patients with AUD.

L. F. Lara (✉)
Division of Digestive Diseases, University of Cincinnati, Cincinnati, OH, USA
e-mail: laralf@ucmail.uc.edu

G. C. Wilson
Division of Surgical Oncology, University of Cincinnati College of Medicine, Cincinnati, OH, USA

S. Chinnakotla et al. (eds.), *Total Pancreatectomy and Islet Auto Transplantation*, https://doi.org/10.1007/978-981-92-0018-4_12

Key Points

1. Alcohol use is prevalent.
2. Alcohol use disorder (AUD) is a major cause of recurrent acute pancreatitis and chronic pancreatitis, of disease progression, and of poorer endoscopic and surgical outcomes.
3. Most centers that perform total pancreatectomy with islet autotransplantation (TPIAT) require at least 6 months of alcohol abstinence, but it is not clear how alcohol abstinence is confirmed or whether absolute abstinence is necessary.
4. Most TPIAT studies include a small number of patients with a history of AUD and do not report the outcomes based on the etiology of pancreatic disease, so the actual outcomes of TPIAT in patients with AUD remain unclear.
5. Alcohol recidivism is common, so patients need long-term follow-up and control of associated psychological factors, which also require long-term follow-up.

12.1 Alcohol Use

According to the World Health Organization, alcohol use disorder (AUD) affects 7% of the world population. In 2019, it was associated with 2.6 million deaths, of which 1.9 million were related to diseases and 700,000 were related to injuries [1]. In the United States, social drinking in adults is common (85%), 23.5% are binge drinkers, and 7.8% are heavy drinkers (defined as >14 alcoholic drinks per week for men and > 7 drinks per week for females), with a similar distribution in both sexes, according to the 2023 National Survey on Drug Use and Health and the Centers for Disease Control [2, 3]. The Diagnostic and Statistical Manual of Mental Disorders (DSM–5) characterizes AUD as the inability to control alcohol use despite adverse consequences, and it can be mild, moderate, or severe [4].

In the United States, a standard drink contains 14 grams or 0.6 fluid ounces of ethanol, which is the equivalent of 12 ounces of 5% alcohol/volume beer or 1.5 ounces of an 80-proof (i.e., 40% alcohol/volume) liquor (Fig. 12.1).

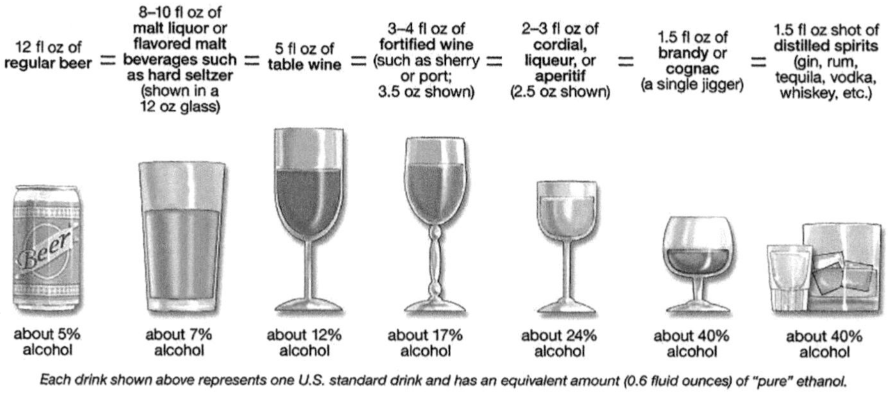

Fig. 12.1 Standard drink equivalents. (Reproduced from [5])

Table 12.1 Recommended amount of alcohol to minimize the risk of disease [2, 3]

	Daily	Weekly	Occasional
Men	2 drinks	14 drinks	4 drinks
Women	1 drink	7 drinks	3 drinks

To minimize alcohol-related risks, the U.S. Dietary Guidelines recommend ≤1 drink a day for females and ≤2 drinks per day for males (Table 12.1) [5].

Alcohol use increases the risk of many diseases, including neoplasia, hepatic diseases, and acute pancreatitis (AP) and chronic pancreatitis (CP) [6].

12.2 The Burden of Acute and Chronic Pancreatitis

Data derived from the Global Burden of Disease Study 2019 [6] showed that new cases of AP are increasing, with an age-standardized rate of 8.7 to 82 cases per 100,000 people [5]. Alcohol and gallstones are the most common causes of AP worldwide; it remains more common in males, and the incidence is spread equally among different sociodemographic groups [7, 8]. Although the total number of deaths associated with AP has increased in the last 20 years, the age-standardized mortality prevalence has decreased to 1.4/100,000 [8]. AP accounts for 5.5% of adult emergency department visits, and the most common etiologies are alcohol and exacerbations of CP [9].

The incidence of CP is between 4 and 12/100,000, with a prevalence of 37 to 99/100,000 people and a slight male predominance. It is frequently associated with alcohol or smoking, and usually with both [10, 11]. CP accounts for frequent emergency department admissions and significant loss of productivity (2.6 billion US dollars per year). At diagnosis, 30% of subjects are already suffering from some disability, and, over time, 50% of subjects become unable to work regularly [11].

The amount and length of alcohol ingestion that result in AP or CP remain unclear, but it appears likely that cumulative dosing >20 g/day over a span of years is necessary [12]. Other environmental factors such as smoking, genetic mutations that affect alcohol metabolism or the susceptibility to pancreatic diseases, and alcohol ingestion concurrent with other etiologies for AP (such as gallstones) may result in a more severe presentation of the disease or an increased risk of progression to CP, eventual endocrine and exocrine pancreatic failure, and associated morbidities. Pain, which has a complex etiology, is the most significant clinical manifestation of the disease and has the most salient effect on quality of life [12–18].

12.3 The Effect of Alcohol on the Pancreas

Alcohol metabolism in the liver has been well described, and it is interesting that many of the mechanisms are present in the human pancreas as well, but the sequence of alcohol interactions that lead to pancreatic inflammation and the necrosis–fibrosis sequence remain unclear [6, 19, 20]. As in the liver, pancreatic alcohol dehydrogenase oxidizes ethanol to acetaldehyde, and, as the dose increases, acetaldehyde accumulates. There is a shift to nonoxidative ethanol metabolism, which overwhelms mitochondrial glutathione and enhances the formation of fatty acid ethyl esters and free radicals (reactive oxygen species). This results in tissue hypoxia; abnormal intracellular calcium signaling; activation of inflammatory transcription factors including NF-κB and AP-1; bacterial endotoxemia possibly due to gut hyperpermeability and translocation; and an enhanced inflammatory response that affects acinar cell stability and causes unstable autophagy, inappropriate activation of digestive and lysosomal enzymes, and stellate cell activation [19, 21–23]. Ethanol also increases secretion of duodenal cholecystokinin (CCK)-releasing factor, which releases acinar pancreatic enzymes and leads to production of a protein-rich pancreatic juice that obstructs pancreatic ductules and intraductal pancreatic enzyme activation; this causes pancreatic autodigestion, fibrosis, and acinar atrophy [24–27]. Over 80% of subjects with AUD also consume tobacco, and tobacco smoke by itself is an important risk factor for pancreatic disease, so together they have a synergistic and potentiating pancreatotoxic effect [14, 28].

12.4 Treatment

The treatment of AP associated with AUD involves ruling out other causes and disease modifiers such as underlying genetic conditions. Continued alcohol use can result in AP recurrences and progression to CP in 13–32% of patients after 3–5 years, and the risk is increased with ongoing tobacco use, so patients require active counseling on remaining sober and abstinent [29–32].

The treatment of CP is reviewed elsewhere in the book (Chaps. 6, 7, and 8). Many institutions have a multidisciplinary patient management conference to chart a usually progressive therapeutic plan for these complex patients [33–35]. Interventions to abstain from alcohol and tobacco should be instituted [36]. The medical history needs to be reviewed for other risk factors, including pancreatotoxic medications. Patients need to be tested for endocrine and exocrine pancreatic dysfunction and treated accordingly [35]. Nutritional deficiencies are not uncommon and need to be addressed. The role of genetic testing remains unclear, but, given the increased availability and affordability, it should be considered because some patients may have an underlying mutation amenable and responsive to treatment [37–39]. Pain management with opioid-sparing medication should be initiated soon, and inclusion in a comprehensive pain management plan is desirable because most patients will eventually require opioids, with the subsequent risk of opioid dependency [36].

Endoscopic retrograde cholangiopancreatography with pancreatic duct cannulation, pancreatic and/or biliary sphincterotomy, pancreatic duct dilation and/or stenting, and removal or lithotripsy of pancreatic duct stones can be performed on a case-by-case basis. The role of endoscopic therapy in small-duct disease without ductal dilation remains controversial [40].

Surgical therapy will be the end point for 25–30% of patients with CP [41]. The surgical approaches can be summarized as gland resection (anatomical resections versus traditional CP resections), ductal drainage procedures (lateral pancreaticojejunostomy or Puestow procedure), combination of resection and drainage (Frey procedure), and subtotal or total pancreatectomy with islet autotransplantation (TPIAT) [42].

12.5 Total Pancreatectomy with Islet Autotransplantation in Patients with Alcohol-Induced Pancreatic Disease

Subjects with CP are considered for treatment with TPIAT, usually as destination therapy, after other medical, endoscopic, and sometimes surgical treatment strategies have failed to control pain and/or AP recurrences and when the disease burden, mostly characterized by pain, is substantial enough to justify the risks of the intervention [43–45]. The decision to pursue TPIAT should be made in a high-volume center with the capacity for a multidisciplinary approach for chronic pancreatitis. When surgical intervention is considered, the morphology of the disease drives surgical decision-making. Patients with focal gland involvement or a dilated pancreatic duct would be considered for resection and/or a drainage procedure [46–48]. When the disease is not amenable to one of the traditional surgical procedures, or if a previous surgical intervention for CP has failed, then TPIAT is considered. Patients with recurrent AP (RAP), idiopathic or primary, can also be selected for TPIAT. Its use for AP has been limited to cases where significant loss of pancreatic parenchyma is expected, and the goal becomes saving islets and decreasing the risk of postintervention diabetes [49]. TPIAT has also been reported for unique conditions of the pancreas like polycystic pancreatic disease, arteriovenous malformations, and others [50].

A major hurdle to identifying the benefits of TPIAT in CP associated with AUD is that most (if not all) centers performing TPIAT exclude subjects who are actively drinking, so it is assumed that patients are sober. Furthermore, studies generally report TPIAT outcomes as a group without distinguishing by etiology, making it impossible to identify differences by cause of the pancreatic disease. Additionally, in the largest available series, less than 10% of patients undergoing TPIAT have a diagnosis of AUD as the etiology of CP [51, 52]. It is likely, and consistent with our institution's clinical practice, that these patients with CP from AUD, in general, are better candidates for traditional CP operations given the frequent calcific disease and dilated pancreatic ducts. Given this, it is difficult to individualize outcomes in patients with alcohol-associated pancreatic disease who undergo TPIAT regarding periprocedural complications, islet yield, metabolic outcomes, quality of life and emotional factors, pain, and opioid use compared to other etiologies of CP, and the rate of alcohol recidivism after TPIAT remains unknown [33, 51, 53]. Little is reported about TPIAT outcomes in children with AUD, but alcohol use is not prevalent in the pancreatitis study cohorts in this population [54]. In most TPIAT studies, alcohol is not the most common etiology associated with pancreatic disease, suggesting a patient-selection bias, or it may indicate that patients with alcohol-induced CP may have inadequate pancreas morphology, liver function, or other characteristics that make them unsuitable for TPIAT [55, 56].

Despite the shortcomings, information from other treatment strategies for alcohol-related CP and the effect of medical, endoscopic, and surgical interventions in these patients can be used to inform the effect that TPIAT may have on outcomes. It is well described that pancreatic disease will progress in subjects who continue to consume alcohol, so it can be expected that TPIAT outcomes are likely poorer in patients who are unable to achieve sobriety. At any rate, TPIAT outcomes that include patients with a history of AUD should be considered highly selective and are probably not representative of the larger population with alcohol-associated RAP or CP who will never be candidates for TPIAT [43].

Endoscopic therapy is less successful in alleviating pain in patients who continue to consume alcohol and/or smoke [57]. In these patients, pancreatic disease progresses, and continued treatment of pancreatic ductal or parenchymal changes with endoscopic drainage, stricture dilation, and stenting may lead to disease that either persists or recurs, which raises the issue of whether it is appropriate to continue to pursue endoscopic treatment or to consider step-up to more definitive surgical interventions including TPIAT in patients who are unable to become or remain sober, given that the disease will almost always progress. The alternate approach would be to consider stopping treatments [57, 58].

Alcohol and smoking affect the postoperative recovery period after pancreatobiliary surgery independent of the underlying pathology and are associated with an increased risk of postoperative complications such as anastomotic dehiscence, pancreatic or biliary duct leak, and delayed wound healing [59]. Alcohol abstinence before pancreatobiliary surgery is ideal, but, unlike heavy alcohol use, which is associated with an increased risk of complications, it is not clear if light-to-moderate alcohol use affects outcomes of pancreatobiliary surgery. It is also not clear if alcohol abstinence, compared to mild, moderate, or heavy alcohol use, influences surgical outcomes specifically for patients with AUD-associated pancreatic disease where other factors, such as concomitant smoking or genetic predisposition, also participate in disease progression [60, 61]. Smoking should be stopped for at least 4 weeks before surgery, as this timeline has a major effect on postsurgical morbidity and outcomes [59]. Regardless of the operation performed, long-term mortality after surgical intervention is worse in patients with alcohol-induced CP [62]. Additionally, the cause of death is more likely to be related to substance abuse and liver disease in these patients than in a similar cohort with other etiologies [62].

Most institutions have adopted the liver transplantation recommendation of requiring sobriety for at least 6 months before considering a TPIAT. Unlike liver transplantation, the extent of preoperative evaluation to rule out ongoing alcohol use prior to TPIAT is poorly studied, and concurrent alcohol use is not systematically tested even in high-risk patients. For example, while phosphatidylethanol (PEth) testing is commonly performed in patients undergoing liver transplant evaluation, it is not common to perform this in patients undergoing TPIAT evaluation [63, 64]. Self-reported alcohol use is unreliable and many times diverges from objective studies, including the PEth level, so it is probable that some patients with alcohol-related pancreatic disease undergoing TPIAT evaluation continue to consume alcohol up to and after the surgical procedure [65]. Patients are advised to quit smoking, but smoking is not an absolute contraindication for TPIAT; however, many surgery programs pursue smoking cessation before TPIAT because of the perisurgical risks of pancreatobiliary surgery associated with continued tobacco use [59]. Unfortunately, long-term smoking cessation has been generally unsuccessful in patients with CP despite enrollment in a directed program [66].

One retrospective study has specifically evaluated the role of TPIAT in the AUD patient population compared to a non-AUD CP cohort. The goal of this study of 100 patients with CP was to optimize patient selection for IAT based on etiology. It compared outcomes between 30 patients with CP and a history of AUD and 70 patients with CP and other etiologies and is the best-phenotyped study to report TPIAT outcomes in this population [67]. Patients with CP and a history of AUD had lower successful islet retrieval and islet yield, and patient-reported quality of life and pain scores did not improve long term in this group compared with patients with non–AUD-associated CP. Unfortunately, there is no information about the duration of alcohol abstinence; how sobriety was confirmed; the outcomes related to other non–AUD-associated CP diagnoses; or the duration of CP, which is known to affect islet yield and metabolic outcomes. Some patients had previous pancreatic resections, and not all patients underwent a total pancreatectomy but rather had segmental pancreatic resections, so the questions of TPIAT selection and metabolic, quality-of-life, and pain outcomes in patients with AUD with CP remain unanswered [44]. The benefits and outcomes in patients with AUD and RAP who undergo TPIAT also remain unclear.

As is the case with most chronic painful diseases, the etiology of pain in CP is complex, with peripheral neuropathic and central pain and an increased burden of psychological diseases, including anxiety and depression, which are exacerbated by concomitant alcohol and tobacco use [33, 68]. The type of pancreatic pain, intermittent (Ammann type 1) or persistent (Ammann type 2), may also determine the pain response to any intervention, including TPIAT [69]. TPIAT is usually not offered to patients with ongoing alcohol use, and efforts are made to curtail smoking, but even previous use of alcohol or tobacco may predict anxiety or depression exacerbations after TPIAT [68]. Pain and opioid use may also persist after TPIAT, so patients need to be followed for recurrence of psychological diseases to help them cope with anxiety and depression, and patients should remain under counseling for alcohol and smoking abstinence to minimize recidivism [68, 70]. The factors that may affect TPIAT outcomes in patients with a history of AUD are described in Box 12.1.

Box 12.1: Factors that may result in poor TPIAT outcomes in patients with alcohol use disorder–associated pancreatic disease

Active alcohol use[a]
Ammann type 2 pain
Duration of disease > 5 years
Tobacco smoking
Previous pancreatic surgery
Presence of glucose intolerance
Islet yield < 5000 IEQ/kg body weight

[a]The effect of mild or moderate alcohol use compared to heavy alcohol use is unknown. *IEQ* islet equivalents

Gene profiling of a small number of patients from tissue obtained during TPIAT suggested biological differences according to whether the etiology of the CP was alcoholic, idiopathic, or hereditary, which in the future may allow for different treatment approaches according to genotype and phenotype [71].

Regardless of etiology, in highly selected patients, TPIAT results in improved pain scores, decreased opioid use, improved quality of life, and decreased resource utilization, as well as insulin independence or adequate glucose control [42, 72, 73].

12.6 Ethics of TPIAT in Alcohol Use Disorder

The discussion by Al-Moussaly et al. is one of the few attempts at reviewing the ethical concerns about continuing to offer endoscopic therapy for CP in subjects who continue to consume alcohol with the premise that the disease is a result of poor choices, yet patient autonomy and the inherent physician interest in helping patients create a therapeutic dilemma [57]. On one side, one can lean on the evidence showing that continuing to consume alcohol (and smoking) leads to disease progression. Also, endoscopic and surgical interventions are less successful and can be associated with increased morbidity and other complications in patients who continue to consume alcohol, so one could defend the futility of further interventions. That reasoning would also justify not performing angioplasty on a patient with an acute myocardial infarction who is poorly compliant with weight management. We need to recognize that addiction is a disease, many times with a family or genetic component, with patient challenges regarding access to counseling, rehabilitation, and long-term care, and that, despite access to these, long-term success remains evasive and recidivism is common [74, 75]. A decision not to treat must be tempered against the presenting symptoms, the possibility that an intervention will help alleviate disease progression or pain, and the potential that continuing interventions for addiction, as well as treating underlying psychosocial factors, may eventually result in abstinence. A multidisciplinary management conference can help delineate an institutional approach that also considers patient autonomy, patient capacity to understand the disease process and personal responsibility when making decisions about interventions, and risks and benefits of offering or withholding treatment [34, 57, 74].

12.7 Conclusions

The role of TPIAT for patients with alcohol-induced CP remains unclear. Treatment of RAP and CP requires a comprehensive approach to understanding the etiology, which should include genetic testing. Patients with AUD and RAP or CP should undergo counseling and treatment for sobriety, as well as underlying psychiatric diseases, which many times coexist with AUD. Smoking is common in subjects with AUD, so it should also be addressed.

Diagnosis and follow-up of AUD in patients being considered for TPIAT need to be confirmed by objective means, such as PEth testing. In appropriately selected patients with RAP and CP, endoscopic and surgical interventions including TPIAT have favorable pain control outcomes, and, in some patients, TPIAT should be considered sooner rather than allowing the disease to progress, but it is not clear if this approach should be expanded to patients with severe alcohol use [76, 77].

References

1. World Health Organization. Alcohol 2024. Available from: https://www.who.int/news-room/fact-sheets/detail/alcohol.
2. Boersma P, Villarroel MA, Vahratian A. Heavy Drinking Among U.S. Adults, 2018. Centers for Disease Control and Prevention, National Center for Health Statistics; 2020. Contract No.: NCHS Data Brief No. 374.
3. National Institute on Alcohol Abuse and Alcoholism. Alcohol use in the united states: age groups and demographic characteristics 2025. Available from: https://www.niaaa.nih.gov/alcohols-effects-health/alcohol-topics-z/alcohol-facts-and-statistics/alcohol-use-united-states-age-groups-and-demographic-characteristics.
4. Diagnostic and statistical manual of mental disorders. 5th edition. American Psychiatric Association; 2013.
5. National Institute on Alcohol Abuse and Alcoholism. The Basics: Defining How Much Alcohol is Too Much 2025 [Available from: https://www.niaaa.nih.gov/health-professionals-communities/core-resource-on-alcohol/basics-defining-how-much-alcohol-too-much#pub-toc0.
6. Meza V, Arnold J, Díaz LA, Ayala Valverde M, Idalsoaga F, Ayares G, et al. Alcohol consumption: medical implications, the liver and beyond. Alcohol Alcohol. 2022;57(3):283–91. https://doi.org/10.1093/alcalc/agac013.
7. Institute for Health Metrics and Evaluation, Global health data exchange. Global burden of disease study 2019 (GBD 2019) Data resources. Available from: https://ghdx.healthdata.org/gbd-2019.
8. Wen Y, Luo Y, Huang Y, Zhang Z, Xiong L, Wang Y. Global, regional, and national pancreatitis burden and health inequality of pancreatitis from 1990 to 2019 with a prediction from 2020 to 2034. BMC Public Health. 2024;24(1) https://doi.org/10.1186/s12889-024-20796-z.

9. Garg SK, Sarvepalli S, Campbell JP, Obaitan I, Singh D, Bazerbachi F, et al. Incidence, admission rates, and predictors, and economic burden of adult emergency visits for acute pancreatitis. J Clin Gastroenterol. 2019;53(3):220–5. https://doi.org/10.1097/mcg.0000000000001030.
10. Yadav D, Lowenfels AB. The epidemiology of pancreatitis and pancreatic cancer. Gastroenterology. 2013;144(6):1252–61. https://doi.org/10.1053/j.gastro.2013.01.068.
11. Conwell DL, Lee LS, Yadav D, Longnecker DS, Miller FH, Mortele KJ, et al. American pancreatic association practice guidelines in chronic pancreatitis. Pancreas. 2014;43(8):1143–62. https://doi.org/10.1097/mpa.0000000000000237.
12. DiMagno MJ. Oktoberfest binge drinking and acute pancreatitis: is there really no relationship? Clin Gastroenterol Hepatol. 2011;9(11):920–2. https://doi.org/10.1016/j.cgh.2011.07.022.
13. Papachristou GI, Papachristou DJ, Morinville VD, Slivka A, Whitcomb DC. Chronic alcohol consumption is a major risk factor for pancreatic necrosis in acute pancreatitis. Am J Gastroenterol. 2006;101(11):2605–10. https://doi.org/10.1111/j.1572-0241.2006.00795.x.
14. Yadav D, Hawes RH, Brand RE, Anderson MA, Money ME, Banks PA, et al. Alcohol consumption, cigarette smoking, and the risk of recurrent acute and chronic pancreatitis. Arch Intern Med. 2009;169(11):1035–45. https://doi.org/10.1001/archinternmed.2009.125.
15. Maisonneuve P, Lowenfels AB, Mullhaupt B, Cavallini G, Lankisch PG, Andersen JR, et al. Cigarette smoking accelerates progression of alcoholic chronic pancreatitis. Gut. 2005;54(4):510–4. https://doi.org/10.1136/gut.2004.039263.
16. Coté GA, Yadav D, Slivka A, Hawes RH, Anderson MA, Burton FR, et al. Alcohol and smoking as risk factors in an epidemiology study of patients with chronic pancreatitis. Clin Gastroenterol Hepatol. 2011;9(3):266–73. https://doi.org/10.1016/j.cgh.2010.10.015.
17. Machicado JD, Amann ST, Anderson MA, Abberbock J, Sherman S, Conwell DL, et al. Quality of life in chronic pancreatitis is determined by constant pain, disability/unemployment, current smoking, and associated co-morbidities. Am J Gastroenterol. 2017;112(4):633–42. https://doi.org/10.1038/ajg.2017.42.
18. Tjora E, Dimcevski G, Haas SL, Erchinger F, Vujasinovic M, Löhr M, et al. Patient reported exposure to smoking and alcohol abuse are associated with pain and other complications in patients with chronic pancreatitis. Pancreatology. 2020;20(5):844–51. https://doi.org/10.1016/j.pan.2020.05.001.
19. Chowdhury P, Gupta P. Pathophysiology of alcoholic pancreatitis: an overview. World J Gastroenterol. 2006;12(46):7421–7. https://doi.org/10.3748/wjg.v12.i46.7421.
20. Rocco A, Compare D, Angrisani D, Sanduzzi Zamparelli M, Nardone G. Alcoholic disease: liver and beyond. World J Gastroenterol. 2014;20(40):14652–9. https://doi.org/10.3748/wjg.v20.i40.14652.
21. Pandol SJ, Periskic S, Gukovsky I, Zaninovic V, Jung Y, Zong Y, et al. Ethanol diet increases the sensitivity of rats to pancreatitis induced by cholecystokinin octapeptide. Gastroenterology. 1999;117(3):706–16. https://doi.org/10.1016/s0016-5085(99)70465-8.
22. Gukovskaya AS, Mouria M, Gukovsky I, Reyes CN, Kasho VN, Faller LD, et al. Ethanol metabolism and transcription factor activation in pancreatic acinar cells in rats. Gastroenterology. 2002;122(1):106–18. https://doi.org/10.1053/gast.2002.30302.
23. Sutton R, Petersen OH, Pandol SJ. Pancreatitis and calcium Signalling. Pancreas. 2008;36(4):e1–e14. https://doi.org/10.1097/mpa.0b013e3181675010.
24. Saluja AK, Bhagat L. Pathophysiology of alcohol-induced pancreatic injury. Pancreas. 2003;27(4):327–31. https://doi.org/10.1097/00006676-200311000-00010.
25. Sarles H. Alcoholism and pancreatitis. Scand J Gastroenterol. 1971;6(3):193–8. https://doi.org/10.3109/00365527109180692.
26. Lankisch PG, Apte M, Banks PA. Acute pancreatitis. Lancet. 2015;386(9988):85–96. https://doi.org/10.1016/s0140-6736(14)60649-8.
27. Clemens DL, Schneider KJ, Arkfeld CK, Grode JR, Wells MA, Singh S. Alcoholic pancreatitis: new insights into the pathogenesis and treatment. World J Gastrointest Pathophysiol. 2016;7(1):48–58. https://doi.org/10.4291/wjgp.v7.i1.48.

28. Batel P, Pessione F, Maitre C, Rueff B. Relationship between alcohol and tobacco dependencies among alcoholics who smoke. Addiction. 1995;90(7):977–80. https://doi.org/10.1111/j.1360-0443.1995.tb03507.x.
29. Nøjgaard C, Becker U, Matzen P, Andersen JR, Holst C, Bendtsen F. Progression from acute to chronic pancreatitis. Pancreas. 2011;40(8):1195–200. https://doi.org/10.1097/mpa.0b013e318221f569.
30. Yadav D, O'Connell M, Papachristou GI. Natural history following the first attack of acute pancreatitis. Am J Gastroenterol. 2012;107(7):1096–103. https://doi.org/10.1038/ajg.2012.126.
31. Gardner TB, Adler DG, Forsmark CE, Sauer BG, Taylor JR, Whitcomb DC. ACG clinical guideline: chronic pancreatitis. Am J Gastroenterol. 2020;115(3):322–39. https://doi.org/10.14309/ajg.0000000000000535.
32. Whitcomb DC, Frulloni L, Garg P, Greer JB, Schneider A, Yadav D, et al. Chronic pancreatitis: an international draft consensus proposal for a new mechanistic definition. Pancreatology. 2016;16(2):218–24. https://doi.org/10.1016/j.pan.2016.02.001.
33. Anderson MA, Akshintala V, Albers KM, Amann ST, Belfer I, Brand R, et al. Mechanism, assessment and management of pain in chronic pancreatitis: recommendations of a multidisciplinary study group. Pancreatology. 2016;16(1):83–94. https://doi.org/10.1016/j.pan.2015.10.015.
34. Lara LF, Takita M, Burdick JS, DC DM, Pimentel RR, Erim T, et al. A study of the clinical utility of a 20-minute secretin-stimulated endoscopic pancreas function test and performance according to clinical variables. Gastrointest Endosc. 2017;86(6):1048–55.e2. https://doi.org/10.1016/j.gie.2017.03.1532.
35. Gariepy CE, Lara LF, Easler JJ, Shaikhkhalil A, Uc A. Pediatric-to-adult transfer of Care in Patients with Pancreas Disease: recommendations for care and research opportunities. Am J Gastroenterol. 2022;118(3):443–51. https://doi.org/10.14309/ajg.0000000000001910.
36. Hart PA, Conwell DL. Chronic pancreatitis: managing a difficult disease. Am J Gastroenterol. 2019;115(1):49–55. https://doi.org/10.14309/ajg.0000000000000421.
37. Ramsey ML, Heald B, Gokun Y, Baker J, Groce JR, Han S, et al. Germline multigene panel testing in acute and chronic pancreatitis. PLoS One. 2024;19(8):e0307076. https://doi.org/10.1371/journal.pone.0307076.
38. Ramsey ML, Li SS, Lara LF, Gokun Y, Akshintala VS, Conwell DL, et al. Cystic fibrosis transmembrane conductance regulator modulators and the exocrine pancreas: a scoping review. J Cyst Fibros. 2023;22(2):193–200. https://doi.org/10.1016/j.jcf.2022.08.008.
39. Ramsey ML, Gokun Y, Sobotka LA, Wellner MR, Porter K, Kirkby SE, et al. Cystic fibrosis transmembrane conductance regulator modulator use is associated with reduced pancreatitis hospitalizations in patients with cystic fibrosis. Am J Gastroenterol. 2021;116(12):2446–54. https://doi.org/10.14309/ajg.0000000000001527.
40. Kitano M, Gress TM, Garg PK, Itoi T, Irisawa A, Isayama H, et al. International consensus guidelines on interventional endoscopy in chronic pancreatitis. Recommendations from the working group for the international consensus guidelines for chronic pancreatitis in collaboration with the International Association of Pancreatology, the American pancreatic association, the Japan pancreas society, and European pancreatic Club. Pancreatology. 2020;20(6):1045–55. https://doi.org/10.1016/j.pan.2020.05.022.
41. Andersen DK, Frey CF. The evolution of the surgical treatment of chronic pancreatitis. Ann Surg. 2010;251(1):18–32. https://doi.org/10.1097/sla.0b013e3181ae3471.
42. Wilson GC, Sutton JM, Smith MT, Schmulewitz N, Salehi M, Choe KA, et al. Completion pancreatectomy and islet cell autotransplantation as salvage therapy for patients failing previous operative interventions for chronic pancreatitis. Surgery. 2015;158(4):872–80. https://doi.org/10.1016/j.surg.2015.04.045.
43. Bellin MD, Abu-El-Haija M, Morgan K, Adams D, Beilman GJ, Chinnakotla S, et al. A multicenter study of total pancreatectomy with islet autotransplantation (TPIAT): POST (prospective observational study of TPIAT). Pancreatology. 2018;18(3):286–90. https://doi.org/10.1016/j.pan.2018.02.001.

44. Takita M, Lara LF, Naziruddin B, Shahbazov R, Lawrence MC, Kim PT, et al. Effect of the duration of chronic pancreatitis on pancreas islet yield and metabolic outcome following islet autotransplantation. J Gastrointest Surg. 2015;19(7):1236–46. https://doi.org/10.1007/s11605-015-2828-x.
45. Abu-El-Haija M, Anazawa T, Beilman GJ, Besselink MG, Del Chiaro M, Demir IE, et al. The role of total pancreatectomy with islet autotransplantation in the treatment of chronic pancreatitis: a report from the international consensus guidelines in chronic pancreatitis. Pancreatology. 2020;20(4):762–71. https://doi.org/10.1016/j.pan.2020.04.005.
46. Izbicki JR, Bloechle C, Broering DC, Knoefel WT, Kuechler T, Broelsch CE. Extended drainage versus resection in surgery for chronic pancreatitis. Ann Surg. 1998;228(6):771–9. https://doi.org/10.1097/00000658-199812000-00008.
47. Frey CF, Amikura K. Local resection of the head of the pancreas combined with longitudinal Pancreaticojejunostomy in the Management of Patients with chronic pancreatitis. Ann Surg. 1994;220(4):492–507. https://doi.org/10.1097/00000658-199410000-00008.
48. Bachmann K, Tomkoetter L, Erbes J, Hofmann B, Reeh M, Perez D, et al. Beger and Frey procedures for treatment of chronic pancreatitis: comparison of outcomes at 16-year follow-up. J Am Coll Surg. 2014;219(2):208–16. https://doi.org/10.1016/j.jamcollsurg.2014.03.040.
49. Jindal RM, Ricordi C, Shriver CD. Autologous pancreatic islet transplantation for severe trauma. N Engl J Med. 2010;362(16):1550. https://doi.org/10.1056/nejmc0912392.
50. Jabłońska B, Mrowiec S. Total Pancreatectomy with autologous islet cell transplantation—the current indications. J Clin Med. 2021;10(12):2723. https://doi.org/10.3390/jcm10122723.
51. Turner KM, Delman AM, Donovan EC, Brunner J, Wahab SA, Dai Y, et al. Total pancreatectomy and islet cell autotransplantation: a 10-year update on outcomes and assessment of long-term durability. HPB. 2022;24(11):2013–21. https://doi.org/10.1016/j.hpb.2022.07.001.
52. Bellin MD, Beilman GJ, Sutherland DER, Ali H, Petersen A, Mongin S, et al. How durable is Total Pancreatectomy and Intraportal islet cell transplantation for treatment of chronic pancreatitis? J Am Coll Surg. 2019;228(4):329–39. https://doi.org/10.1016/j.jamcollsurg.2018.12.019.
53. Bellin MD, Freeman ML, Gelrud A, Slivka A, Clavel A, Humar A, et al. Total pancreatectomy and islet autotransplantation in chronic pancreatitis: recommendations from PancreasFest. Pancreatology. 2014;14(1):27–35. https://doi.org/10.1016/j.pan.2013.10.009.
54. Uc A, Cress GA, Wang F, Abu-El-Haija M, Ellery KM, Fishman DS, et al. Analysis of INSPPIRE-2 cohort. J Pediatr Gastroenterol Nutr. 2022;75(5):643–9. https://doi.org/10.1097/mpg.0000000000003590.
55. Nathan JD, Yang Y, Eaton A, Witkowski P, Wijkstrom M, Walsh M, et al. Surgical approach and short-term outcomes in adults and children undergoing total pancreatectomy with islet autotransplantation: a report from the prospective observational study of TPIAT. Pancreatology. 2022;22(1):1–8. https://doi.org/10.1016/j.pan.2021.09.011.
56. Chinnakotla S, Radosevich DM, Dunn TB, Bellin MD, Freeman ML, Schwarzenberg SJ, et al. Long-term outcomes of Total Pancreatectomy and islet auto transplantation for hereditary/genetic pancreatitis. J Am Coll Surg. 2014;218(4):530–43. https://doi.org/10.1016/j.jamcollsurg.2013.12.037.
57. Al-Moussally F, Fogel EL, Helft PR. An ethical analysis of endoscopic therapy decision-making in patients with refractory substance use disorder and chronic pancreatitis. Pancreatology. 2022;22(6):671–7. https://doi.org/10.1016/j.pan.2022.05.007.
58. Singh VK, Yadav D, Garg PK. Diagnosis and management of chronic pancreatitis. JAMA. 2019;322(24):2422. https://doi.org/10.1001/jama.2019.19411.
59. Melloul E, Lassen K, Roulin D, Grass F, Perinel J, Adham M, et al. Guidelines for perioperative Care for Pancreatoduodenectomy: enhanced recovery after surgery (ERAS) recommendations 2019. World J Surg. 2020;44(7):2056–84. https://doi.org/10.1007/s00268-020-05462-w.
60. Miksch RC, D'Haese JG, Werner J. Surgical therapy of chronic alcoholic pancreatitis: a literature review of current options. Visc Med. 2020;36(3):191–7. https://doi.org/10.1159/000508174.
61. Tønnesen H, Nielsen PR, Lauritzen JB, Møller AM. Smoking and alcohol intervention before surgery: evidence for best practice. Br J Anaesth. 2009;102(3):297–306. https://doi.org/10.1093/bja/aen401.

62. Wilson GC, Turner KM, Delman AM, Wahab S, Ofosu A, Smith MT, et al. Long-term survival outcomes after operative management of chronic pancreatitis: two decades of experience. J Am Coll Surg. 2023; https://doi.org/10.1097/xcs.0000000000000575.
63. Gundlach J-P, Braun F, Mötter F, Bernsmeier A, Barrio P, Ehmke N, et al. Phosphatidylethanol (PEth) for monitoring sobriety in liver transplant candidates: preliminary results of differences between alcohol-related and non-alcohol-related cirrhosis candidates. Ann Transplant. 2022;27 https://doi.org/10.12659/aot.936293.
64. Selim R, Zhou Y, Rupp LB, Trudeau S, Naffouj S, Shamaa O, et al. Availability of PEth testing is associated with reduced eligibility for liver transplant among patients with alcohol-related liver disease. Clin Transpl. 2022;36(5) https://doi.org/10.1111/ctr.14595.
65. Scholten K, Twohig P, Samson K, Brittan K, Fiedler A, Warner J, et al. You can't handle the truth! Comparing serum phosphatidylethanol to self-reported alcohol intake in chronic liver disease patients. Dig Liver Dis. 2024;56(7):1215–9. https://doi.org/10.1016/j.dld.2024.01.195.
66. Han S, Kheder J, Bocelli L, Wassef W. Smoking cessation comparison in chronic pancreatitis patients. Am J Gastroenterol. 2014;109:S71. https://doi.org/10.14309/00000434-201410002-00230.
67. Dunderdale J, McAuliffe JC, McNeal SF, Bryant SMJ, Yancey BD, Flowers G, et al. Should Pancreatectomy with islet cell autotransplantation in patients with chronic alcoholic pancreatitis be abandoned? J Am Coll Surg. 2013;216(4):591–6. https://doi.org/10.1016/j.jamcollsurg.2012.12.043.
68. Lara LF, Wastvedt S, Hodges JS, Witkowski P, Wijkstrom M, Walsh RM, et al. The Association of Smoking and Alcohol Abuse on anxiety and depression in patients with recurrent acute or chronic pancreatitis undergoing Total Pancreatectomy and islet autotransplantation. Pancreas. 2021;50(6):852–8. https://doi.org/10.1097/mpa.0000000000001850.
69. Ammann RW, Muellhaupt B. The natural history of pain in alcoholic chronic pancreatitis. Gastroenterology. 1999;116(5):1132–40. https://doi.org/10.1016/s0016-5085(99)70016-8.
70. Torosian K, Shahrvini B, Johnson WM, Vodkin I, Tincopa M, Lim N, et al. Psychosocial predictors of return to alcohol use after liver transplant: a multicenter cohort study. Alcohol, Clinical and Experimental Research. 2024;48(11):2137–44. https://doi.org/10.1111/acer.15438.
71. Blobner BM, Bellin MD, Beilman GJ, Shelton CA, Park HJ, Whitcomb DC. Gene expression profiling of the pancreas in patients undergoing Total Pancreatectomy with islet autotransplant suggests unique features of alcoholic, idiopathic, and hereditary pancreatitis. Pancreas. 2020;49(8):1037–43. https://doi.org/10.1097/mpa.0000000000001607.
72. Bellin MD, Eaton A, Ramanathan K, Beilman G, Downs E, Schwarzenberg SJ, et al. Long-term islet graft functional assessment in more than 500 patients undergoing Total Pancreatectomy with Intraportal islet autotransplantation. J Am Coll Surg. 2025;240(4):405–13. https://doi.org/10.1097/xcs.0000000000001294.
73. Chinnakotla S, Beilman GJ, Dunn TB, Bellin MD, Freeman ML, Radosevich DM, et al. Factors predicting outcomes after a Total Pancreatectomy and islet autotransplantation lessons learned from over 500 cases. Ann Surg. 2015;262(4):610–22. https://doi.org/10.1097/sla.0000000000001453.
74. Volkow ND, Michaelides M, Baler R. The neuroscience of drug reward and addiction. Physiol Rev. 2019;99(4):2115–40. https://doi.org/10.1152/physrev.00014.2018.
75. Kaner EFS, Beyer FR, Muirhead C, Campbell F, Pienaar ED, Bertholet N, et al. Effectiveness of brief alcohol interventions in primary care populations. Cochrane Database Syst Rev. 2018;2018(6) https://doi.org/10.1002/14651858.cd004148.pub4.
76. Berney T, Rudisuhli T, Oberholzer J, Caulfield A, Morel P. Long-term metabolic results after pancreatic resection for severe chronic pancreatitis. Arch Surg. 2000;135(9):1106–11. https://doi.org/10.1001/archsurg.135.9.1106.
77. Gardner TB, Smith KD. Total Pancreatectomy and islet autotransplant in the treatment of chronic pancreatitis: tread very, Very Carefully. Am J Gastroenterol. 2018;113(3):322–3. https://doi.org/10.1038/ajg.2017.419.

Total Pancreatectomy with Islet Autotransplantation for Hereditary/Genetic Pancreatitis

13

Rosara Bass, Maisam Abu-El-Haija, and A. Jay Freeman

Abstract

Genetic and hereditary etiologies of pancreatitis, which are more common in pediatric patients, impact disease progression, response to conventional surgical approaches, and risk of future malignancy. Thus, consideration of genetic risk may play an important role in determining eligibility for and timing of total pancreatectomy with islet autotransplantation (TPIAT), particularly in children. Multiple genes have been implicated as risk factors for development of acute recurrent and chronic pancreatitis (ARP and CP), including *PRSS1*, *CFTR*, *SPINK1,* and others. Genetic variants may predispose to pancreatitis independently or increase risk of development of pancreatitis in the setting of additional risk factors, such as smoking or the presence of an anatomic variant. Genetic analysis in adults and children with idiopathic ARP or CP can serve a prognostic role, as pancreatitis-associated gene variants are associated with higher risk of recurrent pancreatitis after an initial episode, earlier onset of CP, and often a more severe disease course. Additionally, the presence of a pancreatitis-associated gene variant is associated with decreased efficacy of conventional, pancreas-sparing surgeries, which may delay ultimate TPIAT. Islet yield is an important predictor of insulin independence after TPIAT. Younger age and shorter duration of disease at the time of surgery are associated with higher islet yield, and prior surgical interventions are associated with lower islet yield during TPIAT. Given

R. Bass (✉)
Nationwide Children's Hospital, Colombus, OH, USA
e-mail: rosara.bass@nationwidechildrens.org

M. Abu-El-Haija
Cincinnati Children's Hospital Medical Center, Cincinnati, OH, USA

A. J. Freeman
Nationwide Children's Hospital, Colombus, OH, USA

S. Chinnakotla et al. (eds.), *Total Pancreatectomy and Islet Auto Transplantation*,
https://doi.org/10.1007/978-981-92-0018-4_13

the evidence that alternate surgical approaches for CP are less successful in alleviating symptom burden in patients with hereditary and genetic pancreatitis and may lead to reduced islet yield at the time of TPIAT, pancreas-sparing surgery should be approached with caution in this population.

Key Points

1. Pancreatitis-associated gene variants are associated with higher risk of recurrent pancreatitis after an initial episode, earlier onset of CP, and often a more severe disease course.
2. Consideration of genetic risk may play an important role in determining eligibility for and timing of total pancreatectomy with islet autotransplantation (TPIAT), particularly in children.
3. Genes implicated as risk factors for development of acute recurrent and chronic pancreatitis include *PRSS1*, *CFTR*, *SPINK1*, and others and may predispose to pancreatitis independently or increase risk of development of pancreatitis in the setting of additional risk factors.
4. The presence of a pancreatitis-associated gene variant is associated with decreased efficacy of conventional, pancreas-sparing surgeries, which may delay ultimate TPIAT.
5. Younger age and shorter duration of disease at the time of surgery are associated with higher islet yield, and prior surgical interventions are associated with lower islet yield during TPIAT; thus, pancreas-sparing surgery should be approached with caution in patients with pancreatitis-associated gene variants.

13.1 Hereditary and Genetic Pancreatitis

Total pancreatectomy with islet autotransplantation (TPIAT) is indicated for treatment of intractable pain in patients with impaired quality of life due to acute recurrent pancreatitis (ARP) or chronic pancreatitis (CP) [1]. Genetic and hereditary etiologies of pancreatitis, which are more common in pediatric patients, impact disease progression, response to conventional surgical approaches, and risk of future malignancy [2, 3]. Thus, in addition to pain burden, consideration of genetic risk may also play an important role in determining eligibility for and timing of TPIAT, particularly in children. Multiple genetic mutations impacting pancreatic acinar and ductal cells, as well as calcium regulation, have been implicated in ARP and CP [4, 5]. In this chapter, we specifically examine such genetic etiologies of ARP and CP and their impact on disease course, response to conventional operations, and post-TPIAT outcomes. Because not all patients with ARP or CP undergo genetic testing, hereditary pancreatitis or pancreatitis in the setting of a positive family history of ARP or CP are also considered here. In addition, given the limited genetic testing platforms, a negative genetic etiology does not exclude genetic risk in children.

13.2 Hereditary Pancreatitis and Age

Although ARP and CP are rare in children, the prevalence of both is increasing, and both result in significant morbidity for affected patients that leads to high healthcare utilization requiring chronic, multidisciplinary care [6, 7]. The median numbers of emergency room visits, hospitalizations, and missed days of work or school are similar to those in adults and represent a significant disease burden that negatively impacts quality of life [8]. In pediatrics, the potential presence of endocrine and exocrine insufficiency during critical growth windows can lead to additional complications such as decreased bone density, malnutrition, and growth impairment [9].

Given the significant disease burden and growing prevalence of ARP and CP among children, the INSPPIRE Consortium (INternational Study Group of Pediatric Pancreatitis: In search for a cuRE) was designed to investigate the epidemiology, etiologies, pathogenesis, natural history, and outcomes of pediatric ARP and CP [10, 11]. In contrast with adult ARP and CP, which are often attributable to risk factors such as alcohol and tobacco use, in children, ARP and CP are more commonly associated with an underlying genetic mutation, with up to 70% of participants in the INSPPIRE pediatric registry found to have one or more pancreatitis-predisposing genetic variants [12]; however, this is likely an underestimate because 17% of the cohort had no genetic testing available or had genetic testing limited to a single gene or a limited panel with three or four genes [12]. Genetic variants were more commonly identified in children with CP (73%) than in those with ARP (48%) [13]. Children with an underlying genetic etiology with recurrent or even a single episode of acute pancreatitis (AP) are at increased risk for the development of CP and have an earlier age of onset [13–15]. While genetic mutations are most prevalent in the youngest pancreatitis patients, even in the oldest pediatric age group examined in INSPPIRE (age 12–19 years at onset), over 50% of study participants had at least one pancreatitis-associated gene mutation [16]. A systematic review and meta-analysis of outcomes following TPIAT identified that 74% of children who underwent TPIAT had an underlying genetic etiology of CP [17].

While genetic etiologies in ARP or CP are more prevalent in children, they are commonly identified in adults as well and can impact disease course. Among adults with CP, younger age of onset has been associated with higher overall symptom and healthcare resource burden due to more frequent episodes of ARP prior to development of CP [18]. In adults with ARP or CP who completed germline testing, the prevalence of a positive result for a pancreatitis-associated gene mutation was about 28% in both groups, and the likelihood of a pathogenic variant was highest in younger individuals and those with a family history of pancreatitis [2]. Additionally, an underlying genetic predisposition may result in increased susceptibility to ARP or CP with exposure to additional toxic, metabolic, or medication risk factors [19–21].

13.3 Genetic Etiologies of Pancreatitis and Impact on Disease Course

Multiple genes have been implicated as risk factors for the development of ARP and CP. Additionally, genetic analysis can serve a prognostic role because pancreatitis-associated gene variants are associated with a higher risk of ARP after an initial episode of AP, an earlier onset of CP, and often a more severe disease course [16, 22, 23]. Prognostic information may impact decision-making regarding the timing and type of pancreatic surgery [24]. Current guidelines from the INSPPIRE Consortium recommend genetic testing when positive results would provide clear etiologic information and alter the direction of further causal investigations. Thus, the consensus guidelines strongly recommend genetic testing with *PRSS1* gene analysis and sweat chloride testing for any child who is diagnosed with AP at 5 years of age or younger, has had two or more episodes of AP, or has a strong family history of pancreatitis or pancreatic cancer. Additionally, the INSPPIRE guidelines also recognize that analysis of the *SPINK1*, *CFTR,* and *CTRC* genes may identify risk factors for ARP or CP [22, 25]. Guidelines by the European Pancreatic Club in collaboration with the Hungarian Pancreatic Study Group recommend that any patient with a second episode of idiopathic AP, or a first episode of idiopathic AP and a family history of AP or CP, undergo sweat chloride testing; full sequence analysis of the *PRSS1*, *CPA1*, *SPINK1*, *CTRC,* and *CFTR* gene exons and exon-intron boundaries; and testing for the *CEL* gene pathogenic hybrid allele [25]. A summary of genetic variants implicated in the pathogenesis of ARP and CP and their mechanisms of action is shown in Fig. 13.1 and is described in detail below.

13.3.1 PRSS1

The PRoteaSe Serine 1 (*PRSS1*) gene, which encodes human cationic trypsinogen, is a precursor of trypsin. *PRSS1* is considered to be the most frequent gene involved in autosomal-dominant hereditary pancreatitis, with a high rate of penetrance [26–29]. Over 50 *PRSS1* variants have been reported, but the degree of pathogenicity and penetrance is highly variable. Multiple missense mutations including p.R122H and p.N29I, the two most commonly implicated mutations found in hereditary pancreatitis families, have been shown to cause overproduction of trypsinogen, theoretically leading to its premature activation to trypsin within the pancreas, resulting in pancreatitis [26, 30, 31]. However, other types of genetic variants in the *PRSS1* gene, including gene conversion, copy number, and single nucleotide variants, have also been implicated in hereditary pancreatitis [26]. The presence of *PRSS1* gene variants has been associated with earlier onset of pancreatitis, faster disease progression from ARP to CP, and increased risk of pancreatic malignancy, likely due to increased trypsin activating oncogenes within the pancreas [16, 32–34].

In a cohort of 64 individuals with *PRSS1* gene variants, adverse outcomes following TPIAT, particularly diabetes and persistent opioid use, were associated with older age and prolonged disease [35]. Given the early onset and progression of

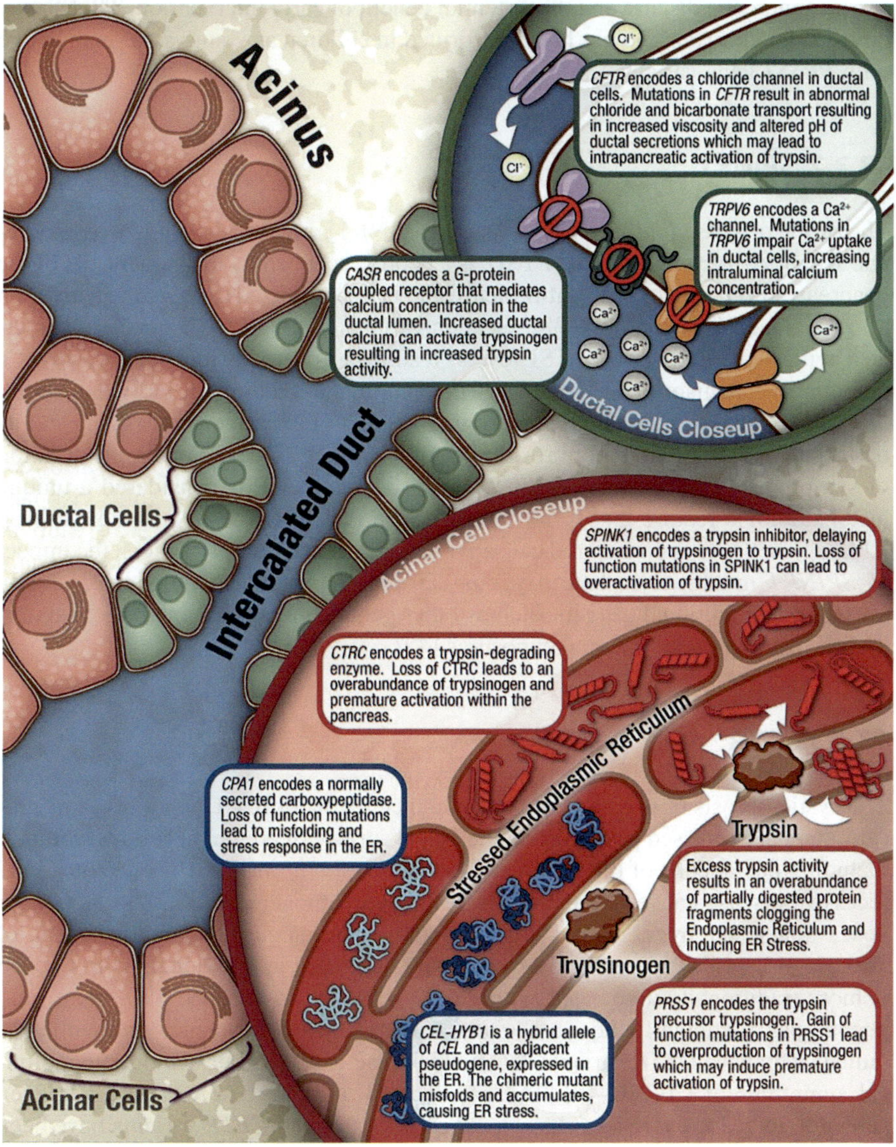

Fig. 13.1 Genetic variants most commonly implicated in hereditary pancreatitis and their proposed mechanisms of action. (Illustrated by Will Ray, PhD, MS)

severe pancreatic disease and the potential benefit of early intervention, TPIAT may be considered earlier and has been performed in children as young as 2 years of age with *PRSS1* gene variants [36].

13.3.2 SPINK1

The serine protease inhibitor Kazal type 1 (SPINK1) protein, also known as pancreatic secretory trypsin inhibitor (PTSI), is a peptide secreted by the acinar cells of the pancreas. SPINK1 acts as an antiprotease and is hypothesized to delay the activation of trypsinogen to trypsin [37, 38]. Genetic variants in the *SPINK1* gene are associated with decreased serum PTSI levels, leading to overactivation of trypsin as a potential mechanism of CP [39, 40]. Histopathologic features of individuals with *SPINK1*-associated CP include the progressive loss of exocrine parenchyma and its replacement with prominent fibrosis, both of which are associated with the duration of symptoms. The fibrosis seen in *SPINK1*-associated CP is considered a unique histopathologic feature that is not seen with *PRSS1*- or *CFTR*-associated CP [41]. Although *SPINK1* is considered causative of CP in homozygous carriers, the impact of *SPINK1* mutations in heterozygous carriers (1% of the population) is likely impacted by additional triggers such as other genetic mutations, anatomical abnormalities, and/or environmental exposures [42].

13.3.3 CFTR

The cystic fibrosis transmembrane conductance regulator (CFTR) protein is a chloride channel expressed primarily on the apical surface of epithelial cell membranes, including ductal cells of the pancreas [43, 44]. Cystic fibrosis (CF) is an autosomal recessive disease caused by the presence of two pathogenic variants in the *CFTR* gene, diagnosed by clinical symptoms and a sweat chloride measurement of >60 mmol/L [45]. Pancreatitis has been well described in individuals with CF, but is more traditionally associated with *CFTR* genotypes associated with more mild phenotypes, particularly those associated with pancreatic sufficiency, and with individuals who have *CFTR* variants detected by genetic testing but without other clinical symptoms of CF [46–49]. The presence of a single *CFTR* variant has been shown to increase the risk of developing ARP or CP, and *CFTR* variants have been the most common genes associated with ARP among children; they have also been associated with ARP in individuals with pancreas divisum [13, 50, 51]. Additionally, ARP or CP may be a presenting symptom of CF disease, and thus a sweat test is recommended in children presenting with ARP or CP to allow for early identification of CF [25]. While genetic variants have historically been used for prognostic purposes in ARP and CP, with *CFTR*, there exists an emerging role for the use of genetic analysis to inform treatment approaches. CFTR correction by modulator therapies, approved for the treatment of CF, has been shown to reduce the risk of pancreatitis in patients with *CFTR* mutations and ARP [52–54].

13.3.4 CTRC

Mutations in chymotrypsin C (CTRC), a trypsin-degrading enzyme, result in loss of function that reduces the enzyme's secretion and activity, resulting in an impaired ability to degrade trypsinogen that leads to harmful trypsinogen activation within the pancreas. Variants in the *CTRC* gene have been found to be overrepresented in adults with CP [55]. *CTRC* variants have also been found to be significantly more likely to occur in children with early-onset pancreatitis than in older pediatric patients with ARP or CP [16]. In transcriptome-wide association studies, differential expression of *CTRC* was suggestively associated with both constant and constant-severe pain, with the greatest effect seen in the pancreas [56].

13.3.5 CASR

The calcium-sensing receptor (CASR) is a G protein-coupled receptor that mediates calcium homeostasis by detecting extracellular calcium levels. Rare *CASR* variants have been described in patients with CP, which may be related to development of hypercalcemia, which is an independent risk factor for pancreatitis [57]. Although heterozygous inactivating mutations in *CASR* are associated with benign familial hypocalciuric hypercalcemia, these mutations may also represent a predisposing factor for the development of ARP and CP with exposure to a second disease-modifying genetic mutation such as *SPINK1* [58].

13.3.6 CPA1

Pathogenic loss-of-function mutations in the carboxypeptidase A1 gene (*CPA1*) have been shown to cause intracellular retention of CPA1 protein, resulting in misfolding of the protein and a stress response within the endoplasmic reticulum as a possible mechanism for predisposition to pancreatitis [59]. In mouse models, this has been associated with increased risk of pancreatitis, which is accelerated with alcohol exposure [60, 61]. In humans, *CPA1* mutations have been associated with hereditary pancreatitis [62].

13.3.7 Other Genes

More recently, other genes have been identified as increasing susceptibility to pancreatitis including *CLDN2* (claudin 2), *MORC4* (MORC family CW-type zinc finger 4), *SEC16A* (Sec16 homolog A, endoplasmic reticulum export factor), *TRPV6* (transient receptor potential cation channel subfamily V member 6), *SBDS* (Shwachman-Bodian-Diamond syndrome protein), *PRSS3*, and *CEL-HYB1* (carboxyl ester lipase) [23, 63–66]. Additionally, genes that may predispose to a specific risk factor for pancreatitis, such as hypertriglyceridemia, may also be considered in the appropriate clinical setting [67].

13.4 "Idiopathic" Pancreatitis

Adults diagnosed with "idiopathic pancreatitis" have a more rapid progression from ARP to CP and a more severe disease course than individuals with ARP or CP secondary to known etiologies (such as alcohol, smoking, or obstruction). While previously attributed to a lack of a treatable cause, the severity of disease seen in idiopathic pancreatitis may, in fact, represent the presence of an undiagnosed genetic predisposition [68]. In a genotype analysis of patients with CP, those with previously diagnosed idiopathic CP had a higher rate of pancreatitis-associated gene detection (57%) than those with alcohol- or smoking-associated CP (40% and 32%, respectively) and had an earlier age of pancreatitis onset [69]. A systematic review and meta-analysis of TPIAT outcomes identified that the majority of TPIATs (49%) were performed in individuals with idiopathic pancreatitis, and 21% were performed in individuals with genetic pancreatitis [17].

13.5 Compounding Risk of Pancreatitis with Genetic Mutations and Nonhereditary Pancreatitis Risk Factors

While the aforementioned genetic variants have all been associated with an increased risk of ARP and CP, wide variability exists in both genotype and phenotype. The presence of certain genes and modifiers may result in a compounding effect, augmenting the phenotype of other pancreatitis-associated gene mutations in the same patient. For example, the presence of a *SPINK1* gene mutation has been associated with faster progression to CP in patients with co-occurring *CFTR* and *PRSS1* mutations [27, 70–72].

The risk of developing ARP and CP may also be additive when a genetic predisposition is combined with exogenous factors that can influence the development of pancreatitis. For example, in the INSPPIRE cohort, 28% of patients diagnosed with drug-associated pancreatitis were also found to have a genetic mutation, suggesting that the underlying predisposition may have increased the risk of pancreatitis when exposed to the drug [21]. Similarly, in adults with hereditary pancreatitis, smoking and alcohol use have been associated with an increased rate of progression from ARP to CP [71–76]. Pancreas divisum is an anatomic variant that has traditionally been considered a risk factor for pancreatitis. However, the relationship between pancreas divisum and pancreatitis may be impacted by genetic variants. Patients with pancreas divisum presenting with pancreatitis had a higher frequency of *SPINK1* gene mutations than healthy controls with pancreas divisum but without pancreatitis [51, 77]. Similarly, in children, a high likelihood of CP has been demonstrated in those with pancreas divisum and genetic variants, but this seemed to be driven by genetic variants, not by pancreas divisum.

Consensus guidelines for the evaluation of pancreatitis in children recognize that multiple risk factors for ARP and CP may be present in the same patient and thus state that anatomic abnormalities, including pancreas divisum and annular pancreas, which are independent risk factors for ARP and CP, should not prevent evaluation for genetic predisposition [22]. In adults, expert consensus guidelines recommend genetic testing for individuals with a positive family history of pancreatic diseases, with persisting disease after therapeutic intervention, or with unclear etiology, particularly in patients <35 years of age [78].

The additive effects of genetic mutations with other risk factors are not limited to pancreatitis—the risk of pancreatic cancer in individuals with *SPINK1, PRSS1,* and *CFTR* mutations has been demonstrated to be augmented in the presence of smoking [79]. Current guidelines by the American Gastroenterological Association recommend consideration of pancreas cancer screening for all patients with hereditary pancreatitis [80]. At this time, it is unknown how pancreatitis-associated genetic variants impact endocrine and exocrine function, although one may postulate that an interactive genetic risk may exist.

13.6 Impact of Pancreatitis-Associated Gene Mutations on Non-TPIAT Interventions for ARP and CP

While TPIAT has the potential to provide relief from intractable pain related to CP and to improve quality of life, careful consideration of alternative therapeutic options must be given prior to surgery, given the irreversible nature of the operation, its potential complications, the subsequent endocrine insufficiency, and the risk of incomplete pain relief. When considering endoscopic and surgical therapies in patients with ARP and CP, it is important to consider not only the potential for benefit from such interventions, but also the implications of prior interventions for subsequent TPIAT outcomes.

13.6.1 Genetic Mutations and ERCP

Given that TPIAT is reserved for patients with ARP or CP who have failed maximal medical and endoscopic management, endoscopic procedures—particularly endoscopic retrograde pancreatic cholangiopancreatography (ERCP)—are nearly universal in the treatment of ARP and CP in patients for whom TPIAT is being considered. ERCP is safe and effective for children and adults, with a trend toward higher rates of primary success in those with ARP as compared with CP [81]. In a single-center retrospective analysis of children and adults with hereditary pancreatitis, therapeutic ERCPs were associated with decreased mean pain scores, hospital visits, and opioid usage [82]. Among the INSPPIRE cohort of pediatric patients with ARP or CP (n = 265, mean age, 12 years), therapeutic ERCP was more commonly performed in patients with CP (66%) than in those with ARP (14%) and in patients with obstructive factors related to pancreatitis than in those with alternate etiologies. No association between the presence of a genetic risk factor and the likelihood of therapeutic ERCP was identified in this cohort. Interventions performed by ERCP included biliary and pancreatic sphincterotomies, stent placement, and stone removal. Among those in the INSPPIRE cohort, therapeutic ERCP was reported to provide symptomatic improvement in 53% of patients with CP and 56% of patients with ARP [83]. Additionally, in a single-center cohort of 20 children with pancreas divisum, 68% of whom had a known genetic variant and who were followed up by telephone, 67% reported symptomatic improvement from ERCP [84]. In adults with genetic mutations that predispose to pancreatic malignancy, endoscopic ultrasound may be used for cancer surveillance [85].

13.6.2 Genetic Mutations and Pancreas-Sparing Surgical Interventions

Surgical interventions for the treatment of CP include conventional operations and TPIAT. Conventional operations can further be divided into drainage procedures and partial resections.

Ductal drainage procedures, such as longitudinal pancreaticojejunostomy (modified Puestow), aim to treat symptoms related to pancreatic ductal dilation. Stasis within a dilated duct can obstruct the flow of secretions, leading to ductal hypertension, or can result in stone formation/obstruction and the development of a pseudocyst or pancreatic ascites. Partial resection procedures, including pancreaticoduodenectomy (Whipple), duodenum-sparing head resection (Berger or Berne), or distal pancreatectomy with splenectomy, are considered for individuals with damage isolated to a specific area of the pancreas, as may be seen with traumatic pancreatitis, inflammatory head mass, malignancy, or obstructive pathology. In some cases, both drainage and resection are indicated and thus combined, for example, a partial resection of pancreatic head combined with longitudinal pancreaticojejunostomy of distal pancreas (Frey) [24]. While conventional operations have been performed safely in children, they have been found to be less effective in achieving sustained pain relief in patients with hereditary pancreatitis [86]. In a single-center retrospective analysis, 92% of patients with hereditary pancreatitis who underwent decompression or resection surgeries developed subsequent complications requiring therapeutic endoscopy [82]. Factors that may limit the success of these operations in hereditary CP are the absence of ductal dilatation and inflammatory head mass, as well as a more predominant neuropathic source of pancreatitis pain in this population [24, 87, 88].

13.6.3 Specific Surgical Interventions for Treatment of Congenital Abnormalities Related to Pediatric ARP and CP

Anatomic and obstructive abnormalities have been found to be present in nearly 20% of children with ARP and over 30% of children with CP. Surgical interventions that directly address congenital abnormalities that contribute to pancreatitis, such as anomalous pancreaticobiliary duct union (long common channel) or annular pancreas, may be appropriate therapies in patients affected by these conditions [5].

An abnormal junction of the pancreatic and common bile ducts occurring outside of the duodenum and forming a long common channel can predispose to choledochal cysts, resulting in ARP as well as cholangiocarcinoma [89, 90]. While familial occurrence of congenital dilation of the common bile duct secondary to pancreaticobiliary maljunction has been reported, identification of traditional genetic risk loci for this condition has been limited by the rarity of the condition [91, 92]. Whole-exome sequencing of patients with congenital dilation of the common bile duct suggests that an oligogenic mechanism may be involved, with implicated genes coinciding with known genes for cancer risk [93]. Specific treatment of the long common channel may include endoscopic stent placement or surgical choledochal cyst excision, often including prophylactic cholecystectomy [94].

Annular pancreas is a rare condition in which tissue from the head of the pancreas partially or completely surrounds the duodenum. Annular pancreas is most often identified in the neonatal period and may be associated with chromosomal abnormalities and other comorbidities including cardiac malformations, esophageal atresia, and tracheoesophageal fistula. The most common presentation of annular pancreas is related to symptoms of duodenal compression, but patients with this abnormality may also be at risk of pancreatitis. Duodenoduodenostomy is the most commonly performed surgical intervention for the treatment of annular pancreas [95, 96].

13.7 TPIAT in Patients with Genetic Risk

13.7.1 Impact of Genetic Risk Factors on Islet Yield in TPIAT

Individuals who undergo TPIAT universally develop exocrine pancreatic insufficiency; however, with IAT, a significant percentage are able to achieve insulin independence [97]. Postoperative insulin independence is directly related to the degree of islet yield during the operation, and this relationship is sustained in the long term [98, 99]. In a long-term follow-up study of patients after TPIAT, islet yield at the time of surgery (islet equivalents per kg >4000) remained the strongest predictor of islet graft function at 10 years [100]. Thus, identification and optimization of preoperative factors that impact islet yield at the time of TPIAT are essential. Unfortunately, individuals with genetic etiologies of CP may have decreased islet yield compared with those who undergo TPIAT for other etiologies. In a single-center study of adults who had undergone TPIAT, individuals with hereditary pancreatitis had lower islet yield and were less likely to achieve insulin independence than those with non-hereditary or genetic causes, although in a multivariate analysis adjusting for pancreas fibrosis, transplant era, years with pancreatitis, and tissue volume, the relationship was no longer significant [100]. In patients with genetically induced pancreatitis, effective optimization of all other modifiable factors is needed because any delay may impact islet yield when TPIAT is performed.

Younger age and shorter duration of disease at the time of surgery are two factors associated with higher islet yield during TPIAT [35, 97]. In a single-center cohort of 17 patients who underwent TPIAT at ages 3–8 years (14/17 with at least one genetic mutation), 82% had a period of postoperative insulin independence during a 1-year postoperative follow-up, compared with 41% in a cohort of children >9 years of age from the same institution [101]. In a single-center cohort of 12 pediatric patients who underwent TPIAT (84% with genetic mutations), insulin independence was also negatively associated with age, as well as with obesity, female gender, and duration of disease [102]. Long-term follow-up has shown that patients who undergo TPIAT in childhood are more likely to have sustained islet function at 10 years than those who undergo the procedure as adults [100].

Another potential benefit of younger age at the time of surgery is the association with decreased postoperative pain and narcotic use. In a cohort of 3- to 8-year-old children who underwent TPIAT, all were able to successfully discontinue opioids postoperatively [101]. In the single-center analysis mentioned above of 12 pediatric patients who underwent TPIAT (84% with genetic mutations), all had improvement in pancreatitis pain after TPIAT, with residual nonpancreatitis pain occurring only in the oldest patients in the cohort [102]. Long-term follow-up has demonstrated that individuals with CP who underwent TPIAT at a younger age (<18 years) had a lower overall prevalence of pain and a lower prevalence of narcotic use 10 years after TPIAT than those who had the procedure at an older age [103]. In addition to improved pain outcomes, a decrease in overall disease burden has been described in pediatric patients who underwent TPIAT—a single-center analysis of TPIAT outcomes in pediatric patients (50% with genetic mutations) found that patients had fewer hospitalizations and invasive procedures after TPIAT than before [104].

13.7.2 Impact of Antecedent Interventions on TPIAT Outcomes

Antecedent surgical interventions have been shown to negatively impact islet yield during TPIAT. Prior surgical drainage and/or resection operations are associated with more rapid decline in beta cell function and glycemic control in people with chronic pancreatitis, as well as with decreased islet yield and a higher risk of insulin dependence in adults undergoing TPIAT [105–107]. Similar outcomes have been seen in children who undergo TPIAT, most commonly for gene variant–associated chronic pancreatitis. In a cohort of pediatric patients undergoing TPIAT, 12/19 with CP attributed to genetic etiology, a history of surgical drainage was associated with lower islet yield and greater incidence of insulin dependence following TPIAT

[108]. Fibrosis and acinar atrophy are negatively correlated with islet yield in hereditary pancreatitis, and prior pancreaticojejunostomy has been associated with more severe fibrosis and lower islet yield [109, 110]. In a study of adults who underwent initial partial pancreatectomy but then ultimately required completion pancreatectomy with IAT for refractory disease, only 22% achieved insulin independence. No association between the type of prior surgical procedure and postoperative insulin requirements was identified [111]. In addition to impact on islet yield, history of prior conventional pancreatic surgery has been associated with use of narcotics 1 year after TPIAT [112].

The impact of antecedent ERCP on islet yield in patients with hereditary and genetic pancreatitis is less conclusive. In a single-center pediatric cohort of 75 patients who underwent TPIAT for chronic pancreatitis (54% due to hereditary/genetic etiology), prior ERCP, sphincterotomy, stent placement, and endoscopic duct drainage were not associated with islet yield at the time of TPIAT [97]. In a multicenter retrospective comparative cohort analysis of data prospectively collected from 230 individuals who underwent TPIAT between January 2017 and September 2019, of whom 29% were children, 76% underwent ERCP prior to TPIAT. In this larger multicenter cohort, it was again demonstrated that prior ERCP, stent placement, or sphincterotomy were not associated with islet yield [113]. While ERCP may provide therapeutic benefit without impacting islet yield, it is not without inherent risk, including infection, pancreatitis, hemorrhage, and perforation [114]. In a single-center retrospective analysis of treatments for CP in patients <21 years of age, having greater than five endoscopic treatments was associated with a lower likelihood of pain relief [115]. A history of ERCP with stent placement and/or sphincterotomy has also been associated with narcotic use 1 year after TPIAT, although this does not represent a causal relationship and may be related to other factors, including duration of disease and overall pain sensitivity [112].

Given the evidence that alternate surgical approaches for CP are less successful in alleviating symptom burden in patients with hereditary and genetic pancreatitis and may lead to reduced islet yield at the time of TPIAT, pancreas-sparing surgery should be approached with caution in this population and only if specifically indicated by an individual patient's disease morphology [24]. Non-TPIAT pancreatic surgery may also delay ultimate TPIAT. Given the understanding that younger age and shorter disease duration are associated with improved islet yield and decreased narcotic use, it is appropriate to consider TPIAT as an initial operative approach in children with genetic etiologies of chronic pancreatitis [24].

13.8 Areas for Future Research

Because many patients who undergo TPIAT for genetic indications are children, future research is warranted to specifically understand how TPIAT early in life impacts long-term growth and development. Guidance for nutritional support following TPIAT has been published, but the impact of pediatric TPIAT on linear growth, body composition, and bone health is unknown [116]. Understanding these factors may inform optimal surveillance and interventions to support skeletal development in this population. Additionally, the impact of TPIAT on neurocognitive development and mental health also warrants consideration in the pediatric age group to support overall longevity and optimal health into adulthood.

Because pain is the primary indication for TPIAT, understanding the influences of genetic risk factors and pancreatitis-associated pain syndromes is also of great importance. Recent genome- and transcriptome-wide association studies have identified risk loci for constant and constant-severe pain in individuals with pancreatitis. The ability to predict not only the risk of developing pancreatitis but also the risk of severe and constant pain related to pancreatitis may also serve as a tool to determine the optimal timing of TPIAT [56].

Finally, as patients with hereditary and genetic etiologies of pancreatitis progress toward adulthood, additional consideration of malignancy risk will be essential. Given the known relationships between genetic causes of ARP and CP and pancreatic malignancy, this risk may also warrant consideration in the TPIAT decision-making process [33, 34, 79].

Bibliography

1. Bellin MD, Freeman ML, Gelrud A, Slivka A, Clavel A, Humar A, et al. Total pancreatectomy and islet autotransplantation in chronic pancreatitis: recommendations from PancreasFest. Pancreatology. 2014;14(1):27–35. https://doi.org/10.1016/j.pan.2013.10.009.
2. Ramsey ML, Heald B, Gokun Y, Baker J, Groce JR, Han S, et al. Germline multigene panel testing in acute and chronic pancreatitis. PLoS One. 2024;19(8):e0307076. https://doi.org/10.1371/journal.pone.0307076.
3. Hasan A, Moscoso DI, Kastrinos F. The role of genetics in pancreatitis. Gastrointest Endosc Clin N Am. 2018;28(4):587–603. https://doi.org/10.1016/j.giec.2018.06.001.
4. LaRusch J, Whitcomb DC. Genetics of pancreatitis. Curr Opin Gastroenterol. 2011;27(5):467–74. https://doi.org/10.1097/MOG.0b013e328349e2f8.
5. Uc A, Cress GA, Wang F, Abu-El-Haija M, Ellery KM, Fishman DS, et al. Analysis of INSPPIRE-2 cohort: risk factors and disease burden in children with acute recurrent or chronic pancreatitis. J Pediatr Gastroenterol Nutr. 2022;75(5):643–9. https://doi.org/10.1097/mpg.0000000000003590.
6. Dike CR, Sellers ZM, Husain SZ, Forsmark CE, Abu-El-Haija M. Multidisciplinary approach to the Care of Children with Acute Recurrent Pancreatitis and Chronic Pancreatitis. Pancreas. 2022;51(3):256–60. https://doi.org/10.1097/mpa.0000000000002008.
7. Ting J, Wilson L, Schwarzenberg SJ, Himes R, Barth B, Bellin MD, et al. Direct costs of acute recurrent and chronic pancreatitis in children in the INSPPIRE registry. J Pediatr Gastroenterol Nutr. 2016;62(3):443–9. https://doi.org/10.1097/mpg.0000000000001057.
8. Schwarzenberg SJ, Uc A, Zimmerman B, Wilschanski M, Wilcox CM, Whitcomb DC, et al. Chronic pancreatitis: pediatric and adult cohorts show similarities in disease Progress despite different risk factors. J Pediatr Gastroenterol Nutr. 2019;68(4):566–73. https://doi.org/10.1097/mpg.0000000000002279.
9. Perito E, Gonska T, Bellin MD, Schwarzenberg SJ. Complications of chronic pancreatitis in children. Curr Opin Gastroenterol. 2021;37(5):498–503. https://doi.org/10.1097/mog.0000000000000762.
10. Uc A, Perito ER, Pohl JF, Shah U, Abu-El-Haija M, Barth B, et al. INternational study Group of Pediatric Pancreatitis: in search for a CuRE cohort study: design and rationale for INSPPIRE 2 from the consortium for the study of chronic pancreatitis, diabetes, and pancreatic cancer. Pancreas. 2018;47(10):1222–8. https://doi.org/10.1097/mpa.0000000000001172.

11. Morinville VD, Lowe ME, Ahuja M, Barth B, Bellin MD, Davis H, et al. Design and implementation of INSPPIRE. J Pediatr Gastroenterol Nutr. 2014;59(3):360–4. https://doi.org/10.1097/mpg.0000000000000417.
12. Schwarzenberg SJ, Bellin M, Husain SZ, Ahuja M, Barth B, Davis H, et al. Pediatric chronic pancreatitis is associated with genetic risk factors and substantial disease burden. J Pediatr. 2015;166(4):890–6.e1. https://doi.org/10.1016/j.jpeds.2014.11.019.
13. Kumar S, Ooi CY, Werlin S, Abu-El-Haija M, Barth B, Bellin MD, et al. Risk factors associated with pediatric acute recurrent and chronic pancreatitis: lessons from INSPPIRE. JAMA Pediatr. 2016;170(6):562–9. https://doi.org/10.1001/jamapediatrics.2015.4955.
14. Abu-El-Haija M, Lowe M, Barth B, Bellin MD, Fishman DS, Freedman S, et al. Pediatric chronic pancreatitis without prior acute or acute recurrent pancreatitis: a report from the INSPPIRE consortium. Pancreatology. 2020;20(4):781–4. https://doi.org/10.1016/j.pan.2020.04.001.
15. Sweeny KF, Lin TK, Nathan JD, Denson LA, Husain SZ, Hornung L, et al. Rapid progression of acute pancreatitis to acute recurrent pancreatitis in children. J Pediatr Gastroenterol Nutr. 2019;68(1):104–9. https://doi.org/10.1097/mpg.0000000000002145.
16. Giefer MJ, Lowe ME, Werlin SL, Zimmerman B, Wilschanski M, Troendle D, et al. Early-onset acute recurrent and chronic pancreatitis is associated with PRSS1 or CTRC gene mutations. J Pediatr. 2017;186:95–100. https://doi.org/10.1016/j.jpeds.2017.03.063.
17. Khazaaleh S, Babar S, Alomari M, Imam Z, Chadalavada P, Gonzalez AJ, et al. Outcomes of total pancreatectomy with islet autotransplantation: a systematic review and meta-analysis. World J Transplant. 2023;13(1):10–24. https://doi.org/10.5500/wjt.v13.i1.10.
18. Shah I, Bocchino R, Ahmed A, Freedman SD, Kothari DJ, Sheth SG. Impact of recurrent acute pancreatitis on the natural history and progression to chronic pancreatitis. Pancreatology. 2022;22(8):1084–90. https://doi.org/10.1016/j.pan.2022.09.237.
19. Husain SZ, Morinville V, Pohl J, Abu-El-Haija M, Bellin MD, Freedman S, et al. Toxic-metabolic risk factors in pediatric pancreatitis: recommendations for diagnosis, management, and future research. J Pediatr Gastroenterol Nutr. 2016;62(4):609–17. https://doi.org/10.1097/mpg.0000000000001035.
20. Uc A, Husain SZ. Pancreatitis in children. Gastroenterology. 2019;156(7):1969–78. https://doi.org/10.1053/j.gastro.2018.12.043.
21. Morinville VD, Husain SZ, Wang F, Cress GA, Abu-El-Haija M, Chugh A, et al. Pediatric drug-associated pancreatitis reveals concomitant risk factors and poor reliability of causality scoring: report from INSPPIRE. J Pediatr Gastroenterol Nutr. 2023;77(4):540–6. https://doi.org/10.1097/mpg.0000000000003898.
22. Gariepy CE, Heyman MB, Lowe ME, Pohl JF, Werlin SL, Wilschanski M, et al. Causal evaluation of acute recurrent and chronic pancreatitis in children: consensus from the INSPPIRE group. J Pediatr Gastroenterol Nutr. 2017;64(1):95–103. https://doi.org/10.1097/mpg.0000000000001446.
23. Masamune A, Kotani H, Sörgel FL, Chen JM, Hamada S, Sakaguchi R, et al. Variants that affect function of Calcium Channel TRPV6 are associated with early-onset chronic pancreatitis. Gastroenterology. 2020;158(6):1626–41.e8. https://doi.org/10.1053/j.gastro.2020.01.005.
24. Nathan JD, Ellery K, Balakrishnan K, Bhatt H, Ganoza A, Husain SZ, et al. The role of surgical Management in Chronic Pancreatitis in children: a position paper from the north American Society for Pediatric Gastroenterology, Hepatology, and nutrition pancreas committee. J Pediatr Gastroenterol Nutr. 2022;74(5):706–19. https://doi.org/10.1097/mpg.0000000000003439.
25. Párniczky A, Abu-El-Haija M, Husain S, Lowe M, Oracz G, Sahin-Tóth M, et al. EPC/HPSG evidence-based guidelines for the management of pediatric pancreatitis. Pancreatology. 2018;18(2):146–60. https://doi.org/10.1016/j.pan.2018.01.001.
26. Girodon E, Rebours V, Chen JM, Pagin A, Levy P, Ferec C, et al. Clinical interpretation of PRSS1 variants in patients with pancreatitis. Clin Res Hepatol Gastroenterol. 2021;45(1):101497. https://doi.org/10.1016/j.clinre.2020.07.004.

27. Pfützer R, Myers E, Applebaum-Shapiro S, Finch R, Ellis I, Neoptolemos J, et al. Novel cationic trypsinogen (PRSS1) N29T and R122C mutations cause autosomal dominant hereditary pancreatitis. Gut. 2002;50(2):271–2. https://doi.org/10.1136/gut.50.2.271.
28. Shelton C, Solomon S, LaRusch J, Whitcomb DC. PRSS1-related hereditary pancreatitis. In: Adam MP, Feldman J, Mirzaa GM, Pagon RA, Wallace SE, Amemiya a, editors. GeneReviews(®). Seattle: University of Washington. Copyright © 1993-2024, University of Washington, Seattle. GeneReviews is a registered trademark of the University of Washington, Seattle. All rights reserved; 1993
29. Rebours V, Boutron-Ruault MC, Schnee M, Férec C, Le Maréchal C, Hentic O, et al. The natural history of hereditary pancreatitis: a national series. Gut. 2009;58(1):97–103. https://doi.org/10.1136/gut.2008.149179.
30. Masson E, Le Maréchal C, Delcenserie R, Chen JM, Férec C. Hereditary pancreatitis caused by a double gain-of-function trypsinogen mutation. Hum Genet. 2008;123(5):521–9. https://doi.org/10.1007/s00439-008-0508-6.
31. Németh BC, Sahin-Tóth M. Human cationic trypsinogen (PRSS1) variants and chronic pancreatitis. Am J Physiol Gastrointest Liver Physiol. 2014;306(6):G466–73. https://doi.org/10.1152/ajpgi.00419.2013.
32. Liu QY, Abu-El-Haija M, Husain SZ, Barth B, Bellin M, Fishman DS, et al. Risk factors for rapid progression from acute recurrent to chronic pancreatitis in children: report from INSPPIRE. J Pediatr Gastroenterol Nutr. 2019;69(2):206–11. https://doi.org/10.1097/mpg.0000000000002405.
33. Shelton CA, Umapathy C, Stello K, Yadav D, Whitcomb DC. Hereditary pancreatitis in the United States: survival and rates of pancreatic cancer. Am J Gastroenterol. 2018;113(9):1376. https://doi.org/10.1038/s41395-018-0194-5.
34. Liu Q, Guo L, Zhang S, Wang J, Lin X, Gao F. PRSS1 mutation: a possible pathomechanism of pancreatic carcinogenesis and pancreatic cancer. Mol Med. 2019;25(1):44. https://doi.org/10.1186/s10020-019-0111-4.
35. Bellin MD, Prokhoda P, Hodges JS, Schwarzenberg SJ, Freeman ML, Dunn TB, et al. Age and disease duration impact outcomes of Total Pancreatectomy and islet autotransplant for PRSS1 hereditary pancreatitis. Pancreas. 2018;47(4):466–70. https://doi.org/10.1097/mpa.0000000000001028.
36. Marfil-Garza BA, Hefler J, Dajani K, Kin T, James Shapiro AM. Total pancreatectomy with islet cell autotransplantation in a 2-year-old child with hereditary pancreatitis due to a PRSS1 mutation. Am J Transplant. 2021;21(11):3790–3. https://doi.org/10.1111/ajt.16723.
37. Kazal LA, Spicer DS, Brahinsky RA. Isolation of a crystalline trypsin inhibitor-anticoagulant protein from pancreas. J Am Chem Soc. 1948;70(9):3034–40. https://doi.org/10.1021/ja01189a060.
38. Pubols MH, Bartelt DC, Greene LJ. Trypsin inhibitor from human pancreas and pancreatic juice. J Biol Chem. 1974;249(7):2235–42.
39. Kume K, Masamune A, Ariga H, Hayashi S, Takikawa T, Miura S, et al. Do genetic variants in the SPINK1 gene affect the level of serum PSTI? J Gastroenterol. 2012;47(11):1267–74. https://doi.org/10.1007/s00535-012-0590-3.
40. Witt H, Luck W, Hennies HC, Classen M, Kage A, Lass U, et al. Mutations in the gene encoding the serine protease inhibitor, Kazal type 1 are associated with chronic pancreatitis. Nat Genet. 2000;25(2):213–6. https://doi.org/10.1038/76088.
41. Jones TE, Bellin MD, Yadav D, Freeman ML, Schwarzenberg SJ, Slivka A, et al. The histopathology of SPINK1-associated chronic pancreatitis. Pancreatology. 2020;20(8):1648–55. https://doi.org/10.1016/j.pan.2020.10.030.
42. Piseddu I, Vielhauer J, Mayerle J. Genetic testing in acute and chronic pancreatitis. Curr Treat Options Gastroenterol. 2022;20:429–44.
43. Goetz D, Ren CL. Review of cystic fibrosis. Pediatr Ann. 2019;48(4):e154–e61. https://doi.org/10.3928/19382359-20190327-01.

44. Strong TV, Boehm K, Collins FS. Localization of cystic fibrosis transmembrane conductance regulator mRNA in the human gastrointestinal tract by in situ hybridization. J Clin Invest. 1994;93(1):347–54. https://doi.org/10.1172/jci116966.
45. Farrell PM, White TB, Ren CL, Hempstead SE, Accurso F, Derichs N, et al. Diagnosis of cystic fibrosis: consensus guidelines from the Cystic Fibrosis Foundation. J Pediatr 2017;181s:S4-S15.e1. doi:https://doi.org/10.1016/j.jpeds.2016.09.064.
46. Ooi CY, Dorfman R, Cipolli M, Gonska T, Castellani C, Keenan K, et al. Type of CFTR mutation determines risk of pancreatitis in patients with cystic fibrosis. Gastroenterology. 2011;140(1):153–61. https://doi.org/10.1053/j.gastro.2010.09.046.
47. Dray X, Fajac I, Bienvenu T, Chryssostalis A, Sogni P, Hubert D. Association of pancreas divisum and recurrent acute pancreatitis with the IVS8-5T-12TG allele of the CFTR gene and CFTR dysfunction. Pancreas. 2007;35(1):90–3. https://doi.org/10.1097/MPA.0b013e318054771f.
48. Augarten A, Ben Tov A, Madgar I, Barak A, Akons H, Laufer J, et al. The changing face of the exocrine pancreas in cystic fibrosis: the correlation between pancreatic status, pancreatitis and cystic fibrosis genotype. Eur J Gastroenterol Hepatol 2008;20(3):164–168. doi:https://doi.org/10.1097/MEG.0b013e3282f36d04.
49. Cohn JA, Friedman KJ, Noone PG, Knowles MR, Silverman LM, Jowell PS. Relation between mutations of the cystic fibrosis gene and idiopathic pancreatitis. N Engl J Med. 1998;339(10):653–8. https://doi.org/10.1056/nejm199809033391002.
50. Gelrud A, Sheth S, Banerjee S, Weed D, Shea J, Chuttani R, et al. Analysis of cystic fibrosis gener product (CFTR) function in patients with pancreas divisum and recurrent acute pancreatitis. Am J Gastroenterol. 2004;99(8):1557–62. https://doi.org/10.1111/j.1572-0241.2004.30834.x.
51. Garg PK, Khajuria R, Kabra M, Shastri SS. Association of SPINK1 gene mutation and CFTR gene polymorphisms in patients with pancreas divisum presenting with idiopathic pancreatitis. J Clin Gastroenterol. 2009;43(9):848–52. https://doi.org/10.1097/MCG.0b013e3181a4e772.
52. Freeman AJ, Ng K, Wang F, Abu-El-Haija MA, Chugh A, Cress GA, et al. Pancreatic enzyme use reduces pancreatitis frequency in children with acute recurrent or chronic pancreatitis: a report from INSPPIRE. Am J Gastroenterol. 2024;119(10):2094–102. https://doi.org/10.14309/ajg.0000000000002772.
53. Mun KS, Nathan JD, Jegga AG, Wikenheiser-Brokamp KA, Abu-El-Haija M, Naren AP. Personalized medicine approaches in cystic fibrosis related pancreatitis. Am J Transl Res. 2022;14(10):7612–20.
54. Phadke MY, Sellers ZM. Current clinical opinion on CFTR dysfunction and patient risk of pancreatitis: diagnostic and therapeutic considerations. Expert Rev Gastroenterol Hepatol. 2022;16(6):499–509. https://doi.org/10.1080/17474124.2022.2084072.
55. Rosendahl J, Witt H, Szmola R, Bhatia E, Ozsvári B, Landt O, et al. Chymotrypsin C (CTRC) variants that diminish activity or secretion are associated with chronic pancreatitis. Nat Genet. 2008;40(1):78–82. https://doi.org/10.1038/ng.2007.44.
56. Dunbar EK, Greer PJ, Saloman JL, Albers KM, Yadav D, Whitcomb DC, et al. Genetics of constant and severe pain in the NAPS2 cohort of recurrent acute and chronic pancreatitis patients. J Pain. 2024:104754. https://doi.org/10.1016/j.jpain.2024.104754.
57. Ewers M, Canaff L, Weh AE, Masson E, Eiseler K, Chen JM, et al. The three common polymorphisms p.A986S, p.R990G and p.Q1011E in the calcium sensing receptor (CASR) are not associated with chronic pancreatitis. Pancreatology. 2021;21(7):1299–304. https://doi.org/10.1016/j.pan.2021.08.008.
58. Felderbauer P, Hoffmann P, Einwächter H, Bulut K, Ansorge N, Schmitz F, et al. A novel mutation of the calcium sensing receptor gene is associated with chronic pancreatitis in a family with heterozygous SPINK1 mutations. BMC Gastroenterol. 2003;3:34. https://doi.org/10.1186/1471-230x-3-34.
59. Sándor M, Thiel FG, Schmid M, Demcsák A, Morales Granda NC, Németh BC, et al. Novel p.G250A mutation associated with chronic pancreatitis highlights Misfolding-prone region in carboxypeptidase A1 (CPA1). Int J Mol Sci. 2022;23(24) https://doi.org/10.3390/ijms232415463.

60. Hegyi E, Sahin-Tóth M. Human CPA1 mutation causes digestive enzyme misfolding and chronic pancreatitis in mice. Gut. 2019;68(2):301–12. https://doi.org/10.1136/gutjnl-2018-315994.
61. Orekhova A, Geisz A, Sahin-Tóth M. Ethanol feeding accelerates pancreatitis progression in CPA1 N256K mutant mice. Am J Physiol Gastrointest Liver Physiol. 2020;318(4):G694–g704. https://doi.org/10.1152/ajpgi.00007.2020.
62. Lin JH, Boulling A, Masson E, Cooper DN, Li ZS, Férec C, et al. Most unambiguous loss-of-function CPA1 mutations are unlikely to predispose to chronic pancreatitis. Gut. 2020;69(4):785–6. https://doi.org/10.1136/gutjnl-2019-318564.
63. Derikx MH, Kovacs P, Scholz M, Masson E, Chen JM, Ruffert C, et al. Polymorphisms at PRSS1-PRSS2 and CLDN2-MORC4 loci associate with alcoholic and non-alcoholic chronic pancreatitis in a European replication study. Gut. 2015;64(9):1426–33. https://doi.org/10.1136/gutjnl-2014-307453.
64. Deng Y, Li Z. Effects of PRSS1-PRSS2 rs10273639, CLDN2 rs7057398 and MORC4 rs12688220 polymorphisms on individual susceptibility to pancreatitis: a meta-analysis. Genomics. 2020;112(1):848–52. https://doi.org/10.1016/j.ygeno.2019.05.025.
65. Johansson BB, Fjeld K, El Jellas K, Gravdal A, Dalva M, Tjora E, et al. The role of the carboxyl ester lipase (CEL) gene in pancreatic disease. Pancreatology. 2018;18(1):12–9. https://doi.org/10.1016/j.pan.2017.12.001.
66. Wang MJ, Wang YC, Masson E, Wang YH, Yu D, Qian YY, et al. SEC16A variants predispose to chronic pancreatitis by impairing ER-to-Golgi transport and inducing ER stress. Adv Sci (Weinh). 2024;11(38):e2402550. https://doi.org/10.1002/advs.202402550.
67. Theodoropoulos P, Fanaropoulou NM, Manessis A. Unmasking a rare genetic mutation: the importance of genetic testing in refractory hypertriglyceridemia. AACE Clin Case Rep. 2024;10(6):240–3. https://doi.org/10.1016/j.aace.2024.08.006.
68. Tao H, Xu J, Li N, Chang H, Duan L. Early identification of high-risk patients with recurrent acute pancreatitis progression to chronic pancreatitis. Arch Med Sci. 2022;18(2):535–9. https://doi.org/10.5114/aoms/146262.
69. Zou WB, Tang XY, Zhou DZ, Qian YY, Hu LH, Yu FF, et al. SPINK1, PRSS1, CTRC, and CFTR genotypes influence disease onset and clinical outcomes in chronic pancreatitis. Clin Transl Gastroenterol. 2018;9(11):204. https://doi.org/10.1038/s41424-018-0069-5.
70. Schneider A, Larusch J, Sun X, Aloe A, Lamb J, Hawes R, et al. Combined bicarbonate conductance-impairing variants in CFTR and SPINK1 variants are associated with chronic pancreatitis in patients without cystic fibrosis. Gastroenterology. 2011;140(1):162–71. https://doi.org/10.1053/j.gastro.2010.10.045.
71. Pfützer RH, Whitcomb DC. SPINK1 mutations are associated with multiple phenotypes. Pancreatology. 2001;1(5):457–60. https://doi.org/10.1159/000055847.
72. Drenth JP, te Morsche R, Jansen JB. Mutations in serine protease inhibitor Kazal type 1 are strongly associated with chronic pancreatitis. Gut. 2002;50(5):687–92. https://doi.org/10.1136/gut.50.5.687.
73. Dike CR, Kao SC, Uc A. Progression from acute to chronic pancreatitis associated with CFTR and SPINK1 mutations. Pancreatology. 2020;20(5):1019–20. https://doi.org/10.1016/j.pan.2020.05.012.
74. Wang YC, Zou WB, Tang DH, Wang L, Hu LH, Qian YY, et al. High clinical and genetic similarity between chronic pancreatitis associated with light-to-moderate alcohol consumption and classical alcoholic chronic pancreatitis. Gastro Hep Adv. 2023;2(2):186–95. https://doi.org/10.1016/j.gastha.2022.09.009.
75. Hegyi P, Wilschanski M, Muallem S, Lukacs GL, Sahin-Tóth M, Uc A, et al. CFTR: a new horizon in the Pathomechanism and treatment of pancreatitis. Rev Physiol Biochem Pharmacol. 2016;170:37–66. https://doi.org/10.1007/112_2015_5002.
76. Lin TK, Abu-El-Haija M, Nathan JD, Palermo JP, Barth B, Bellin M, et al. Pancreas Divisum in pediatric acute recurrent and chronic pancreatitis: report from INSPPIRE. J Clin Gastroenterol. 2019;53(6):e232–e8. https://doi.org/10.1097/mcg.0000000000001063.

77. Bertin C, Pelletier AL, Vullierme MP, Bienvenu T, Rebours V, Hentic O, et al. Pancreas divisum is not a cause of pancreatitis by itself but acts as a partner of genetic mutations. Am J Gastroenterol. 2012;107(2):311–7. https://doi.org/10.1038/ajg.2011.424.
78. Gardner TB, Adler DG, Forsmark CE, Sauer BG, Taylor JR, Whitcomb DC. ACG clinical guideline: chronic pancreatitis. Am J Gastroenterol. 2020;115(3):322–39. https://doi.org/10.14309/ajg.0000000000000535.
79. Grigorescu RR, Husar-Sburlan IA, Gheorghe C. Pancreatic cancer: a review of risk factors. Life (Basel). 2024;14(8) https://doi.org/10.3390/life14080980.
80. Aslanian HR, Lee JH, Canto MI. AGA clinical practice update on pancreas cancer screening in high-risk individuals: expert review. Gastroenterology. 2020;159(1):358–62. https://doi.org/10.1053/j.gastro.2020.03.088.
81. Wen J, Li T, Liu L, Bie LK, Gong B. Long-term outcomes of therapeutic ERCP in pediatric patients with pancreas divisum presenting with acute recurrent or chronic pancreatitis. Pancreatology. 2019;19(6):834–41. https://doi.org/10.1016/j.pan.2019.08.004.
82. Dever JB, Irani S, Brandabur J, Traverso LW, Kozarek R. Outcomes of interventional ERCP in hereditary pancreatitis. J Clin Gastroenterol. 2010;44(1):46–51. https://doi.org/10.1097/01.mcg.0000360462.64261.55.
83. Troendle DM, Fishman DS, Barth BA, Giefer MJ, Lin TK, Liu QY, et al. Therapeutic endoscopic retrograde Cholangiopancreatography in pediatric patients with acute recurrent and chronic pancreatitis: data from the INSPPIRE (INternational study group of pediatric pancreatitis: in search for a cuRE) study. Pancreas. 2017;46(6):764–9. https://doi.org/10.1097/mpa.0000000000000848.
84. Lin TK, Pathak SJ, Hornung LN, Vitale DS, Nathan JD, Abu-El-Haija M. Clinical outcomes following therapeutic endoscopic retrograde Cholangiopancreatography in children with pancreas Divisum. J Pediatr Gastroenterol Nutr. 2021;72(2):300–5. https://doi.org/10.1097/mpg.0000000000002996.
85. Goggins M, Overbeek KA, Brand R, Syngal S, Del Chiaro M, Bartsch DK, et al. Management of patients with increased risk for familial pancreatic cancer: updated recommendations from the International cancer of the pancreas screening (CAPS) consortium. Gut. 2020;69(1):7–17. https://doi.org/10.1136/gutjnl-2019-319352.
86. Laje P, Adzick NS. Modified Puestow procedure for the management of chronic pancreatitis in children. J Pediatr Surg. 2013;48(11):2271–5. https://doi.org/10.1016/j.jpedsurg.2013.03.048.
87. Vardanyan M, Rilo HL. Pathogenesis of chronic pancreatitis-induced pain. Discov Med. 2010;9(47):304–10.
88. Abu-El-Haija M, Nathan JD. Pediatric chronic pancreatitis: updates in the 21st century. Pancreatology. 2018;18(4):354–9. https://doi.org/10.1016/j.pan.2018.04.013.
89. Roukounakis NE, Kuhn JA, McCarty TM. Association of an abnormal pancreaticobiliary junction with biliary tract cancers. Proc (Bayl Univ Med Cent). 2000;13(1):11–3. https://doi.org/10.1080/08998280.2000.11927636.
90. Kamisawa T, Tu Y, Nakajima H, Egawa N, Tsuruta K, Okamoto A, et al. Acute pancreatitis and a long common channel. Abdom Imaging. 2007;32(3):365–9. https://doi.org/10.1007/s00261-006-9057-4.
91. Iwasaki J, Ogura Y, Nakagawa S, Kato K, Kondo A, Shiraki K. Familial occurrence of congenital bile duct dilatation. World J Gastroenterol. 2008;14(6):941–3. https://doi.org/10.3748/wjg.14.941.
92. Iwama T, Iwata S, Murakami S, Ishida H, Mishima Y. Congenital bile duct dilatation--possibly an hereditary condition. Jpn J Surg. 1985;15(6):501–5. https://doi.org/10.1007/bf02470098.
93. Wong JK, Campbell D, Ngo ND, Yeung F, Cheng G, Tang CS, et al. Genetic study of congenital bile-duct dilatation identifies de novo and inherited variants in functionally related genes. BMC Med Genet. 2016;9(1):75. https://doi.org/10.1186/s12920-016-0236-z.
94. Sundaram S, Kale AP, Giri S, Ramani N, Dodmani M, Shukla A. Anomalous Pancreatobiliary ductal union presenting as recurrent acute and chronic pancreatitis in children and adolescents with response to Endotherapy. Cureus. 2023;15(2):e35046. https://doi.org/10.7759/cureus.35046.

95. Jimenez JC, Emil S, Podnos Y, Nguyen N. Annular pancreas in children: a recent decade's experience. J Pediatr Surg. 2004;39(11):1654–7. https://doi.org/10.1016/j.jpedsurg.2004.07.003.
96. Huddleston VS, Lippuner V, Dyer AW. Annular pancreas in an adult presenting with acute pancreatitis. J Radiol Case Rep. 2018;12(10):11–6. https://doi.org/10.3941/jrcr.v12i10.3461.
97. Chinnakotla S, Bellin MD, Schwarzenberg SJ, Radosevich DM, Cook M, Dunn TB, et al. Total pancreatectomy and islet autotransplantation in children for chronic pancreatitis: indication, surgical techniques, postoperative management, and long-term outcomes. Ann Surg. 2014;260(1):56–64. https://doi.org/10.1097/sla.0000000000000569.
98. Colling KP, Bellin MD, Schwarzenberg SJ, Berry L, Wilhelm JJ, Dunn T, et al. Total Pancreatectomy with Intraportal islet autotransplantation as a treatment of chronic pancreatitis in patients with CFTR mutations. Pancreas. 2018;47(2):238–44. https://doi.org/10.1097/mpa.0000000000000968.
99. Wahoff DC, Paplois BE, Najarian JS, Farney AC, Leonard AS, Kendall DM, et al. Islet autotransplantation after total pancreatectomy in a child. J Pediatr Surg. 1996;31(1):132–5.; discussion 5–6. https://doi.org/10.1016/s0022-3468(96)90335-8.
100. Chinnakotla S, Radosevich DM, Dunn TB, Bellin MD, Freeman ML, Schwarzenberg SJ, et al. Long-term outcomes of total pancreatectomy and islet auto transplantation for hereditary/genetic pancreatitis. J Am Coll Surg. 2014;218(4):530–43. https://doi.org/10.1016/j.jamcollsurg.2013.12.037.
101. Bellin MD, Forlenza GP, Majumder K, Berger M, Freeman ML, Beilman GJ, et al. Total Pancreatectomy with islet autotransplantation resolves pain in young children with severe chronic pancreatitis. J Pediatr Gastroenterol Nutr. 2017;64(3):440–5. https://doi.org/10.1097/mpg.0000000000001314.
102. Grybowski D, Bachul PJ, Pyda JS, Kijek M, Fillman N, Perez-Gutierrez A, et al. Pain resolution and glucose control in pediatric patients with chronic pancreatitis after total pancreatectomy with islet auto-transplantation. Pediatr Surg Int. 2021;37(10):1383–92. https://doi.org/10.1007/s00383-021-04956-5.
103. Bellin MD, Beilman GJ, Sutherland DE, Ali H, Petersen A, Mongin S, et al. How durable is Total Pancreatectomy and Intraportal islet cell transplantation for treatment of chronic pancreatitis? J Am Coll Surg. 2019;228(4):329–39. https://doi.org/10.1016/j.jamcollsurg.2018.12.019.
104. Kassam AF, Cortez AR, Johnston ME, Zang H, Fei L, Lin TK, et al. Total pancreatectomy with islet autotransplantation reduces resource utilization in pediatric patients. Am J Surg. 2021;222(4):786–92. https://doi.org/10.1016/j.amjsurg.2021.01.030.
105. Gruessner RW, Sutherland DE, Dunn DL, Najarian JS, Jie T, Hering BJ, et al. Transplant options for patients undergoing total pancreatectomy for chronic pancreatitis. J Am Coll Surg 2004;198(4):559–567; discussion 68–9. doi:https://doi.org/10.1016/j.jamcollsurg.2003.11.024.
106. Gutama BW, Yang Y, Beilman GJ, Freeman ML, Kirchner VA, Pruett TL, et al. Risk factors associated with progression toward endocrine insufficiency in chronic pancreatitis. Pancreas. 2019;48(9):1160–6. https://doi.org/10.1097/mpa.0000000000001394.
107. Wang H, Desai KD, Dong H, Owzarski S, Romagnuolo J, Morgan KA, et al. Prior surgery determines islet yield and insulin requirement in patients with chronic pancreatitis. Transplantation. 2013;95(8):1051–7. https://doi.org/10.1097/TP.0b013e3182845fbb.
108. Bellin MD, Freeman ML, Schwarzenberg SJ, Dunn TB, Beilman GJ, Vickers SM, et al. Quality of life improves for pediatric patients after total pancreatectomy and islet autotransplant for chronic pancreatitis. Clin Gastroenterol Hepatol. 2011;9(9):793–9. https://doi.org/10.1016/j.cgh.2011.04.024.
109. Bellin MD, Sutherland DE. Pediatric islet autotransplantation: indication, technique, and outcome. Curr Diab Rep. 2010;10(5):326–31. https://doi.org/10.1007/s11892-010-0140-4.

110. Kobayashi T, Manivel JC, Bellin MD, Carlson AM, Moran A, Freeman ML, et al. Correlation of pancreatic histopathologic findings and islet yield in children with chronic pancreatitis undergoing total pancreatectomy and islet autotransplantation. Pancreas. 2010;39(1):57–63. https://doi.org/10.1097/MPA.0b013e3181b8ff71.
111. Wilson GC, Sutton JM, Smith MT, Schmulewitz N, Salehi M, Choe KA, et al. Completion pancreatectomy and islet cell autotransplantation as salvage therapy for patients failing previous operative interventions for chronic pancreatitis. Surgery. 2015;158(4):872–8.; discussion 9–80. https://doi.org/10.1016/j.surg.2015.04.045.
112. Chinnakotla S, Beilman GJ, Dunn TB, Bellin MD, Freeman ML, Radosevich DM, et al. Factors predicting outcomes after a Total Pancreatectomy and islet autotransplantation lessons learned from over 500 cases. Ann Surg. 2015;262(4):610–22. https://doi.org/10.1097/sla.0000000000001453.
113. Trikudanathan G, Elmunzer BJ, Yang Y, Abu-El-Haija M, Adams D, Ahmad S, et al. Preoperative ERCP has no impact on islet yield following total pancreatectomy and islet autotransplantation (TPIAT): results from the prospective observational study of TPIAT (POST) cohort. Pancreatology. 2021;21(1):275–81. https://doi.org/10.1016/j.pan.2020.11.008.
114. Szary NM, Al-Kawas FH. Complications of endoscopic retrograde cholangiopancreatography: how to avoid and manage them. Gastroenterol Hepatol (N Y). 2013;9(8):496–504.
115. Sacco Casamassima MG, Goldstein SD, Yang J, Gause CD, Abdullah F, Meoded A, et al. The impact of surgical strategies on outcomes for pediatric chronic pancreatitis. Pediatr Surg Int. 2017;33(1):75–83. https://doi.org/10.1007/s00383-016-3999-6.
116. Downs EM, Brun A, Bellin MD. Nutrition support in the pediatric total pancreatectomy with islet autotransplantation recipient. Nutr Clin Pract. 2024;39(1):100–8. https://doi.org/10.1002/ncp.11101.

14 Total Pancreatectomy with Islet Autotransplantation for Chronic Pancreatitis in Children: Surgical Techniques and Outcomes

Srinath Chinnakotla

Abstract

Chronic pancreatitis in affected children is often progressive, resulting in debilitating pain, opioid use, recurrent hospitalization, missed school, and poor quality of life (QoL). The etiology in children is primarily genetic due to *PRSS1, SPINK1*, and *CFTR* mutations. A number of surgical procedures (partial resection/drainage) have been used, but due to diffuse gland involvement, pain recurs in >50% of patients. Total pancreatectomy with islet autotransplantation (TPIAT) is now increasingly being used to treat children with chronic pancreatitis refractory to medical and endoscopic treatment. TP is the only procedure that removes the root cause of the pain and theoretically eliminates the risk of pancreatic cancer. The islets of Langerhans are infused back into the patient's liver, where they engraft in the sinusoids of the liver and produce insulin and prevent brittle diabetes. TPIAT surgery, even in very young children, is safe, with a low operative mortality (0–1%). Surgical complications occur in 20% of patients and include intra-abdominal bleeding (5.3%), bowel obstruction (5.3%), abdominal abscess (4%), enteric leak (2.6%), biliary leak (1.3%), and wound infection (1.3%). Pancreatitis-type pain and the severity of pain significantly improve in >90% of patients following TPIAT, and at 10 year follow-up, opioid use is <20%. Approximately 50% of children achieve insulin independence long term, and 90.3% of these patients do so within 1 year. Younger children (<12 years) are more likely to achieve insulin independence than older children (12–18) (56.0% versus 40.5%; $p = 0.05$). Quality of life improves dramatically after TPIAT, with most children reporting improved ability to participate in school and play activities with reduced days of missed school.

S. Chinnakotla (✉)
Department of Surgery, University of Minnesota Medical School and University of Minnesota Masonic Children's Hospital, Minneapolis, MN, USA
e-mail: chinni@umn.edu

S. Chinnakotla et al. (eds.), *Total Pancreatectomy and Islet Auto Transplantation*,
https://doi.org/10.1007/978-981-92-0018-4_14

Key Points

- TPIAT is considered in children who have impaired quality of life due to painful chronic pancreatitis refractory to medical and endoscopic therapies.
- During the surgery, a key step is to carefully preserve the blood vessels supplying the pancreas to the very end to minimize warm ischemia time and to maximize islet cell preservation.
- Pylorus preservation, use of a Roux-en-Y loop for duodenojejunostomy, and avoidance of small-vessel injury or spasm are important surgical components.
- During islet cell infusion, portal pressure should be monitored every 3 min and paused if it goes above 25 cm saline. If the pressure does not decrease below this threshold after 15 min, the islets should be implanted in the peritoneal cavity as a thin film, rather than through a portal infusion.
- Young age (e.g., 3 years old) is not a contraindication to TPIAT, as long as the total liver volume is >400 ml.

14.1 Introduction

Chronic pancreatitis (CP) is a rare diagnosis in children, with an estimated incidence of less than one case per 200,000 [1]. The etiology of CP in children is most often mutations in the *PRSS1*, *SPINK1*, and/or *CFTR* genes [2, 3]. A recent study demonstrated a genetic etiology in 67% of cases, with obstructive etiology—including biliary calculi and congenital anatomic abnormalities—in 33% [3]. Some of these children had both genetic and obstructive etiologies, and in 11% of patients, no risk factors could be identified (idiopathic CP). Anatomic abnormalities associated with pancreatitis include pancreas divisum, annular pancreas, intestinal duplication cysts, anomalous pancreaticobiliary junction, and choledochal cysts [4–8].

The first line of treatment for childhood CP is medical management, which includes narcotic analgesics; pancreatic enzyme supplementation to minimize pancreatic stimulation; nerve block procedures for pain relief; and endoscopic decompression of obstructive disease by stone extraction, sphincterotomy, stricture dilation, and stent placement [9, 10]. Children who fail medical or endoscopic interventions are surgical candidates. The traditional surgical interventions include partial resections (Whipple's procedure, distal pancreatectomy) and drainage procedures such as lateral pancreaticojejunostomy (Puestow) or its variants (such as Frey, Beger, or Duval procedures) [11]. Patients can obtain transient pain relief from these procedures, but due to the diffuse nature of CP, pain eventually recurs in up to 50% of patients [12–17]. Despite the aforementioned interventions, exocrine and endocrine insufficiency can still develop in these children over time [18].

A novel approach to treatment of CP was developed in 1977, when the first human total pancreatectomy with islet autotransplantation (TPIAT) was performed. The first pediatric case was performed in 1989 at the University of Minnesota [19, 20]. TP removes the source of the pain and theoretically eliminates the risk of pancreatic cancer. In isolation, however, a total pancreatectomy can lead to a lifetime of brittle diabetes. The goal of IAT is to prevent or minimize TP-related brittle diabetes. Isolated islets of Langerhans are infused back into the patient, most typically via the portal vein, and eventually engraft in the sinusoids of the liver [19]. Following success at our institution, TPIAT is now increasingly being used to treat children with CP refractory to medical and endoscopic treatment. To date, over 400 cases have been performed worldwide [21–23]. This chapter will review the indications, surgical procedure, islet isolation, and early postoperative care in children.

14.2 Selection of Patients for TPIAT

TPIAT is considered in children when medical and endoscopic therapy have failed and children have pain requiring daily narcotics or have impaired quality of life (QoL) as indicated by the inability to attend school or participate in daily activities [21–26]. To justify the major surgical procedure and the potential complication of lifelong diabetes, patients must be carefully selected to ensure that TPIAT will provide more benefit than harm. Robust family support and treatment of any associated mental health comorbidities are essential for successful postoperative outcomes in children [25].

The child should have a confirmed diagnosis of CP before receiving TPIAT. At our institution, the Minnesota Criteria [21, 25] guide selection of appropriate patients (Box 14.1). Each patient is discussed by a multidisciplinary committee, and surgery is scheduled only after approval from the committee.

Box 14.1: Criteria for TPIAT, University of Minnesota

Indications for TPIAT

Chronic pancreatitis (CP)

Chronic abdominal pain, lasting more than 6 months; features consistent with CP; and evidence of CP by at least one of the following:

1. Morphologic or functional evidence of CP (per computed tomography [CT] of the abdomen indicating calcifications, or per endoscopic retrograde cholangiopancreatography [ERCP])
2. At least six of nine criteria positive for CP per endoscopic ultrasound (EUS)
3. At least two of the following:
   (a) Findings suggestive of CP (abnormal duct or side branch) per secretin-enhanced magnetic resonance cholangiopancreatography (sMRCP) or magnetic resonance imaging (MRI) T1 evidence of fibrosis
   (b) At least four of nine criteria positive for CP per EUS
   (c) Abnormal exocrine pancreatic function test results (peak bicarbonate <80)

(continued)

Box 14.1 (continued)

Or

Relapsing acute pancreatitis (relapsing AP)

1. Three or more episodes of documented AP (elevated amylase or lipase, CT evidence) with ongoing episodes for more than 6 months and with disabling interval pain similar to AP pain
2. No evidence of current gallstone disease (patients with gallstones should undergo cholecystectomy) and no evidence of other correctable conditions

Documented hereditary pancreatitis with compatible clinical history

All of the criteria below:

1. Documented CP or relapsing AP with chronic or severe abdominal pain, directly resulting in at least one of the following:
   (a) Chronic narcotic dependence (narcotics required on a daily or near-daily basis for >3 months)
   (b) Impaired quality of life per the RAND medical outcomes study 36-item short form (SF-36) health survey
2. Complete evaluation with no reversible cause of CP or relapsing AP present or untreated
3. Unresponsiveness to maximal medical therapy and endoscopic therapy
4. Ongoing abdominal pain requiring routine narcotics for CP or relapsing AP
5. Adequate islet function (i.e., either no diabetes or non–insulin-requiring diabetes with positive C-peptide levels)

Contraindications for TPIAT

1. Active alcoholism (to be considered for a TPIAT, patient must be abstinent for 6 months with documented success of therapy)
2. Pancreatic cancer
3. End-stage pulmonary disease, cirrhosis, or severe arteriosclerotic heart disease.
4. Poorly controlled psychiatric illness
5. Inability to comply with postoperative regimen
6. Intraductal papillary mucinous neoplasia (patient should undergo IAT only as part of a clinical trial)
7. Illegal drug use (to be considered for TPIAT, patient must be abstinent for 6 months with documented success of therapy)

Apart from the surgical preoperative evaluation for a major surgical procedure, all patients must have assessment of islet function, which should include fasting glucose, hemoglobin A1c, C-peptide levels, and oral or intravenous stimulatory tests [22, 24]. Such information may help estimate the likelihood of successful islet isolation [27]. All children should have a computed tomography (CT) scan of the abdomen with intravenous contrast to assess the vascular anatomy. In younger children (age <8 years), volumetrics of the liver are necessary to assess adequacy of liver volume for intraportal islet transplantation. A total liver volume of >400 ml is acceptable for intraportal IAT.

14.3 Surgical Considerations in Pediatric Patients

The extent of the surgical resection is shown in Fig. 14.1. The main variation in the surgical technique for children receiving an IAT is carefully preserving the blood supply to the pancreas until the resection is completed, thus minimizing warm ischemia time and maximizing islet cell preservation [22]. In addition, important surgical steps in the pediatric patient include special attention to avoid any inadvertent injury or spasm of the small vessels to the pancreas, preservation of the pylorus, and use of a Roux-en-Y loop for duodenojejunostomy (Fig. 14.2) to minimize postoperative gastrointestinal complications such as bile reflux gastritis. The procedure can be performed via an open technique or a laparoscopic approach. For the open procedure, we use a midline incision, which is associated with less pain than a bilateral subcostal incision [21, 22]. After opening the abdominal cavity and performing any necessary adhesion lysis, a Kocher maneuver is performed to completely mobilize the duodenum and the pancreatic head until the left renal vein and the superior mesenteric artery are well visualized. The peritoneum on the anterior surface of the

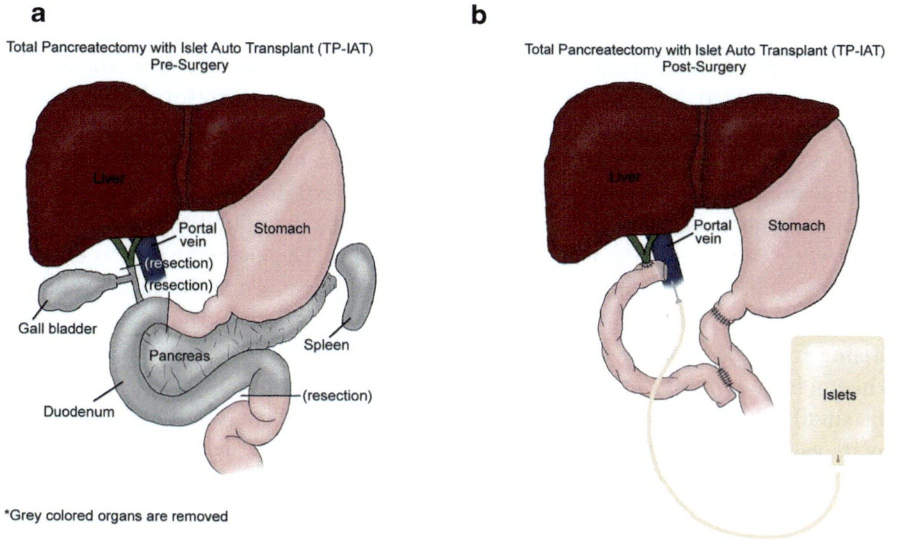

Fig. 14.1 Total pancreatectomy with islet autotransplantation (TPIAT). (**a**) The anatomy before surgery is shown, with the organs to be removed colored gray. (**b**) The anatomy after pancreatectomy and Roux-en-Y reconstruction is shown. Purified islets are shown being injected into the portal vein

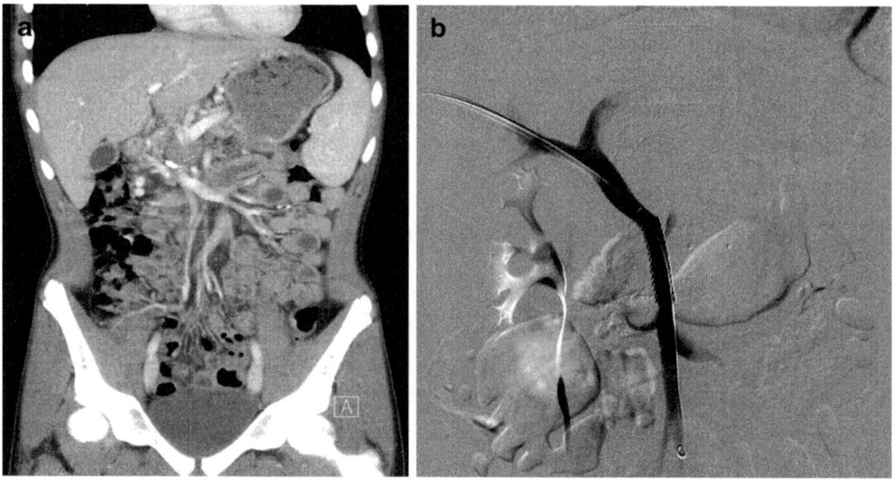

Fig. 14.2 (**a**) CT scan showing complete portal vein thrombosis. (**b**) Portovenogram showing successful placement of a stent opening the portal vein occlusion

portal triad is opened; the gastroduodenal artery is dissected and looped. Papaverine (1%) is sprayed on the artery to prevent spasm [21, 22]. Next, the short gastric vessels are divided; the spleen is mobilized by dividing the splenorenal and splenocolic ligaments. Using the spleen as a handle, the tail and body of the pancreas are mobilized all the way medially to the level of the superior mesenteric vein. The fibrofatty tissue both in front of and behind the splenic artery and splenic vein is dissected; the splenic artery is identified and looped on the superior border of the pancreas. The splenic vein is looped distal to the entry of the inferior mesenteric vein. The duodenum is transected 3 cm distal to the pylorus using a gastrointestinal anastomosis (GIA) stapler (1 Proximate, reloadable linear cutter stapler, 55 mm, Ethicon Endo-Surgery, USA). The right gastric and gastroepiploic blood vessels are preserved, and the stomach is reflected upward and laterally to expose the head and body of the pancreas. The distal duodenum is transected at the ligament of Treitz. The superior mesenteric vein is identified and carefully dissected. The pancreatic neck is elevated off the portal vein. The bile duct is identified and transected at the superior border of the pancreas. Careful examination identifies any accessory right hepatic artery arising from the superior mesenteric artery; if one exists, it is carefully preserved. The uncinate process of the pancreas is mobilized off the portal vein by dividing all the small tributaries to the portal vein. At this stage, the pancreas is connected only by its vascular structures, and the islet cell isolation team is alerted [21, 22].

The vascular structures are divided in the following order: gastroduodenal artery, splenic artery, and splenic vein. The pancreas is then immediately placed in cold sterile preservative solution and transported to the islet isolation laboratory. While processing of the pancreas is continued in the laboratory, gastrointestinal reconstruction is initiated as follows: the proximal jejunum is mobilized and brought into the infrahepatic region on the right side. An end-to-side choledochojejunostomy (end of bile duct to the side of jejunum) is constructed using multiple interrupted absorbable sutures. Twenty centimeters downstream, the jejunum is divided using a GIA stapler. A 40-cm Roux-en-Y limb is fashioned. A duodenojejunostomy is constructed in an end-to-side fashion in two layers using multiple absorbable interrupted sutures. A gastrojejunostomy (GJ) tube is placed in the stomach using the Stamm technique, and the tip of the jejunal tube is placed in the distal jejunum.

We have recently started performing this procedure with laparoscopic assistance. In a case-controlled study where 21 patients receiving a laparoscopic procedure were compared to matched controls, the surgical complications and islet graft outcomes were similar. The laparoscopic approach allows for a smaller incision and better scar satisfaction [28].

14.4 Special Considerations

14.4.1 Recent Episode of Acute Pancreatitis

In an acute attack of pancreatitis in a child, the surgical planes are very inflamed. The portal vein can be friable, and dissection of the hepatic artery, superior mesenteric artery, and celiac artery off the pancreas can be treacherous. It is our practice to avoid TPIAT in a child in the setting of an acute episode of pancreatitis due to the additional risk of injury to the vascular structures (portal vein, superior mesenteric artery and vein). Ideally, we wait for 4–6 weeks after an episode of acute pancreatitis to allow the inflammation to resolve and to often confirm this with a CT scan of the abdomen.

14.4.2 Portal Vein Thrombosis

Severe pancreatic inflammation and pseudocyst formation are complications of hereditary pancreatitis that affect >10% of children. In some of these children, the pancreatitis/pseudocyst formation can result in portal vein thrombosis, portal vein stenosis, and/or superior mesenteric vein thrombosis or even a fistulous communication with the portal vein. These children develop cavernous transformation of the portal vein and can present with gastrointestinal bleeding. Dissection of the pancreas can be difficult, and the vascular collaterals around the pancreas are friable, which can result in severe blood loss. For such patients, we elect to stent the portal vein preoperatively by employing a transhepatic approach with an iCAST (Atrium Medical Corporation, Hudson, NJ) balloon-expandable polytetrafluoroethylene-covered stent across the thrombosis (Fig. 14.2a, b) [29]. This maneuver reduces the portal vein pressure and makes the pancreatectomy easier. After the pancreatectomy, we obtain proximal control of the superior mesenteric artery by placing a vascular clamp and distal control by placing a vascular bulldog clamp on the portal vein. The stent is removed, and the portal vein is reconstructed with a splenic graft patch that can be prepared on the back table from the resected pancreas specimen (Fig. 14.3). Another alternative for the jump graft could be a cryopreserved vein.

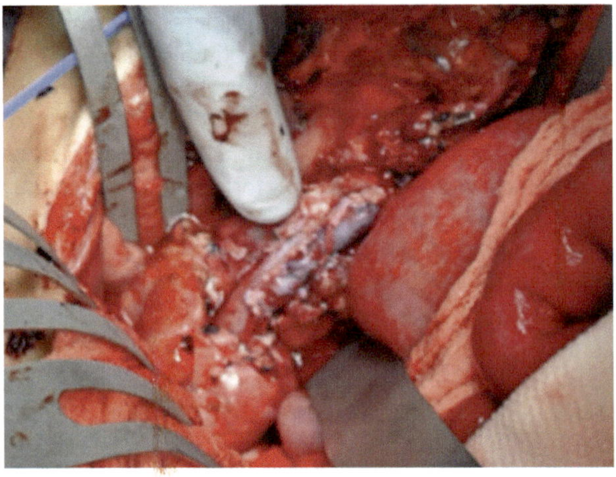

Fig. 14.3 Portal vein reconstruction with a splenic graft patch from the resected pancreas specimen

14.4.3 Microbial Contamination of the Islet Preparation

Microorganisms that colonize the diseased pancreas are not eliminated during islet processing before transplantation, so the final islet preparation that is infused into the patient's portal vein is often contaminated with bacteria. In one study of 86 pediatric patients, the final islet preparation was positive for microbiologic growth in 44 (51.2%) [30].

The bacterial species commonly isolated were *Streptococcus*, *Staphylococcus*, and *Enterobacter* species and *Escherichia coli*. Previous pancreatic surgery or multiple previous ERCP and stent placements were associated with increased risk of contamination. In addition to the perioperative antibiotics, patients with positive microbial cultures should receive additional directed antimicrobial therapy for 7 days. While a positive microbial culture of the islet preparation is not associated with increased post-IAT infections, it can have a higher risk of graft failure at 2 years. The plausible explanation is that transplanting microbes into the portal system results in an inflammatory response that hinders islet engraftment, leading to a greater incidence of graft failure. Microbial contamination of the final islet preparation does not appear to compromise safety and should not preclude IAT in children undergoing total pancreatectomy for CP.

14.5 Islet Isolation

The pediatric pancreata are small and often very fibrotic. To obtain a low tissue volume and a high yield of islets, the recommended enzyme mixture is a high proportion of intact class 1 (C1) and class 2 (C2) collagenases combined with neutral proteases, all derived from the organism *Clostridium histolyticum*. The methods employed for success include minimal mechanical disruption during digestion, warm enzymatic digestion using the special enzyme mixture, and extended distention and trimming time during isolation. This specialized enzyme mixture has been shown to improve islet yields from pediatric pancreata without compromising their functional capacity in vivo [31, 32]. After ductal perfusion of the enzymes, the pancreas is digested by using a modified Ricordi's semiautomated method [24, 33]. Of note, younger patients benefit from a prolonged stationary digestion time prior to mechanical digestion compared with the time used for adults [24, 31]. The digested tissue is typically not purified for autologous transplantation unless it exceeds 0.25 cc/kg of the patient's body weight. Despite the small size of the pediatric pancreas, consistently higher islet yield per gram of pancreas can be obtained in children than in adults [24, 31, 34]. Following isolation, the islet product is suspended in albumin-based medium, with added antibiotics, and returned to the operating room for infusion.

14.6 Islet Cell Infusion

Children have smaller portal veins and intrahepatic vessels compared with adults; thus, higher degrees of anticoagulation and slower rates of infusion of islets into the liver are necessary to allow the islets to evenly distribute within the liver and prevent portal vein thrombosis. Prior to starting islet infusion, the patient is given a bolus intravenously 35 units heparin per kilogram, and the heparin is allowed to circulate for at least 3 min. The islet product also contains 35 units heparin per kilogram. The patient is also started on dextran 0.5 cc per kilogram to a maximum of 10 cc per hour continuous infusion. Dextran specifically inhibits the extrinsic pathway of coagulation and helps prevent platelet plugs [21]. During the islet infusion, it is not uncommon to have transient hypotension, which is successfully managed by use of vasopressors.

We prefer to infuse the islets in the operating room concurrently with the TP procedure. The splenic vein stump or the middle colic vein is cannulated using a micropuncture catheter and attached to pressure tubing with an inline manometer. The manometer is zeroed prior to starting the infusion. The islet preparation is infused by gravity into the portal venous system. We prefer to see the drops slowly trickling rather than a steady stream of infusate. Baseline portal pressure is first recorded, and the pressure is measured every 3 min. If the pressure increases to greater than 25 cm of saline, the infusion is paused for 10 min to allow the portal pressure to autoregulate, and the pressure is then rechecked. Most of the time, autoregulation causes the portal pressure to decrease. Infusion is restarted, and pressures are again measured at 3-min intervals. It is important to closely monitor pressure changes at 3-min intervals in children. If the pressure is less than 25 cm saline, the infusion is restarted. If the pressure persistently remains more than 25 cm saline after 10 min of waiting for autoregulation, or if the total tissue volume exceeds 0.25 cc/kg of recipient body weight, the portal infusion is terminated, and the rest of the islet preparation is implanted in the peritoneal cavity as a thin film. It can alternatively be placed in an omental pocket. It is critical to infuse the islets slowly and not rush the process. The total time spent on infusing islets ranges from 60 to 110 min [21].

14.7 Postoperative Care

Patients are admitted to the pediatric intensive care unit for postoperative monitoring, including frequent blood glucose checks [21–23]. A continuous infusion of insulin is adjusted to maintain strict blood glucose control between 80 and 120 mg/dl; this range of blood glucoses avoids stress on the engrafting islets and aids in improved long-term islet graft function. Tube feeds via the jejunal part of the GJ tube are initiated at 48 h postoperatively. The gastrostomy (G) tube is vented for the first few weeks until gastric motility returns. Once the patient achieves target nutritional goals, insulin is converted to the subcutaneous route, which is continued on discharge. A recent randomized study in 14 children showed that the use of continuous glucose monitoring systems gave better glycemic control in children [34]. Tube feeds are cycled, and diet is advanced as gastric emptying improves. Tube feeds are stopped when the child can demonstrate adequate oral intake of calories and protein. Mean duration of hospitalization is 16–21 days.

Regular use of digestive enzymes is required after total pancreatectomy. The target dose is 1400 lipase units/kg per meal and half this amount for snacks [21]. Patients also take fat-soluble vitamin supplementation (AquADEKs®) and are counseled to consume a low-oxalate diet to prevent kidney stones [21].

Nearly all pediatric patients receive exogenous insulin during the first 3 months after TPIAT to relieve functional stress on beta cells during the engraftment (neovascularization) stage [23, 35–38]. During this time, islets rely on diffusion to obtain nutrients and oxygen and are particularly at risk of injury from hyperglycemia in a hypoxic environment. Subsequently, insulin is gradually discontinued, provided that blood glucose levels remain within a near-normal target range. The target range is a fasting glucose of <125 mg/dl, postprandial glucose of <180 mg/dl, and glycosylated hemoglobin $\leq 6.5\%$ [25]. If these parameters are not met, then the patients must continue insulin use. Corticosteroids and other medications that induce hyperglycemia should be avoided whenever possible [38].

14.8 Pain Management

A dedicated pediatric pain team is mandatory to manage postoperative pain in children post-TPIAT. Paravertebral blocks placed prior to surgery can improve pain management and reduce narcotic use [39]. The paravertebral catheters can be left in place for 7 days. Patients are postoperatively started on intravenous narcotics, and as they resume gastrointestinal function, oral narcotics are started. Nonsteroidal anti-inflammatory agents like Ketorolac can be started intravenously after postoperative day 2 (when the risk of bleeding decreases) for a maximum of 5 days to augment pain relief. Patients are weaned off narcotics in the outpatient clinics.

14.9 Splenectomy Management

Although spleen-preserving TPIAT procedures have been described, most children who undergo TPIAT will have their spleen removed as part of the procedure, due to the technical difficulty of spleen preservation in this population and the risk of postoperative splenic congestion [21–23]. To prevent overwhelming postsplenectomy sepsis, vaccination is completed at least 2 weeks preoperatively and includes *Haemophilus influenzae* type b, meningococcal, and pneumococcal vaccines. All children are maintained on prophylactic antibiotics for 1 year postoperatively [21]. This differs from adults, who do not undergo antibiotic prophylaxis following TPIAT. Pediatric patients and their caretakers also receive counseling regarding the risks of infection following splenectomy and strategies for risk reduction (see more on counseling in Chap. 3).

14.10 Surgical Morbidity and Mortality

Despite TPIAT being a major surgery with prolonged operative times, operative mortality after TPIAT in pediatric patients is very low, and it is safe even in small children (0–1%) [21–24]. In a review of 75 patients, surgical complications occurred in 15 patients (20%) and included abdominal bleeding (5.3%), bowel obstruction (5.3%), abdominal abscess (4%), enteric leak (2.6%), biliary leak (1.3%), and wound infection (1.3%) [21]. Of note, in this series, the complication rate was significantly lower in younger children (<12 years of age; $p = 0.041$). Interestingly, all four patients who developed intra-abdominal bleeding had elevated islet infusion portal pressures (>25 mmHg), highlighting the need to maintain low portal pressures during islet cell infusion into the liver. In another series, complications included acute respiratory distress syndrome, pneumonia, urinary tract infection, and central line–associated bloodstream infection [23]. None of the patients had long-term sequelae from their complications. Gastrojejunostomy tube malfunction and dislocation are very common, occurring in 20–30% of patients in the Minnesota experience, requiring interventional radiology or endoscopy to replace them.

Postsplenectomy thrombocytosis (platelet count >$10^6/\mu L$) occurs in 40% of patients and is managed with hydroxyurea [21]. Although there is a risk of portal vein thrombosis with islet infusion, no pediatric cases have been reported thus far. Portal vein stenosis requiring a surgical shunt for correction has been reported in one patient [21].

14.11 Narcotic Use and Pain After TPIAT

Pain relief after TPIAT in children is excellent, and the benefits are sustained long term. Following their operation, patients remain on narcotics for acute postoperative pain, and the dose is gradually tapered over 2–12 weeks. Narcotics can be discontinued in the majority of patients, with 79–90% reported as narcotic-free on follow-up [21–23]. On postoperative surveys, patients report that pancreatitis-type pain and the severity of pain significantly improve over time following TPIAT ($p < 0.001$) [21]. Long-term opioid use (at 10-year follow-up) is reported to be about 10–20%.

14.12 Islet Function After TPIAT

Children have higher rates of insulin independence and partial graft function compared with adults. In one reported series of pediatric patients, 41.3% achieved insulin independence following TPIAT, and 90.3% of these patients did so within 1 year [21, 22]. Younger children (<12 years) are more likely to achieve insulin independence compared with older children (12–18 years) (56.0% versus 40.5%; $p = 0.05$) [21]. In another series, 29% were insulin independent, and an additional 57% required less than 20 U of insulin daily [22]. Insulin independence has been observed for longer than 12 years after TPIAT [21].

It is important to remember that, even without pancreatectomy, 30–50% of pediatric CP patients will develop diabetes in their lifetime solely from progression of their disease [18]. Even children who have partial function and must use some insulin on a daily basis often have hypoglycemic awareness and have been shown to have improved quality of life compared with their pre-TPIAT status [21, 40].

14.13 Factors Predicting Insulin Independence

The most important predictor of insulin independence after TPIAT is the islet yield from the pancreas. Patient factors associated with a higher probability of insulin independence include younger age, lack of prior Puestow procedure, lower body surface area, higher islet equivalents (IEQ)/kg of body weight, and total IEQ transplanted [21–24]. Total IEQ infused into the liver is by far the factor most strongly associated with insulin independence (odds ratio = 2.62; $p < 0.001$) [21]. Children who received the most islets, >5000 IEQ/kg body weight, had the highest insulin independence rate of 76% at 2 years after TPIAT. The lowest insulin independence rate was seen in children who received <2500 IEQ/kg [21].

Prior pancreatic surgery has been shown to have a significant impact on outcomes of TPIAT. Drainage procedures such as the Puestow procedure lead to significantly lower islet yields, as the ability to isolate islets in the laboratory by duct infusion of enzymes is lost and the risk of post-TPIAT diabetes and insulin requirements is increased [21, 41]. Parents should be counseled accordingly when considering TPIAT after surgical drainage procedures.

14.14 How Young Is Too Young for TPIAT?

Fear of major surgery and risk of long-term diabetes can deter referral of younger children for TPIAT. Some of these children can end up suffering from intractable pain and poor quality of life. We evaluated outcomes in our youngest TPIAT recipients and noted that they in fact do well. Among 17 children aged 3–8 years who received TPIAT, all (100%) had relief of pain and all 17 were off narcotics [42]. Fourteen of the seventeen (82%) were insulin independent, higher than the 41% rate observed in patients older than 8 years [42]. There was no operative mortality. Although the decision to proceed with TPIAT must be carefully considered in the management of young children with CP, with the risks of major surgery taken into consideration, the age and size of the child do not negatively affect outcomes. Younger age is not a contraindication to referral [41].

14.15 Conclusions

Chronic pancreatitis is rare in children, often genetic in etiology. For affected children, it is often a debilitating disease that leads to very poor quality of life due to severe abdominal pain, pancreatic insufficiency, loss of school days, and narcotic dependence. Rare though it may be, pancreatitis is increasingly recognized as a cause of chronic abdominal pain in children [43]. Ongoing pain, such as that experienced by children with CP, has been associated with mental health issues such as anxiety, depression, and low self-esteem and also with chronic physical health problems [44, 45]. If medical or endoscopic interventions do not provide adequate relief for pediatric patients, a provider should consider referral for TP to remove the root cause of the patient's pain.

With improvements in islet isolation, infusion, and engraftment, the complication of brittle diabetes can be avoided or minimized. As a rule, most pediatric patients experience sustained pain relief and acceptable long-term glycemic control. Quality of life improves dramatically after TPIAT, with most children reporting full-time return to school. Early referral to an experienced center allows for evaluation and surgical treatment before extensive damage to the pancreas has occurred. Further advances in islet isolation techniques will allow increasing numbers of patients to remain insulin independent.

References

1. Spanier B, Bruno MJ, Dijkgraaf MG. Incidence and mortality of acute and chronic pancreatitis in The Netherlands: a nationwide record-linked cohort study for the years 1995-2005. World J Gastroenterol. 2013;19(20):3018–26.
2. Schmitt F, Le Henaff G, Piloquet H, Leclair MD, David A, Heloury Y, et al. Hereditary pancreatitis in children: surgical implications with special regard to genetic background. J Pediatr Surg. 2009;44(11):2078–82.
3. Schwarzenberg SJ, Bellin M, Husain SZ, Ahuja M, Barth B, Davis H, et al. Pediatric chronic pancreatitis is associated with genetic risk factors and substantial disease burden. J Pediatr. 2015;166(4):890–6.e1.
4. Jaunin-Stalder N, Stahelin-Massik J, Knuchel J, Gnehm HE. A pair of monozygotic twins with anomalous pancreaticobiliary junction and pancreatitis. J Pediatr Surg. 2002;37(10):1485–7.
5. Ozel A, Uysal E, Tufaner O, Erturk SM, Yalcin M, Basak M. Duodenal duplication cyst: a rare cause of acute pancreatitis in children. J Clin Ultrasound. 2008;36(9):584–6.
6. Urushihara N, Fukumoto K, Fukuzawa H, Suzuki K, Matsuoka T, Kawashima S, et al. Recurrent pancreatitis caused by pancreatobiliary anomalies in children with annular pancreas. J Pediatr Surg. 2010;45(4):741–6.
7. Neblett WW 3rd, O'Neill JA Jr. Surgical management of recurrent pancreatitis in children with pancreas divisum. Ann Surg. 2000;231(6):899–908.
8. Fujishiro J, Masumoto K, Urita Y, Shinkai T, Gotoh C. Pancreatic complications in pediatric choledochal cysts. J Pediatr Surg. 2013;48(9):1897–902.
9. Ammann RW. Diagnosis and management of chronic pancreatitis: current knowledge. Swiss Med Wkly. 2006;136(11–12):166–74.
10. Choudari CP, Nickl NJ, Fogel E, Lehman GA, Sherman S. Hereditary pancreatitis: clinical presentation, ERCP findings, and outcome of endoscopic therapy. Gastrointest Endosc. 2002;56(1):66–71.
11. Clifton MS, Pelayo JC, Cortes RA, Grethel EJ, Wagner AJ, Lee H, et al. Surgical treatment of childhood recurrent pancreatitis. J Pediatr Surg. 2007;42(7):1203–7.
12. Gachago C, Draganov PV. Pain management in chronic pancreatitis. World J Gastroenterol. 2008;14(20):3137–48.
13. Holmberg JT, Isaksson G, Ihse I. Long term results of pancreaticojejunostomy in chronic pancreatitis. Surg Gynecol Obstet. 1985;160(4):339–46.
14. Bradley EL 3rd. Long-term results of pancreatojejunostomy in patients with chronic pancreatitis. Am J Surg. 1987;153(2):207–13.
15. Markowitz JS, Rattner DW, Warshaw AL. Failure of symptomatic relief after pancreaticojejunal decompression for chronic pancreatitis. Strategies for salvage. Arch Surg. 1994;129(4):374–9. discussion 9–80
16. O'Neil SJ, Aranha GV. Lateral pancreaticojejunostomy for chronic pancreatitis. World J Surg. 2003;27(11):1196–202.
17. Cahen DL, Gouma DJ, Nio Y, Rauws EA, Boermeester MA, Busch OR, et al. Endoscopic versus surgical drainage of the pancreatic duct in chronic pancreatitis. N Engl J Med. 2007;356(7):676–84.
18. Sasikala M, Talukdar R, Pavan kumar P, Radhika G, Rao GV, Pradeep R, et al. Beta-cell dysfunction in chronic pancreatitis. Dig Dis Sci. 2012;57(7):1764–72.
19. Blondet JJ, Carlson AM, Kobayashi T, Jie T, Bellin M, Hering BJ, et al. The role of total pancreatectomy and islet autotransplantation for chronic pancreatitis. Surg Clin North Am. 2007;87(6):1477–501. x
20. Wahoff DC, Paplois BE, Najarian JS, Farney AC, Leonard AS, Kendall DM, et al. Islet autotransplantation after total pancreatectomy in a child. J Pediatr Surg 1996;31(1):132–135; discussion 5–6.
21. Chinnakotla S, Bellin MD, Schwarzenberg SJ, Radosevich DM, Cook M, Dunn TB, et al. Total pancreatectomy and islet autotransplantation in children for chronic pancreatitis: indi-

cation, surgical techniques, postoperative management, and long-term outcomes. Ann Surg. 2014;260(1):56–64.

22. Florek E, Chinnakotla S. Total Pancreatectomy and islet auto-transplantation for chronic pancreatitis children: pre-surgical evaluation, patient selection, the surgical procedures, islet isolation procedure, and the early inpatient management. In: Shapiro R, Sarwal MM, Raina R, Sethi SK, editors. Pediatric solid organ transplantation. Singapore: Springer; 2023. https://doi.org/10.1007/978-981-19-6909-6_25.
23. Wilson GC, Sutton JM, Salehi M, Schmulewitz N, Smith MT, Kucera S, et al. Surgical outcomes after total pancreatectomy and islet cell autotransplantation in pediatric patients. Surgery. 2013;154(4):777–83. discussion 83–4
24. Bottino R, Bertera S, Grupillo M, Melvin PR, Humar A, Mazariegos G, et al. Isolation of human islets for autologous islet transplantation in children and adolescents with chronic pancreatitis. J Transp Secur. 2012;2012:642787.
25. Bellin MD, Schwarzenberg SJ, Cook M, Sutherland DE, Chinnakotla S. Pediatric autologous islet transplantation. Curr Diab Rep. 2015;15(10):639.
26. Sutherland DE, Radosevich DM, Bellin MD, Hering BJ, Beilman GJ, Dunn TB, et al. Total pancreatectomy and islet autotransplantation for chronic pancreatitis. J Am Coll Surg 2012;214(4):409–424; discussion 24–6.
27. Lundberg R, Beilman GJ, Dunn TB, Pruett TL, Chinnakotla SC, Radosevich DM, et al. Metabolic assessment prior to total pancreatectomy and islet autotransplant: utility, limitations and potential. Am J Transplant. 2013;13(10):2664–71.
28. Berger M, Bellin MD, Kirchner V, Schwarzenberg SJ, Chinnakotla S. Laparoscopic-assisted versus open total pancreatectomy and islet autotransplantation: a case-matched study of pediatric patients. J Pediatr Surg. 2020;55(3):558–63.
29. Peterson KJ, Serrano OK, Flanagan S, Chinnakotla S. Vascular reconstruction technique of a perforated portal vein during a pediatric total pancreatectomy and islet autotransplant. Am J Transplant. 2018;18(9):2342–6.
30. Berger MG, Majumder K, Hodges JS, Bellin MD, Schwarzenberg SJ, Gupta S, et al. Microbial contamination of transplant solutions during pancreatic islet autotransplants is not associated with clinical infection in a pediatric population. Pancreatology. 2016;16(4):555–62.
31. Balamurugan AN, Chang Y, Bertera S, Sands A, Shankar V, Trucco M, et al. Suitability of human juvenile pancreatic islets for clinical use. Diabetologia. 2006;49(8):1845–54.
32. Wilhelm JJ, Balamurugan AN, Bellin MD, Hodges JS, Diaz J, Jane Schwarzenberg S, et al. Progress in individualizing autologous islet isolation techniques for pediatric islet autotransplantation after total pancreatectomy in children for chronic pancreatitis. Am J Transplant. 2021;21(2):776–86.
33. Ricordi C, Lacy PE, Finke EH, Olack BJ, Scharp DW. Automated method for isolation of human pancreatic islets. Diabetes. 1988;37(4):413–20.
34. Balamurugan AN, Loganathan G, Bellin MD, Wilhelm JJ, Harmon J, Anazawa T, et al. A new enzyme mixture to increase the yield and transplant rate of autologous and allogeneic human islet products. Transplantation. 2012;93(7):693–702.
35. Finzi G, Davalli A, Placidi C, Usellini L, La Rosa S, Folli F, et al. Morphological and ultrastructural features of human islet grafts performed in diabetic nude mice. Ultrastruct Pathol. 2005;29(6):525–33.
36. Biarnes M, Montolio M, Nacher V, Raurell M, Soler J, Montanya E. Beta-cell death and mass in syngeneically transplanted islets exposed to short- and long-term hyperglycemia. Diabetes. 2002;51(1):66–72.
37. Davalli AM, Scaglia L, Zangen DH, Hollister J, Bonner-Weir S, Weir GC. Vulnerability of islets in the immediate posttransplantation period. Dynamic changes in structure and function. Diabetes. 1996;45(9):1161–7.
38. Juang JH, Bonner-Weir S, Wu YJ, Weir GC. Beneficial influence of glycemic control upon the growth and function of transplanted islets. Diabetes. 1994;43(11):1334–9.

39. Hutchins J, Castro C, Wang Q, Chinnakotla S. Postoperative pain control with paravertebral catheters after pediatric total pancreatectomy and islet autotransplantation: a retrospective cohort study. Paediatr Anaesth. 2016;26(3):315–20.
40. Bellin MD, Freeman ML, Schwarzenberg SJ, Dunn TB, Beilman GJ, Vickers SM, et al. Quality of life improves for pediatric patients after total pancreatectomy and islet autotransplant for chronic pancreatitis. Clin Gastroenterol Hepatol. 2011;9(9):793–9.
41. Ahmad SA, Lowy AM, Wray CJ, D'Alessio D, Choe KA, James LE, et al. Factors associated with insulin and narcotic independence after islet autotransplantation in patients with severe chronic pancreatitis. J Am Coll Surg. 2005;201(5):680–7.
42. Bellin MD, Forlenza GP, Majumder K, Berger M, Freeman ML, Beilman GJ, et al. Total Pancreatectomy with islet autotransplantation resolves pain in young children with severe chronic pancreatitis. J Pediatr Gastroenterol Nutr. 2017;64(3):440–5.
43. Werlin SL, Kugathasan S, Frautschy BC. Pancreatitis in children. J Pediatr Gastroenterol Nutr. 2003;37(5):591–5.
44. Walker SM. Pain in children: recent advances and ongoing challenges. Br J Anaesth. 2008;101(1):101–10.
45. King S, Chambers CT, Huguet A, MacNevin RC, McGrath PJ, Parker L, et al. The epidemiology of chronic pain in children and adolescents revisited: a systematic review. Pain. 2011;152(12):2729–38.

Pancreatectomy and Islet Autotransplantation for Intraductal Papillary Mucinous Neoplasms and Pancreatic Neoplasms

15

Francesca Aleotti and Lorenzo Piemonti

Abstract

Total pancreatectomy with islet autotransplantation (TPIAT) has traditionally been employed for patients with chronic pancreatitis, but its use has increasingly expanded to include specific cases of pancreatic neoplasms. The Milan protocol has systematically extended TPIAT indications to both malignant and nonmalignant pancreatic lesions, provided that multifocality is excluded preoperatively and confirmed with negative intraoperative frozen section margins. This procedure is also being explored for patients undergoing salvage completion pancreatectomy after severe postoperative pancreatic fistula (POPF) following pancreaticoduodenectomy, as well as for those at high risk of developing POPF, offering a potential alternative to pancreaticoduodenectomy. Recent randomized studies have demonstrated that TPIAT is both feasible and safe in these contexts, with metabolic outcomes similar to those observed in patients with chronic pancreatitis. However, the application of TPIAT for intraductal papillary mucinous neoplasms (IPMNs) remains limited, with scarce data and no prospective trials specifically addressing this indication. The increasing detection of IPMNs, particularly as incidental findings, and their potential for multifocality underscore the need for further investigation into the role of TPIAT in this setting. Despite TPIAT's relatively niche status for pancreatic neoplasms, largely due to the limited availability of islet processing centers, existing evidence supports its use in carefully selected cases. Although concerns regarding tumor spread after TPIAT in oncologic contexts persist, available data suggest that the procedure can be

F. Aleotti
Pancreatic and Transplant Surgery Unit, IRCCS Ospedale San Raffaele, Milan, Italy

L. Piemonti (✉)
Diabetes Research Institute, IRCCS Ospedale San Raffaele and University "Vita Salute San Raffaele", Milan, Italy
e-mail: piemonti.lorenzo@hsr.it

S. Chinnakotla et al. (eds.), *Total Pancreatectomy and Islet Auto Transplantation*,
https://doi.org/10.1007/978-981-92-0018-4_15

performed safely, offering a significant improvement in the quality of life for patients following total pancreatectomy. In conclusion, while TPIAT for pancreatic neoplasms remains an emerging application, it holds promise as a strategy to address diabetes following pancreatectomy. As the understanding of its safety and efficacy in this context continues to evolve, further research is needed to clarify its role, particularly in the management of IPMNs and other pancreatic malignancies.

Key Points

- Total pancreatectomy with islet autotransplantation (TPIAT) is a viable option for select patients with pancreatic neoplasms, including IPMNs and malignant tumors, when rigorous oncologic precautions are taken. Careful patient selection, preoperative imaging, and intraoperative frozen section analysis are essential to ensure safety.
- The risk of malignant cell dissemination in IAT remains a concern, particularly in IPMN cases due to their premalignant and multifocal nature. While evidence suggests minimal risk with proper purification techniques and negative-margin requirements, further research is needed to confirm long-term oncologic safety.
- Metabolic outcomes after TPIAT in patients with pancreatic neoplasms are generally comparable to those in patients with chronic pancreatitis, despite lower islet yields due to oncologic constraints. Achieving insulin independence depends on islet mass, and optimizing transplantation protocols remains crucial.
- TPIAT has shown success not only in planned procedures but also as a salvage option in high-risk surgical scenarios, such as completion pancreatectomy for severe postoperative pancreatic fistula. These cases highlight its role in complex pancreatic surgery.
- Prospective studies are needed to refine patient selection criteria, evaluate long-term outcomes, and explore alternatives such as islet allotransplantation for patients ineligible for IAT. Standardizing protocols will be key to ensuring both metabolic benefits and oncologic safety.

15.1 Introduction

Islet autotransplantation (IAT) following pancreatectomy has evolved from its initial application in managing chronic pancreatitis to becoming a potential therapeutic option for patients with various pancreatic neoplasms. These include intraductal papillary mucinous neoplasms (IPMNs), malignant pancreatic tumors, and other nonmalignant pancreatic conditions. While the primary aim of IAT was initially to prevent diabetes after pancreatectomy for chronic pancreatitis, its utility has grown as clinical experience expands. This chapter will review current evidence and experiences with IAT in the context of IPMNs, malignant pancreatic tumors, and other pancreatic neoplasms. We will examine metabolic outcomes, oncologic safety, and quality of life for patients undergoing IAT and identify critical gaps in knowledge. By doing so, we aim to enhance understanding of the evolving role of IAT in treating both malignant and nonmalignant pancreatic diseases.

15.2 Current Clinical Evidence and Experiences

15.2.1 Intraductal Papillary Mucinous Neoplasms

IPMNs represent a unique and challenging clinical context for IAT. A search of scientific databases, such as PubMed, for terms including "islet autotransplantation" (and its variations) and "IPMN" reveals a striking absence of studies. While the lack of research on IAT in certain clinical scenarios is unsurprising, the complete void in the literature connecting these two topics underscores a significant gap. This absence is especially noteworthy in light of the rapid expansion of scientific publications in recent years and emphasizes the need for targeted investigations. The lack of studies addressing IAT in IPMNs raises a fundamental question: why has this area remained unexplored? To address this issue, it is crucial to examine the biological characteristics of IPMNs and their impact on patient suitability for IAT. IPMNs represent premalignant lesions of the pancreas, which can be broadly categorized into two groups [31]. The first category consists of lesions with low malignant potential, which may serve as ideal tissue for islet isolation. However, these lesions typically require management through radiologic or endoscopic surveillance rather than surgical intervention, thereby limiting their availability for IAT [31]. The second category includes high-risk IPMNs, characterized by main pancreatic duct involvement or the presence of concerning features such as mural nodules, rapid cyst growth, or pancreatic duct dilation [31]. These lesions often necessitate surgical resection, thereby providing tissue for IAT. Nevertheless, their inherent risk of malignancy complicates their use in islet transplantation. A critical unresolved question in this context is whether the neoplastic potential of an IPMN, present at its native site, is preserved after undergoing enzymatic digestion, partial purification, and infusion into the liver during IAT. In preclinical models, we modeled the risk of iatrogenic pancreatic cancer metastasis after islet infusion [14], using the KPC mouse model (LSL-KrasG12D/+; LSL-Trp53R172H/+; Pdx1-Cre), which develops pancreatic ductal adenocarcinoma with 100% penetrance. We implanted pancreatic exocrine tissue with varying degrees of purity, derived from mice that had not yet developed cancer, into syngeneic wild-type diabetic recipients via the portal vein. Over a 13-month follow-up period, no liver metastases were observed. These results suggest that exocrine tissue from KPC mice, which retains a 100% probability of transforming into cancer in the native pancreatic environment, completely loses this ability when transplanted into a syngeneic diabetic recipient via portal vein infusion. It remains uncertain whether the malignant potential of IPMNs, characteristic of their original location, is retained following the processing steps and implantation in humans. Further complicating the suitability of IPMNs for IAT are two additional challenges. The first pertains to the multifocal nature of these lesions, often associated with skip areas exhibiting varying degrees of dysplasia. This heterogeneity complicates the identification and isolation of healthy tissue from diseased regions, increasing the risk of inadvertently preserving undetected foci of IPMN. This issue is particularly pronounced in tissue regions that initially appear healthy, presenting significant obstacles to the feasibility of IAT even when imaging suggests that the IPMN is predominantly focal. The second challenge stems from the risk of synchronous or metachronous malignancies. The pancreatic parenchyma affected by IPMNs may harbor or develop pancreatic ductal adenocarcinoma, either simultaneously or at a later stage. Mitigating this risk requires meticulous preoperative evaluations, including advanced imaging techniques and intraoperative frozen section analyses, to detect and exclude any synchronous malignant lesions. However, this may conflict with the need to preserve pancreatic tissue necessary for digestion and islet isolation. Thus, the primary issue in utilizing IPMNs for IAT lies in balancing the need to address high-risk (pre)malignant lesions while preserving the functional pancreatic tissue critical for digestion and for the isolation of islets, which are essential for glucose regulation.

These challenges help clarify why the two primary protocols for autologous islet transplantation, the Minnesota [13] and Milan [3] protocols, both list IPMN as a contraindication for IAT outside of clinical trials. Both protocols recognize the risks involved in using pancreatic tissue from IPMN patients for IAT, given the complex nature of IPMNs and the difficulties in ensuring the complete removal of malignant or premalignant cells. However, the Milan protocol is somewhat more permissive, stating that IAT may be performed in cases of IPMN if multifocal lesions can be definitively ruled out through endoscopic ultrasound. This increased risk is counterbalanced by the fact that, unlike the Minnesota protocol, the Milan protocol includes a purification step, significantly reducing the volume of exocrine tissue infused. Furthermore, the Milan protocol requires a minimum 1-cm negative margin during surgery to minimize the risk of leaving behind transformed cells. A closer examination of the literature reveals a few reported cases of partial pancreatectomy (e.g., extended distal pancreatectomy) with IAT in patients who underwent pancreatic resection for IPMN at the Samsung Medical Center in Korea (see Table 15.1) [20, 21, 25]. In all cases, the authors described the steps taken to minimize the risk of disease spread and recurrence, including preoperative computed tomography (CT) and endoscopic retrograde cholangiopancreatography (ERCP) evaluations of the entire pancreas to exclude multifocality, along with intraoperative frozen section analysis. A histopathologic review of the cases [25] showed that the ductal epithelium of IPMN primarily exhibited moderate dysplasia, with a background adenomatous lesion also identified. These findings suggest that the risk of malignant potential in these cases was not high. In these rare instances, no cases of disease recurrence or new-onset pancreatic ductal adenocarcinoma (PDAC) unrelated to IPMN were reported, although the follow-up duration varied. To our knowledge, only one article describes patients ($n = 2$) who underwent total pancreatectomy with IAT for localized IPMN [26]. Unfortunately, the authors did not provide final histopathological details, including the grade of dysplasia or subtype analysis. However, they did report that both patients were alive at the last follow-up, with a median

Table 15.1 Cases of partial or total pancreatectomy with IAT in patients with IPMN

Site	N	Type of resection	Follow-up	Ref.
Samsung medical center, Sungkyunkwan University School of Medicine, Seoul, South Korea	3	Extended distal pancreatectomy	No recurrence at 5, 6, and 9 years, respectively	[20, 21, 25]
University hospital Carl Gustav Carus, Technische Universität Dresden, Dresden, Germany	2	Total pancreatectomy	Alive at last follow-up	[26]
Diabetes research institute, IRCCS Ospedale san Raffaele, Milan, Italy	5	Extended distal pancreatectomy	All alive and without recurrence at 7, 7, 8, 8, and 9 years	[32]
	2	Completion pancreatectomy after POPF	One died after 6 days due to surgical complications; one alive without recurrence at 12 years	

POPF postoperative pancreatic fistula

follow-up of 46 ± 5.7 months. Our group has recently reported on the outcomes of patients who underwent IAT at San Raffaele Scientific Institute, along with four other hospitals in surrounding regions of Italy that rely on our Islet Processing Facility [32]. Among the five patients who underwent extended distal pancreatectomy for localized IPMN, all are alive and disease-free at follow-up intervals of 7, 7, 8, 8, and 9 years. These results underscore the possibility of achieving excellent long-term outcomes when patients are carefully selected and appropriate precautions are taken. In the two cases where completion pancreatectomy was performed following postoperative pancreatic fistula (POPF) after an initial pancreaticoduodenectomy for IPMN, the outcomes were mixed. One patient unfortunately passed away 6 days postoperatively due to surgical complications. However, the other patient has had a remarkably positive outcome, remaining alive and free of disease recurrence 12 years after the procedure. These findings underscore the potential for achieving favorable long-term survival and effective disease control in IPMN patients undergoing IAT, particularly when careful attention is given to surgical technique and patient selection. While complications, such as those encountered in the completion pancreatectomy case, remain a significant consideration, the overall outcomes suggest that IAT can be a viable option for appropriately chosen IPMN patients, providing promising long-term results.

Another point of discussion is whether patients who undergo pancreatectomy for IPMN might be suitable candidates for islet allotransplantation. As early as 2008, Sakata et al. [37] proposed that patients with IPMN—even those with IPMN-associated adenocarcinoma—could be considered ideal candidates for total pancreatectomy followed by potential islet allotransplantation, given their relatively better prognosis than patients with non-IPMN-associated PDACs [3]. In their study, the authors ruled out the option of IAT due to concerns over the potential for malignant dissemination. However, they acknowledged the risk of disease recurrence under immunosuppressive therapy, highlighting a critical trade-off in the context of allotransplantation.

In conclusion, while IPMNs pose a considerable challenge for IAT, they should not be viewed as an absolute contraindication when stringent precautions are implemented. However, there remains a pressing need for additional data—especially from prospective or randomized studies—to further validate these findings and refine the criteria for selecting the most suitable candidates for IAT.

15.2.2 Pancreatic Neoplasms: Periampullary Cancer and Ductal Carcinoma

Given the limited information on IAT in premalignant conditions like IPMN, one might expect a complete lack of data on its application in other pancreatic neoplasms, including malignant ones. This assumption is not correct, but the available data on IAT in these contexts primarily come from single case reports or case series, typically in extreme clinical situations. Many of these cases involve patients with severe POPF who underwent completion pancreatectomy after pancreaticoduodenectomy as a life-saving procedure. Some of these cases (summarized in Table 15.2) are related to pancreatic resection performed for pancreatic ductal adenocarcinoma or so-called periampullary carcinomas, which include carcinomas of the ampulla, Vater's papilla, and the distal bile duct. These types of carcinomas are often challenging to distinguish preoperatively.

The primary concern regarding IAT in malignant cases, as in IPMN, is the risk of malignant dissemination through islet transplantation. While only a few, albeit notable, cases point to this possibility, it remains a widespread concern. This fear was heightened by a report from Muratore et al. [29] that documented liver metastases in a patient who underwent total pancreatectomy with IAT for chronic pancreatitis, a condition that inherently increases the risk of developing PDAC. Similarly, Savari et al. [38] reported a case of preemptive total pancreatectomy with IAT in a patient at high risk for POPF due to severe post-ERCP pancreatitis. The patient passed away at 6 months due to disease recurrence in the skin, locally, and in the liver. These cases raise important questions about the safety and effectiveness of total pancreatectomy with IAT in malignant contexts. However, accumulating evidence suggests this risk is minimal [1, 12]. First, islet isolation is performed on pancreatic tissue that has been thoroughly evaluated preoperatively and deemed free of disease, meaning that this tissue would not have been removed in the absence of malignancy-associated surgical indications. Supporting this, several studies have demonstrated no survival advantage (disease-free or disease-specific) with total pancreatectomy over partial pancreatectomy for PDAC, challenging the assumption that more extensive resection is inherently safer [15, 18, 24, 33, 34, 40]. Second, animal models have demonstrated that islet transplantation does not promote malignant dissemination. For example, studies showed no tumor formation when (a) nontumoral exocrine and endocrine cells isolated from PDAC patients were transplanted into immunodeficient mice [35] or (b) islets from KPC mice (which have a 100%

Table 15.2 Case reports and series of IAT after pancreatectomy in malignant neoplasms

Site	N, neoplasm	Type of resection	Follow-up	Ref.
Tachikawa general hospital, Nagaoka, Japan	1 PDAC	Completion pancreatectomy after local recurrence	Disease-free at 20 months	[22]
University of Rostock, Rostock, Germany	1 PDAC	Completion pancreatectomy after POPF	Died at 2.5 years due to disease recurrence; no liver metastases	[16]
University of Alberta, Edmonton, Alberta, Canada	1 ampullary cancer	Completion pancreatectomy after POPF	Disease-free at 1 year	[2]
University of Minnesota, Minneapolis, MN, USA	1 ampullary cancer	Total pancreatectomy	Disease-free at 3 months	[19]
Institute for Clinical and Experimental Medicine, Prague, Czech Republic	2 PDACs, 2 papillary cancers, 1 cholangiocarcinoma	Completion pancreatectomy after POPF	One postoperative death; one PDAC case disease-free at 9 months; others experienced recurrence at varying times	[23]
University of Chicago, Chicago, IL, USA	1 ampullary cancer	Total pancreatectomy	Died at 6 months with recurrence in the liver, skin, and locally	[38]
University hospital Carl Gustav Carus, Technische Universität Dresden, Dresden, Germany	2 duodenal cancers, 2 papillary tumors	Total/completion pancreatectomy	One died of postoperative MOF; others died of disease progression	[26]
Diabetes research institute, IRCCS Ospedale san Raffaele, Milan, Italy	24 PDACs, 4 ampullary cancers, 9 duodenal cancers, 19 cholangiocarcinomas	Total pancreatectomy	No difference in recurrence rate or location compared with the standard pancreaticoduodenectomy group	[32]

MOF multisystem organ failure, *PDAC* pancreatic ductal adenocarcinoma, *POPF* postoperative pancreatic fistula

PDAC penetrance rate) were transplanted into syngeneic diabetic mice [14]. Third, the majority of the reported experiences have excluded any additional specific risk of malignant dissemination. In all of the cases presented in Table 15.2, the authors acknowledge the potential risk of malignant dissemination and detail the precautions taken to reduce it. These precautions include comprehensive preoperative evaluations to rule out multifocality, as well as frozen section examination of the resection margins and additional resections of safety margins distal to these. Furthermore, both disease-free survival and disease-specific/overall survival are reported, with no patients experiencing recurrence exclusively in the liver (the site of islet implantation), where these data are available. A paradigmatic, albeit somewhat unusual, case report by Kobayashi et al. [22] further supports the safety of the procedure when proper precautions are observed. In this case, a completion pancreatectomy was performed not immediately after surgery for complications but rather 3 years later due to a local recurrence of ampullary carcinoma at the pancreatic anastomosis. The authors used the entire distal pancreas, taken 3 cm from the lesion, with negative intraoperative frozen sections, for a heterotopic autotransplantation. The patient remained disease-free at the 20-month follow-up, highlighting the potential success of partial pancreatic autotransplantation even in the context of malignant disease when adequate precautions are taken. The most significant evidence supporting IAT safety in malignant contexts comes from our group's prospective, randomized clinical trial (NCT01346098) [9]. Early observations at our center indicated that the risk of disease dissemination following IAT was minimal [3–5, 7, 8]. Among 31 patients who underwent IAT after either extended distal pancreatectomy or total pancreatectomy for malignant disease (including salvage completion pancreatectomy after POPF and as prophylaxis for POPF in high-risk patients), only three developed de novo liver metastasis [3, 6]. Additionally, both overall and disease-free survival rates were more favorable in these patients than in those who underwent surgery without IAT during the same period. These initial data prompted the design of a controlled clinical trial to further evaluate these outcomes. The NCT01346098 trial enrolled patients at very high risk for pancreatic anastomosis leakage, regardless of the underlying pathology, including malignancy. High risk was characterized by soft pancreatic parenchyma and duct diameter $\leq$ 3 mm as assessed through preoperative imaging and confirmed intraoperatively by experienced pancreatic surgeons [9]. These patients were then randomly assigned in a 1:1 ratio to either standard pancreaticoduodenectomy or total pancreatectomy with IAT. The results showed no statistically significant difference in overall survival, disease-specific survival, or disease-free survival between the two groups, in both intent-to-treat and per-protocol analyses. Moreover, for those with disease recurrence, there was no difference in the site of first recurrence, including the rate of liver metastasis as the initial site.

Having established the safety of total pancreatectomy with IAT in the context of pancreatic or periampullary malignancy, it is also important to discuss the islet isolation and transplantation process, as well as the resulting metabolic outcomes. Regarding the technical procedures for islet preparation, the steps taken are largely the same as those for patients undergoing total pancreatectomy with IAT for chronic pancreatitis, aside from the previously discussed safety measures, such as the frozen section examination of pancreatic resection margins. In addition to the standard processes of digestion, isolation, and purification (the latter not being universally used), islet preparations at our center are often cultured overnight and then infused into the patient's portal vein the following day during an angiographic procedure. This practice, which has been highlighted elsewhere [3], is not universally available, particularly in centers in the USA, where the islet culture time exceeds the limits established by the Food and Drug Administration [10]. It is important to note that, due to the need to remove the tumor and ensure negative margins, the amount of pancreatic tissue available for islet extraction is reduced, resulting in a somewhat lower number of islets infused than in patients with chronic pancreatitis. However, the 1-year metabolic outcomes in these patients appear to be comparable to those observed in a large cohort of individuals undergoing IAT for chronic pancreatitis, when considering the same dose of islets received [27, 28, 32]. Differences in isolation outcomes are noted in the case of completion pancreatectomy performed as a salvage procedure after severe complications from pancreatic surgery. Balzano et al. described the experience at our center, comparing patients undergoing a priori IAT for high-risk anastomosis with those who underwent IAT following salvage completion pancreatectomy [7]. Fewer patients in the salvage IAT group received islet infusion (59.1%) than in the simultaneous IAT group (88.9%; $p = 0.008$). The reasons for this difference included inadequate islet preparations due to low islet count or bacterial contamination.

15.2.3 Pancreatic Neoplasms: Other Types

Another category of pancreatic neoplasms to consider for IAT includes benign or borderline lesions, such as cystic neoplasms (excluding IPMNs) and neuroendocrine tumors (NETs). When these tumors are located in the proximal body or isthmus of the pancreas, extended distal pancreatectomy with IAT is often a preferred alternative to intermediate pancreatectomy, which is associated with a higher risk of POPF. Conversely, lesions situated in the pancreatic head are frequently ideal candidates for preemptive total pancreatectomy with IAT. Unlike periampullary cancers and ductal carcinoma, benign or borderline pancreatic tumors generally do not cause retrograde dilation of the pancreatic duct or distal parenchymal atrophy, which increases the risk of POPF [11]. Pancreatic resections with IAT for benign or borderline pancreatic lesions are summarized in Table 15.3. The data clearly indicate that IAT is more frequently performed in conjunction with extended distal pancreatectomy. This is not unexpected, given the significant impact of total pancreatectomy on postoperative mortality, morbidity, and long-term metabolic outcomes—without providing oncological benefits—leading surgeons to approach total pancreatectomy with caution in cases of nonmalignant lesions. Nevertheless, IAT should always be considered when total pancreatectomy is required for patients with a very high risk of POPF. This consideration is especially relevant as emerging research continues to highlight the links between diabetes and an elevated risk of

Table 15.3 Cases of IAT following extended distal pancreatectomy or total pancreatectomy in patients with benign/borderline pancreatic neoplasms and miscellaneous lesions

Site	N, neoplasm	Type of resection	Follow-up	Ref.
Geneva University Hospitals and University of Geneva School of Medicine, Geneva, Switzerland	2 NETs (insulinomas)	Extended distal pancreatectomy	No recurrence at 3 and 6 years	[30]
	6 SCAs, 4 MCNs, 4 NETs	Extended distal pancreatectomy	Median follow-up of 90 months; no recurrence	[36]
Samsung Medical Center, Sungkyunkwan University School of Medicine, Seoul, South Korea	5 SPPNs, 2 MCNs, 8 SCAs, 1 NET	Extended distal pancreatectomy	Median follow-up of the entire IAT cohort (20 patients): 61 months; no recurrence	[20, 21, 25]
University of Alberta, Edmonton, Alberta, Canada	1 multifocal metastasis from renal cell carcinoma	Total pancreatectomy	No recurrence at 1 year	[17]
University Hospital Carl Gustav Carus, Technische Universität Dresden, Dresden, Germany	1 NET, 1 dendritic sarcoma, 1 mesenchymal mediastinal sarcoma	Total pancreatectomy	Median follow-up of 46 ± 5.7 months; no recurrence	[26]
Diabetes Research Institute, IRCCS Ospedale San Raffaele, Milan, Italy	4 NETs, 2 SCAs, 4 ampullary adenomas	Total pancreatectomy	Median follow-up of 11.5 ± 0.2 years: NET G3 with local recurrence and liver metastases at 3 months; NET G3 with liver metastases at 1.7 years; NET G3 with liver and bone metastases at 2.1 years	[32]
	18 NETs, 9 SPPNs, 4 MCNs, 4 SCAs	Extended distal pancreatectomy	Median follow-up of 5.6 ± 1.5 years; no recurrence	
	3 NETs, 1 SPPN, 2 ampullary adenomas	Completion pancreatectomy after POPF	Median follow-up 11.6 ± 3.3 years; no recurrence	

MCN mucinous cystic neoplasm; *NET* neuroendocrine tumor; *POPF* postoperative pancreatic fistula; *SCA* serous cystadenoma; *SPPN* solid pseudopapillary neoplasm

cancer [39]. Notably, among the cases documented in the literature, no disease recurrence has been observed, except for three NET G3 cases [32].

15.3 Insights Gained from the Experience with IAT for IPMN and Pancreatic Neoplasms

The use of IAT in patients undergoing pancreatectomy for IPMN has significantly advanced our understanding of the procedure's feasibility, safety, and potential benefits (Table 15.4). Once considered controversial, IAT in the context of neoplasms is now viewed as a viable option to mitigate postpancreatectomy diabetes, provided it is implemented with a rigorous and cautious approach [10]. This growing body of clinical experience has challenged traditional contraindications, reshaping how surgeons and multidisciplinary teams approach these complex cases. One of the most significant shifts in perspective has been the reconsideration of neoplasms as an absolute contraindication for IAT. Historically, there were substantial concerns about the potential dissemination of tumor cells during the preparation and infusion of islets. However, accumulating evidence suggests that this risk is lower than previously assumed when appropriate precautions are taken [32]. For patients with both benign and malignant pancreatic neoplasms, IAT is no longer automatically excluded as part of their treatment plan. Instead, it is now recognized as a potentially valuable tool for preserving beta-cell function and preventing pancreatogenic diabetes, which can have a profound impact on long-term quality of life. To safely implement IAT in these patients, certain essential precautions have been emphasized [3]. A comprehensive preoperative assessment is critical to exclude multifocal disease or advanced malignancies. Imaging modalities such as CT and endoscopic ultrasound play a key role in this phase. During surgery, intraoperative histological analysis, including frozen section examinations, ensures that resection margins are negative and that no tumor cells are present in the pancreatic tissue selected for islet isolation. The islet purification process further reduces the risk of contamination by separating endocrine from exocrine cells, although it does not entirely eliminate the possibility of residual malignant cells. In some cases, genetic testing of the islets—targeting markers such as *SMAD4*, *CDKN2A*, *USP9X*, *TP53*, and *KRAS*—could provide an additional safeguard by identifying any residual malignant cells in the preparation. However, the practical feasibility and routine applicability of such testing have yet to be fully established. These precautions are particularly relevant in the context of IPMNs, which were once considered a contraindication for IAT. Today, IPMNs are increasingly regarded as a manageable risk under specific circumstances. When the disease is localized, surgical margins are negative, and preoperative assessments exclude multifocality, IAT can be performed with a favorable risk–benefit profile. The type of IPMN also influences decision-making, as subtypes such as the gastric variant are associated with a lower risk of malignant transformation than the intestinal and pancreatobiliary subtypes [31]. However, even low-grade gastric IPMNs are not entirely without risk, as they can progress to high-grade lesions in some cases. Preventing diabetes after pancreatectomy remains a primary goal in

Table 15.4 Summary of key insights on islet autotransplantation (IAT) in pancreatic neoplasms

Topic	Insights	Implications
IAT and neoplasms	The diagnosis of pancreatic neoplasms, whether benign or malignant, is no longer considered an absolute contraindication for IAT. Studies show that the risk of tumor dissemination with islet infusion is lower than initially anticipated	Expands the indications for IAT, allowing its application in patients previously considered unsuitable for the procedure
Essential precautions	Stringent precautions are required to minimize the risk of tumor spread. These include preoperative evaluation using CT and endoscopic ultrasound, intraoperative histological analysis with frozen sections, islet purification, and perhaps genetic marker analysis	Ensures the safety of the procedure and reduces the risk of tumor cell dissemination during islet infusion
IPMN and IAT	IPMNs are not an absolute contraindication for IAT, especially when the tumor is localized, with negative resection margins and no evidence of multifocality during preoperative assessment	Facilitates the use of IAT in patients with IPMN, potentially improving metabolic outcomes after pancreatectomy
Types of IPMN	Different IPMN subtypes exhibit varying prognoses. Gastric-type IPMN is often low grade, while intestinal and pancreatobiliary subtypes carry a higher risk of progression to carcinoma. Gastric lesions with low-grade dysplasia are considered precursors of high-grade lesions	Informs therapeutic decision-making based on the specific subtype of IPMN and its potential for malignancy
Postpancreatectomy diabetes	The primary goal of IAT is to prevent postpancreatectomy diabetes by preserving beta-cell function and enhancing glycemic control	Improves quality of life and survival in patients following pancreatectomy, reducing the burden of diabetes
Oncological considerations	While early data suggest that IAT does not increase the risk of metastasis compared to non-IAT procedures, long-term studies are necessary to fully assess oncological safety	Calls for continued oncological follow-up and the need for further research to confirm the long-term oncological safety of IAT in pancreatic neoplasm patients
IAT and postoperative pancreatic fistula (POPF)	IAT has been successfully employed in emergency situations, such as in the management of severe POPFs. Salvage IAT after completion pancreatectomy has shown positive metabolic outcomes. Infection at the time of islet infusion does not necessarily correlate with increased clinical risk	Broadens the scope of IAT applications, particularly in urgent cases involving postsurgical complications such as POPF

(continued)

Table 15.4 (continued)

Topic	Insights	Implications
Need for further studies	Prospective, randomized clinical trials are required to confirm preliminary findings, refine patient selection criteria, and optimize treatment protocols	Directs future research efforts to enhance clinical practice by providing clearer evidence on the efficacy and safety of IAT
Importance of islet yield	Adequate islet yield is crucial for achieving optimal metabolic outcomes after IAT. Islet doses exceeding 3000 IEQ/kg are associated with better results. Islet yield is influenced by factors such as age, BMI, and the presence of pancreatic atrophy	Optimizes transplant strategies and preoperative planning, ensuring that adequate islet quantities are harvested for successful outcomes
Extent of pancreatectomy	The extent of pancreatectomy, whether total or partial, significantly impacts the achievement of optimal metabolic results post-IAT	Guides surgical decision-making and the tailoring of treatment approaches to individual patient needs, optimizing metabolic outcomes

BMI body mass index, *CT* computed tomography, *IAT* islet autotransplantation, *IEQ* islet equivalents, *IPMN* intraductal papillary mucinous neoplasms

these patients, given the profound impact that diabetes can have on survival and overall well-being. IAT has shown consistent success in preserving beta-cell function and improving glycemic control, even when complete independence from exogenous insulin is not achieved. For many patients, the procedure significantly reduces insulin requirements and stabilizes glycemic levels, mitigating the severe metabolic challenges associated with total or distal pancreatectomy. Despite the encouraging outcomes, oncological safety remains a key area of ongoing research. Early data suggest that the metastasis rates in patients undergoing IAT for malignant tumors are comparable to those of patients not receiving the procedure. While this finding is reassuring, the limited long-term follow-up available underscores the need for further studies to fully evaluate the procedure's safety in this context. This is particularly important given the variability in tumor biology and the inherent risks associated with handling malignant pancreatic tissue. Another notable application of IAT has emerged in emergency scenarios, such as cases of severe POPF. In these situations, salvage IAT after completion pancreatectomy has been shown to improve metabolic outcomes, even in the presence of complications such as infections. This underscores the versatility of IAT as a tool for managing not only planned surgical cases but also unanticipated challenges that arise during the postoperative course. Looking ahead, further research is essential to refine the use of IAT in patients with pancreatic neoplasms. Prospective, randomized studies will help identify the ideal candidates for the procedure, optimize islet isolation techniques, and confirm the long-term safety of IAT in both benign and malignant cases. Advances in genetic and molecular testing, as well as innovations in islet processing, hold promise for improving outcomes and further minimizing risks.

15.4 Conclusions

Although the majority of data on pancreatectomy with IAT for pancreatic neoplasms are derived from small case series, the findings suggest that this procedure may have a role in carefully selected patients. Larger studies and prospective clinical trials are needed to confirm these conclusions and to refine patient selection criteria, ensuring that those who are most likely to benefit from total pancreatectomy with islet auto-transplantation (TPIAT) are identified.

Authorship FA: Conceptualization, writing—original draft; LP: Conceptualization, formal analysis, project administration, writing—review and editing.

Disclosure The authors of this manuscript have no conflicts of interest to disclose.

References

1. Aleotti F, Nano R, Piemonti L, Falconi M, Balzano G. Total pancreatectomy sequelae and quality of life: results of islet autotransplantation as a possible mitigation strategy. Updat Surg. 2021;73:1237–46.
2. Alsaif F, Molinari M, Al-Masloom A, Lakey JR, Kin T, Shapiro AM. Pancreatic islet auto-transplantation with completion pancreatectomy in the management of uncontrolled pancreatic fistula after whipple resection for ampullary adenocarcinoma. Pancreas. 2006;32:430–1.
3. Balzano G, Piemonti L. Autologous islet transplantation in patients requiring pancreatectomy for neoplasm. Curr Diab Rep. 2014;14:512.
4. Balzano G, Maffi P, Nano R, Zerbi A, Venturini M, Melzi R, et al. Extending indications for islet autotransplantation in pancreatic surgery. Ann Surg. 2013;258:210–8.
5. Balzano G, Carvello M, Piemonti L, Nano R, Ariotti R, Mercalli A, et al. Combined laparoscopic spleen-preserving distal pancreatectomy and islet autotransplantation for benign pancreatic neoplasm. World J Gastroenterol. 2014;20:4030–6.
6. Balzano G, Maffi P, Nano R, Mercalli A, Melzi R, Aleotti F, et al. Autologous islet transplantation in patients requiring Pancreatectomy: a broader Spectrum of indications beyond chronic pancreatitis. Am J Transplant. 2016;16:1812–26.
7. Balzano G, Nano R, Maffi P, Mercalli A, Melzi R, Aleotti F, et al. Salvage islet auto transplantation after relaparatomy. Transplantation. 2017;101:2492–500.
8. Balzano G, Maffi P, Nano R, Mercalli A, Melzi R, Aleotti F, et al. Diabetes-free survival after extended distal pancreatectomy and islet auto transplantation for benign or borderline/malignant lesions of the pancreas. Am J Transplant. 2019;19:920–8.
9. Balzano G, Zerbi A, Aleotti F, Capretti G, Melzi R, Pecorelli N, et al. Total Pancreatectomy with islet autotransplantation as an alternative to high-risk pancreatojejunostomy after Pancreaticoduodenectomy: a prospective randomized trial. Ann Surg. 2023;277:894–903.
10. Bellin MD. Success with islet autotransplantation for pancreatic neoplasia using a careful approach. Transplantation. 2024;108:1830–1.
11. Callery MP, Pratt WB, Kent TS, Chaikof EL, Vollmer CM Jr. A prospectively validated clinical risk score accurately predicts pancreatic fistula after pancreatoduodenectomy. J Am Coll Surg. 2013;216:1–14.
12. Chaouch MA, Leon P, Cassese G, Aguilhon C, Khayat S, Panaro F. Total pancreatectomy with intraportal islet autotransplantation for pancreatic malignancies: a literature overview. Expert Opin Biol Ther. 2022;22:491–7.

13. Dudeja V, Beilman GJ, Vickers SM. Total Pancreatectomy with islet autotransplantation in patients with malignancy: are we there yet? Ann Surg. 2013;258:219–20.
14. Dugnani E, Pasquale V, Liberati D, Citro A, Cantarelli E, Pellegrini S, et al. Modeling the iatrogenic pancreatic cancer risk after islet autotransplantation in mouse. Am J Transplant. 2017;17:2720–7.
15. Ferrone CR, Brennan MF, Gonen M, Coit DG, Fong Y, Chung S, et al. Pancreatic adenocarcinoma: the actual 5-year survivors. J Gastrointest Surg. 2008;12:701–6.
16. Forster S, Liu X, Adam U, Schareck WD, Hopt UT. Islet autotransplantation combined with pancreatectomy for treatment of pancreatic adenocarcinoma: a case report. Transplant Proc. 2004;36:1125–6.
17. Gala-Lopez BL, Semlacher E, Manouchehri N, Kin T, Shapiro AM. Autologous islet transplantation after total pancreatectomy for renal cell carcinoma metastases. Am J Transplant. 2013;13:2487–91.
18. Grace PA, Pitt HA, Tompkins RK, DenBesten L, Longmire WP Jr. Decreased morbidity and mortality after pancreatoduodenectomy. Am J Surg. 1986;151:141–9.
19. Iyegha UP, Asghar JA, Beilman GJ. Total pancreatectomy and islet auto-transplantation as treatment for ampullary adenocarcinoma in the setting of pancreatic ductal disruption secondary to acute necrotizing pancreatitis. A case report. Jop. 2012;13:239–42.
20. Jin SM, Oh SH, Kim SK, Jung HS, Choi SH, Jang KT, et al. Diabetes-free survival in patients who underwent islet autotransplantation after 50% to 60% distal partial pancreatectomy for benign pancreatic tumors. Transplantation. 2013;95:1396–403.
21. Jung HS, Choi SH, Kim SJ, Choi DW, Heo JS, Lee KT, et al. Delayed improvement of insulin secretion after autologous islet transplantation in partially pancreatectomized patients. Metabolism. 2009;58:1629–35.
22. Kobayashi T, Sato Y, Hirukawa H, Soeno M, Shimoda T, Matsuoka H, et al. Total pancreatectomy combined with partial pancreas autotransplantation for recurrent pancreatic cancer: a case report. Transplant Proc. 2012;44:1176–9.
23. Kocik M, Lipar K, Saudek F, Girman P, Boucek P, Kucera M, et al. Pancreatic islet autotransplantation after completion pancreatectomy for pancreatic fistula after hemipancreatoduodenectomy for carcinoma. Transplant Proc. 2014;46:1996–8.
24. Latenstein AE, Scholten L, Al-Saffar HA, Björnsson B, Butturini G, Capretti G, et al. Clinical outcomes after total pancreatectomy: a prospective multicenter pan-European snapshot study. Ann Surg. 2022;276:e536–e43.
25. Lee BW, Jee JH, Heo JS, Choi SH, Jang KT, Noh JH, et al. The favorable outcome of human islet transplantation in Korea: experiences of 10 autologous transplantations. Transplantation. 2005;79:1568–74.
26. Ludwig S, Distler M, Schubert U, Schmid J, Thies H, Welsch T, et al. Quality of life and metabolic outcomes after total pancreatectomy and simultaneous islet autotransplantation. Commun Med. 2022;2:24.
27. Mattke J, Eaton A, Wijkstrom M, Witkowski P, Trikudanathan G, Singh VK, et al. Islet isolation outcomes in patients undergoing Total Pancreatectomy with islet autotransplantation in the POST consortium. Transplantation. 2025;109:207–16.
28. McEachron KR, Yang Y, Hodges JS, Beilman GJ, Kirchner VA, Pruett TL, et al. Performance of modified Igls criteria to evaluate islet autograft function after total pancreatectomy with islet autotransplantation–a retrospective study. Transpl Int. 2021;34:87–96.
29. Muratore S, Zeng X, Korc M, McElyea S, Wilhelm J, Bellin M, et al. Metastatic pancreatic adenocarcinoma after Total Pancreatectomy islet autotransplantation for chronic pancreatitis. Am J Transplant. 2016;16:2747–52.
30. Oberholzer J, Mathe Z, Bucher P, Triponez F, Bosco D, Fournier B, et al. Islet autotransplantation after left pancreatectomy for non-enucleable insulinoma. Am J Transplant. 2003;3:1302–7.
31. Ohtsuka T, Fernandez-Del Castillo C, Furukawa T, Hijioka S, Jang JY, Lennon AM, et al. International evidence-based Kyoto guidelines for the management of intraductal papillary mucinous neoplasm of the pancreas. Pancreatology. 2024;24:255–70.

32. Piemonti L, Melzi R, Aleotti F, Capretti G, Nano R, Mercalli A, et al. Autologous pancreatic islet cell transplantation following Pancreatectomy for pancreas diseases other than chronic pancreatitis: a 15-Y study of the Milan protocol. Transplantation. 2024;108:1962.
33. Pulvirenti A, Pea A, Rezaee N, Gasparini C, Malleo G, Weiss MJ, et al. Perioperative outcomes and long-term quality of life after total pancreatectomy. Br J Surg. 2019;106:1819–28.
34. Reddy S, Wolfgang CL, Cameron JL, Eckhauser F, Choti MA, Schulick RD, et al. Total Pancreatectomy for pancreatic adenocarcinoma: evaluation of morbidity and long-term survival. Ann Surg. 2009;250:282–7.
35. Renaud F, Chetboun M, Thevenet J, Delalleau N, Gmyr V, Hubert T, et al. Safety of islet autotransplantation after Pancreatectomy for adenocarcinoma. Transplantation. 2019;103:177–81.
36. Ris F, Niclauss N, Morel P, Demuylder-Mischler S, Muller Y, Meier R, et al. Islet autotransplantation after extended pancreatectomy for focal benign disease of the pancreas. Transplantation. 2011;91:895–901.
37. Sakata N, Egawa S, Motoi F, Mikami Y, Ishida M, Aoki T, et al. Institutional indications for islet transplantation after total pancreatectomy. J Hepato-Biliary-Pancreat Surg. 2008;15:488–92.
38. Savari O, Golab K, Solomina J, Konsur E, Cieply K, Ramachandran S, et al. Total Pancreatectomy with islet autotransplantation for the Ampullary cancer. A Case Report. J Gastrointest Cancer. 2019;50:543–7.
39. Wu D, Hu D, Chen H, Shi G, Fetahu IS, Wu F, et al. Glucose-regulated phosphorylation of TET2 by AMPK reveals a pathway linking diabetes to cancer. Nature. 2018;559:637–41.
40. Zhu J, Jiang Z, Xie B, Fu C, Xiao W, Li Y. Comparison of oncologic outcomes between pancreaticoduodenectomy and total pancreatectomy for pancreatic adenocarcinoma. Surg Endosc. 2023;37:109–19.

Long-Term Outcomes and Follow-Up After Total Pancreatectomy with Islet Autotransplantation (TPIAT)

16

Melena D. Bellin

Abstract

Total pancreatectomy with islet autotransplantation (TPIAT) is performed to relieve pain and allow for a better quality of life for patients with the most severe and disabling manifestations of recurrent acute and chronic pancreatitis. Several large centers have now reported data on outcomes at 5–10 years after TPIAT. In the largest series, long-term survival is 85% at 10 years after TPIAT. Opioid use decreases over time, with approximately 70% of individuals off opioids at 10 years after surgery and over 80% of individuals reporting pain reduction and robust improvements in quality of life that are sustained over time. Pain relief and opioid discontinuation are greatest in the youngest patients (children) and oldest patients (>50 years). A successful IAT procedure results in higher quality of life and reduced diabetes distress than TP alone. In the first 5 years after TPIAT, most patients have islet graft function, with 20–30% of patients completely off insulin, and even 10 years after TPIAT, more than 10% of patients remain off insulin. Young children have higher rates of insulin independence and better sustained islet function. Those individuals receiving >5000 islet equivalents per kilogram of body weight have better islet function and glycemic control and are more likely to be off insulin through 10 years of follow-up than those with a lower islet mass transplanted.

M. D. Bellin (✉)
Division of Pediatric Endocrinology, Department of Pediatrics, University of Minnesota Medical School, Minneapolis, MN, USA
e-mail: bell0130@umn.edu

S. Chinnakotla et al. (eds.), *Total Pancreatectomy and Islet Auto Transplantation*, https://doi.org/10.1007/978-981-92-0018-4_16

Key Points

1. Relief from pancreatitis pain is sustained long term in over 80% of patients, with 70% off opioids even 10 years after TPIAT. Some patients will develop new abdominal pain, which warrants evaluation for potential treatable causes.
2. Health-related quality of life measures improve robustly after TPIAT, and this benefit to quality of life is sustained long term.
3. Between 1 and 5 years after TPIAT, 20–30% of patients are off insulin; at 10 years, just over 10% of patients are off insulin. Most individuals retain some beta-cell function, as measured by C-peptide, even if using insulin. Young children and those with high islet mass generally have better long-term islet function.
4. Insulin independence after IAT has been associated with higher general health-related quality-of-life scores and significantly lower diabetes distress.
5. The 10-year Kaplan–Meier–estimated survival after TPIAT is 85%. Common causes of death long term include infection/sepsis, intestinal complications of surgery, diabetes complications, liver failure, malabsorption, and suicide or overdose.

16.1 Introduction

The earlier chapters in this textbook have detailed the patient population, surgical procedure, medical management, and early outcomes of total pancreatectomy with islet autotransplantation (TPIAT) performed to treat recurrent acute pancreatitis (RAP) or chronic pancreatitis (CP). It has only been more recently that long-term outcomes—defined here as 5 years or longer after TPIAT—have been reported. In this chapter, we will focus on what is known about patients' long-term outcomes after TPIAT, with a focus on more recent literature reporting pain symptoms, quality of life (QoL), diabetes, and survival at ~5–10 years after TPIAT.

16.2 Long-Term Patient Survival After TPIAT

Because RAP and CP are heterogeneous syndromes, with various causes, complications, and treatments, the exact life expectancy for individuals with CP is difficult to quantify and varies among studies. However, mortality in CP is estimated to be around fourfold higher than that of an age-matched general population, with mortality rates of 20–40% after 10 years with the disease [1–3]. Thus, individuals with CP who present for TPIAT already have compromised health and worse long-term survival than the general population.

Multiple studies have reported on long-term mortality after TPIAT (Table 16.1) [4–10]. Estimates for survival after TPIAT have varied depending on the patient population included, with 10-year actuarial survival rates ranging from 62% to 90%

Table 16.1 Long-term survival reported in patients undergoing TPIAT

Article	Year published	N	Total deaths (n)	Kaplan–Meier survival	Additional details
Chinnakotla et al. [4]	2014	484	NR	90% at 5 years 84% at 10 years	Compared 80 patients with genetic pancreatitis to 404 with nongenetic pancreatitis, with similar survival
Wilson et al. [5]	2014	112	6	98% at 1 year 96% at 3 years 95% at 5 years	
Chinnakotla et al. [6]	2014	75	3		Only included children (based on age at TPIAT)
Morgan et al. [7]	2017	195	13	92% at 5 years ~90% at 10 years	
Bellin et al. [8]	2019	215	50	95% at 1 year 72% at 10 years	Limited to patients who had TPIAT >10 years prior; predictors of mortality were obesity (ninefold increase) and short (<5 years) or long (5–10 years) duration of pancreatitis
Turner et al. [9]	2022	142	59	96% at 1 year 80% at 5 years 73% at 7.5 years 62% at 10 years	Median 9.4-year follow-up; infection was the most common known cause of death, but most causes of death were unknown
Hooks et al. [10]	2024	693	89	93% at 5 years 85% at 10 years 76% at 15 years	53 deaths deemed possibly TPIAT related; older age, earlier year of TPIAT, longer duration of pancreatitis, and alcohol-related pancreatitis all increased risk of death related to TPIAT

NR not reported, *TPIAT* total pancreatectomy with islet autotransplantation

[7–10]; in the largest reported series, 85% survived for 10 years [10]. Mortality is lowest in individuals undergoing TPIAT as children, which is not surprising given that mortality is closely related to age, and children often have fewer comorbidities and lower rates of postoperative diabetes. In children, 10-year survival exceeds 90% [6, 10]. Potential risk factors identified for mortality include obesity (up to a ninefold increased risk of death in one study), earlier era at surgery, alcoholic pancreatitis, and shorter duration of disease before TPIAT [8, 10].

Because patients with TPIAT often are referred from diverse geographic areas of the USA and are only seen at surgical centers for surgery and TPIAT-specific follow-up, causes of death were often unknown in early publications. More recently, we were able to use a combination of electronic health records and data from the National Death Index to more specifically detail long-term causes of mortality in this population [10]. Some causes of death are entirely unrelated to TPIAT and pancreatitis history (e.g., nonpancreatic cancer). We noted a high rate of suicide and accidental overdoses in this population, and depression, anxiety, and substance overuse are common comorbidities for those with painful CP [11, 12]. The most common causes of death that were deemed possibly related to TPIAT were infection/sepsis, intestinal complications of surgery, diabetes complications, liver failure, malabsorption, bleeding, and metastatic pancreatic adenocarcinoma [10]. Of note, infections were considered possibly related to the surgical interventions because of increased risk for sepsis with asplenia and also known risks of enteric bacterial sepsis (e.g., cholangitis) [13]. About 1.5% of deaths were noted to occur from liver failure, which was a new finding in TPIAT. Because there are no known cases of liver failure related to intraportal infusion of allogeneic islets for type 1 diabetes, the relationship between the transplant procedure and liver failure is not clear. Notably, at least half of the individuals with liver failure had other clear risk factors (e.g., alcohol abuse, cystic fibrosis).

16.3 Pain and Opioid Use Outcomes

Multiple studies across several large centers have reported outcomes at 5–10 years after TPIAT for pain, QoL, and diabetes [4–9, 14–22]. Collectively, these single-center studies suggest a significant reduction in pancreatitis pain, pain scores, and use of opioid pain medications. In a cohort of >200 patients, all ≥10 years out from TPIAT, pain was reported by participants in standardized questionnaires as improved in 75% at 5 years and in 82% at 10 years after TPIAT, with 68% of individuals off all opioids at 10 years postoperatively [8]. This is very similar to reports from other centers, which have noted declines in pain symptoms and opioid use, with another large center with 10 years of follow-up reporting 75% off opioids at 10 years after TPIAT [9]. Average daily morphine equivalents are also reduced long term [7].

In the first large cohort reported in pediatrics, of 75 children undergoing TPIAT, pancreatitis pain and opioid use were reported in <20% of the cohort at yearly follow-up through at least 10 years after the procedure [6]. Notably, pain and opioid use have been reported to be lowest in those in the youngest (<18 years old) or oldest (>50 years old) age groups [8]. In two different published cohorts, patients with hereditary or genetic pancreatitis (inclusive of adults and children) tended to have lower pain scores before TPIAT and to have somewhat lower long-term pain scores and opioid use than those with nongenetic disease [4, 15].

Of note, although relief of pancreatitis pain is common, having some other abdominal pain is also often reported [8]. Typically, this is identified as a new pain of much lower severity than the original pancreatitis. The reasons for this can be highly variable. In some cases, this may represent residual neuropathic pain. However, other specific causes including (but not limited to) gastrointestinal dysmotility, marginal ulcer or gastric ulcer, small intestinal bacterial overgrowth, partial bowel obstruction, and constipation need to be considered in the evaluation because these causes of pain may respond to specific interventions. Recurrent abdominal pain and its management are covered in greater detail in an earlier chapter.

16.4 Quality-of-Life Outcomes

Perhaps more important than simple pain relief and freedom from opioid medications, health-related QoL robustly improves for many patients, and these improvements are sustained long term [4–9, 14, 18–20]. The instruments most widely used to assess health-related QoL in this population are the Short Form 36 (SF-36) or the SF-12. Studies with long-term data have demonstrated robust improvements at ≥5 years after transplant compared to the pre-TPIAT baseline [7–9]. Both physical component summary (PCS) and mental component summary (MCS) scores increase by as much as 1 standard deviation (equivalent to 10 points in the standardized scoring) (Fig. 16.1). In addition, most or all subscales improve long term, with the greatest improvements in bodily pain scores [8]. The European Organisation for Research

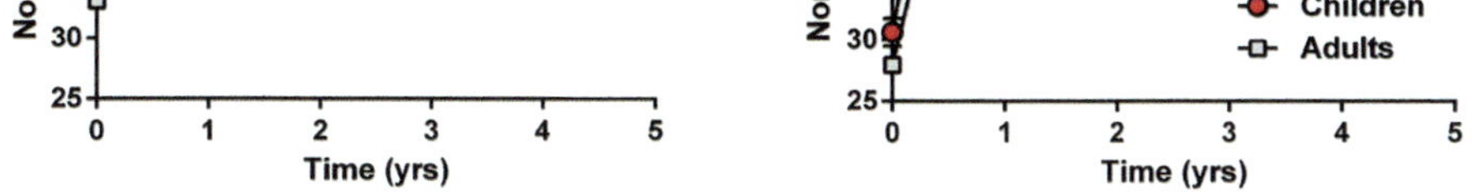

Fig. 16.1 Quality of life in children and adults from internal data at the University of Minnesota. Data were obtained using 1494 SF-36 responses from 483 patients (106 children, 377 adults, based on age at TPIAT). Both groups had robust improvements in quality of life, with children having higher physical component summary (PCS) and mental component summary (MCS) scores at the pre-TPIAT baseline ($p = 0.02$ and 0.03, respectively) and higher PCS and MCS at every time after TPIAT ($p \leq 0.003$ at all times for PCS; $p \leq 0.025$ at all times for MCS) Internal data originally presented at the International Symposium on Chronic Pancreatitis, Kiawah, South Carolina, 2014

and Treatment of Cancer Quality of Life Questionnaire has also been used in a smaller cohort of 116 patients and similarly demonstrated improved QoL and reduced pain and digestive symptoms, though patients were only assessed up to 3 years in that cohort [14].

Patients who have RAP without CP have similar improvements in pain and QoL measures [20]. Children tend to have more robust improvements, with mean PCS and MCS near the population normal value after TPIAT (Fig. 16.1). In children, school attendance improves, and the number of days limited by health problems decreases by 80% after TPIAT [6, 23]. One small study of cost-effectiveness in adult TPIAT recipients reported that the cost of continued medical management was \$196,042 per 11.5 quality-adjusted life years (QALYs) vs. \$153,576 per 14.9 QALYs for TPIAT [19].

Most of this improvement in long-term QoL is attributed to the reduced pain burden. However, a successful IAT adds benefit in health-related QoL outcomes. In 564 patients with >2100 QoL assessments (42% collected at >5 years and 17% collected at >10 years after TPIAT), PCS scores were approximately 3 points higher in patients off insulin, and most of the 8 subscores in the SF-36 were higher in insulin-independent patients, a difference that was still statistically and clinically significant even after adjusting for opioid use, pain, and age [18].

Generalized health-related QoL scores may be insufficient to detect disease-specific burdens, particularly for diabetes. Our group at the University of Minnesota has incorporated measures of diabetes distress (the Diabetes Distress Scale [DDS], also known as the Problem Areas in Diabetes scale) in our post-TPIAT follow-up assessments [24]. In an early analysis of these diabetes-specific data, out of 189 patients who completed questionnaires 1 year after TPIAT, 80% reported no or low diabetes distress, as defined by a DDS score <2. Although DDS tends to increase over time after surgery (Fig. 16.2a), it remains relatively low on average even at 7 years after surgery. Not surprisingly, those individuals who are off insulin after a successful IAT have much lower DDS than those who require insulin (Fig. 16.2b). Better glycemic control by HbA1c measures was also associated with reduced DDS. Thus, adding IAT to TP may benefit long-term QoL, both for generalized health-related QoL measures and disease-specific burdens related to diabetes [24].

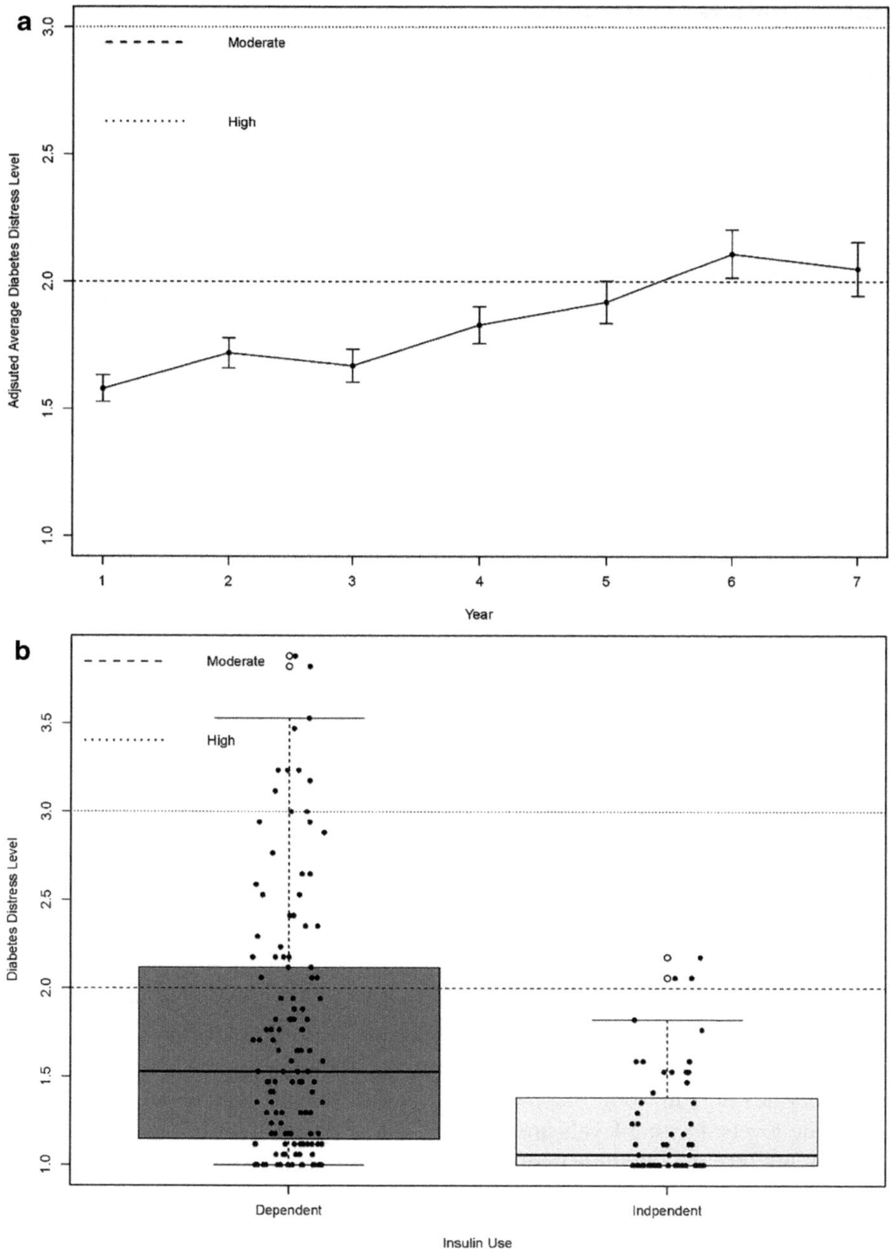

Fig. 16.2 Diabetes distress scores in TPIAT recipients. (**a**) Diabetes distress increases over time but remains low through 7 years of follow-up. (**b**) Diabetes distress was significantly lower with insulin independence. A diabetes distress score below 2 indicates no to mild distress, 2 to <3 is moderate distress, and 3 or above is severe distress. (Adapted with permission from Lane et al., Clinical Transplantation, 2018 [24])

16.5 Diabetes Outcomes

While the TP portion of the surgery is performed to treat and relieve the pain of the underlying RAP or CP, the IAT portion is designed to reduce the burden of the diabetes that would result from a TP alone [25]. As detailed in an earlier chapter on endocrine management (Chap. 8), all patients undergoing TPIAT are initially started on insulin therapy while islets are engrafting, then weaned from insulin gradually after surgery. The major outcome measures studied in IAT are insulin independence, islet graft function, and glycemic control.

Insulin independence is the outcome reported most often because it is often relatively easy to assess whether someone is taking insulin or not. The largest reports across multiple centers are consistent in their findings. With a mean transplanted islet mass that is most often around ~3500–4000 islet equivalents/kg body weight (IEQ/kg), large centers report insulin independence rates of 22–29% at 1 year, 22–28% at 5 years, and 11–13% at 10 years after TPIAT [7–9, 14]. Although islet attrition occurs over time, insulin independence is sustained >10 years post-TPIAT in a number of individuals [8].

Factors that appear to be particularly important in achieving and sustaining insulin independence are high islet mass transplanted and young age [8, 17, 26]. Individuals with genetic or hereditary pancreatitis may have slightly lower rates of insulin independence at 1 year postoperatively, but once independence is achieved, they seem to sustain it at a similar rate long term [4, 15, 27]. Insulin resistance before surgery (assessed with the Homeostatic Model Assessment of Insulin Resistance [HOMA-IR]) and obesity have been associated with a lower chance of insulin independence, as has having prediabetes or diabetes before surgery [26]. Patients with diabetes before TPIAT are nearly always on insulin after TPIAT (with a goal in these cases only to preserve some endogenous islet function) [28]. Early postoperative function assessed by beta-2 scores at 3 months after surgery also predicts later insulin independence [21]. In pediatric patients, insulin-independent rates may exceed 40% or higher if limited to young (preadolescent) children [6, 23, 29–31].

Islet graft function is an important outcome but is more nuanced to assess. Ideally, islet graft function should be assessed by C-peptide levels—a direct measure of endogenous beta-cell function—but this requires patients to come in for laboratory testing. In addition, the conditions at the time of testing will affect C-peptide levels. Fasting levels are useful in that they are standardized and easy to perform, but fasting C-peptide may be low, especially in insulin-treated patients and those with low-normal glucose or hypoglycemia at the time of testing. Stimulated C-peptide testing can be performed by administering a standardized meal (Boost or similar nutritional shake), oral glucose, or an intravenous stimulus like glucose or arginine as a more sensitive marker for islet function [17, 32–34]. The C-peptide results from these various testing protocols cannot be used interchangeably because responses will vary with the stimulus used, but all may be appropriate methods for assessing islet function, and when the same method is used repeatedly, the results can be used to follow patients' graft function over time in TPIAT. At our center, we use a meal beverage stimulus (Boost HP) with fasting and stimulated C-peptide over 2 h as a measure of islet function.

When C-peptide is not available, insulin dose has been used to make assumptions about islet graft function. In some cases, the need for multiple daily injections (a basal–bolus regimen) has been used as an indication of islet graft failure, and, in other cases, insulin dose under a threshold (e.g., <20 units/day) has been used as a proxy measure of islet graft function [8, 9]. When reading the literature, it is important to note that using insulin dosing to make assumptions about islet graft function usually overestimates islet graft failure; we now know from ongoing studies that most patients on basal–bolus insulin or using >20 units/day of insulin do have islet graft function as measured with C-peptide.

Within these inherent limitations, the published literature has suggested an islet function rate of around 70% at ≥5 years after TPIAT [4, 8, 9]. Most of these studies have relied in part (or entirely) on insulin dosing in the absence of C-peptide data [8]. In fact, when we specifically assess patients 5–20 years out from TPIAT with mixed-meal tolerance testing in one of our ongoing studies, over 90% have meaningful islet graft function by C-peptide, even if they were told they had islet failure based on insulin use (Bellin et al. [8] unpublished data). Similar to insulin independence, islet graft function is strongly associated with transplanted islet mass, with islet failure much more common in those with <2000–2500 IEQ/kg transplanted [6, 35]. Importantly, having islet function may be protective against acute and chronic diabetes complications, with the type 1 diabetes literature suggesting a clear benefit in outcomes when C-peptide is 0.6 ng/mL or higher [36]. In TPIAT, HbA1c is substantially lower (better) when any islet function is present than in the context of islet failure. Multiple studies have shown stability of C-peptide over time when it is measured [18].

Although there is an attrition of islet function over time, we have shown that islet function by mixed-meal C-peptide assessments is sustained better in young children and in those with higher transplanted islet mass (Fig. 16.3) [17, 31]. In terms of glycemic control, most studies report average HbA1c levels of 7.0–7.5%, even through 10 years of follow-up [9, 14, 15, 20]. Around 12% of patients report one or more severe hypoglycemic episodes [18]. Chronic diabetes complications are sparsely reported to date; in one study based on medical records, at 10 years after TPIAT, 37% reported neuropathy symptoms, but only 3.9% had retinopathy, and 20% had albuminuria [9].

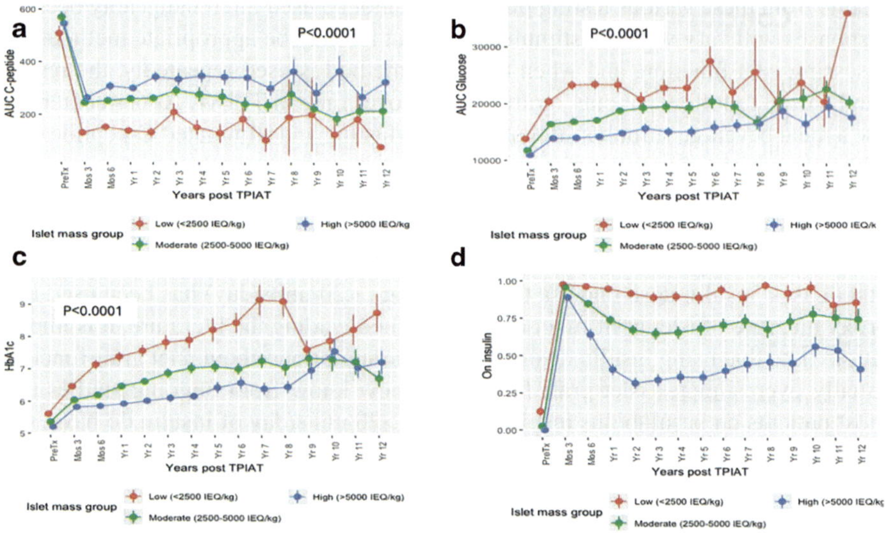

Fig. 16.3 Relationship of islet mass transplanted to long-term islet function. Data from 500 TPIAT recipients were used to assess (**a**) C-peptide and (**b**) glucose from mixed-meal tolerance testing (MMTT), (**c**) hemoglobin A1c level, and (**d**) insulin dependence. C-peptide, glucose, HbA1c, and insulin levels were all associated with the number of islets transplanted, with more islets corresponding to better islet function. Used with permission from Bellin et al., Journal of the American College of Surgeons, 2025 [17]

16.6 Other Long-Term Morbidity

While most of the outcomes research has focused on efficacy of the procedure for treating pain and reversing diabetes, there are long-term morbidities that require monitoring, including gastroparesis, vitamin deficiencies, nephrolithiasis, and osteoporosis. These are largely covered in other chapters in this textbook on the management of TPIAT recipients (Chaps. 7, 8, 10, and 11). It is worth noting that patients usually have surgical asplenia, and historically we have anecdotally observed a few cases of meningococcal meningitis and pneumococcal sepsis in our large ~900-patient cohort, highlighting the importance of immunization compliance over the long term. Patients require lifelong pancreatic enzyme supplementation and are at risk for malnutrition and micronutrient deficiency, particularly for vitamins A, D, E, and K [37, 38]. We have described loss of bone mineral density after TPIAT in adults [39]. We have recently described a high risk of calcium oxalate stones presumed to be secondary to enteric hyperoxaluria that occurs in malabsorption syndromes, with around one-third of TPIAT patients having at least one kidney stone episode by 15 years after TPIAT [40]. Monitoring and, where feasible, taking steps to prevent long-term adverse events should be a priority in the long-term management of the TPIAT recipient.

16.7 Conclusion

Large cohorts from multiple centers now demonstrate the overall long-term durability of TPIAT with sustained pain reduction and QoL improvement in many or most patients out to at least 5–10 years. Despite islet attrition over time, most patients appear to have islet function when specifically assessed by C-peptide, a few (~10%) remain off insulin even at 10 years, and glycemic control is overall good in this population of patients.

References

1. Yadav D, Lowenfels AB. The epidemiology of pancreatitis and pancreatic cancer. Gastroenterology. 2013;144(6):1252–61. https://doi.org/10.1053/j.gastro.2013.01.068.
2. Bang UC, Watanabe T, Bendtsen F. The relationship between the use of statins and mortality, severity, and pancreatic cancer in Danish patients with chronic pancreatitis. Eur J Gastroenterol Hepatol. 2018;30(3):346–51. https://doi.org/10.1097/meg.0000000000001060.
3. Nøjgaard C, Bendtsen F, Becker U, Andersen JR, Holst C, Matzen P. Danish patients with chronic pancreatitis have a four-fold higher mortality rate than the Danish population. Clin Gastroenterol Hepatol. 2010;8(4):384–90. https://doi.org/10.1016/j.cgh.2009.12.016.
4. Chinnakotla S, Radosevich DM, Dunn TB, Bellin MD, Freeman ML, Schwarzenberg SJ, et al. Long-term outcomes of total pancreatectomy and islet auto transplantation for hereditary/genetic pancreatitis. J Am Coll Surg. 2014;218(4):530–43. https://doi.org/10.1016/j.jamcollsurg.2013.12.037.
5. Wilson GC, Sutton JM, Abbott DE, Smith MT, Lowy AM, Matthews JB, et al. Long-term outcomes after total pancreatectomy and islet cell autotransplantation: is it a durable operation? Ann Surg. 2014;260(4):659–65.; discussion 65–7. https://doi.org/10.1097/sla.0000000000000920.
6. Chinnakotla S, Bellin MD, Schwarzenberg SJ, Radosevich DM, Cook M, Dunn TB, et al. Total pancreatectomy and islet autotransplantation in children for chronic pancreatitis: indication, surgical techniques, postoperative management, and long-term outcomes. Ann Surg. 2014;260(1):56–64. https://doi.org/10.1097/sla.0000000000000569.
7. Morgan KA, Lancaster WP, Owczarski SM, Wang H, Borckardt J, Adams DB. Patient selection for Total Pancreatectomy with islet autotransplantation in the surgical Management of Chronic Pancreatitis. J Am Coll Surg. 2018;226(4):446–51. https://doi.org/10.1016/j.jamcollsurg.2017.12.018.
8. Bellin MD, Beilman GJ, Sutherland DE, Ali H, Petersen A, Mongin S, et al. How durable is Total Pancreatectomy and Intraportal islet cell transplantation for treatment of chronic pancreatitis? J Am Coll Surg. 2019;228(4):329–39. https://doi.org/10.1016/j.jamcollsurg.2018.12.019.
9. Turner KM, Delman AM, Donovan EC, Brunner J, Wahab SA, Dai Y, et al. Total pancreatectomy and islet cell autotransplantation: a 10-year update on outcomes and assessment of long-term durability. HPB (Oxford). 2022;24(11):2013–21. https://doi.org/10.1016/j.hpb.2022.07.001.
10. Hooks G, Lu H, Eaton A, Trikudanathan G, Downs E, Freeman ML, et al. Addressing long-term mortality risk in patients undergoing total pancreatectomy with islet autotransplant (TPIAT): causes of death and risk factors. HPB (Oxford). 2024;26(5):664–73. https://doi.org/10.1016/j.hpb.2024.02.002.
11. Lara LF, Wastvedt S, Hodges JS, Witkowski P, Wijkstrom M, Walsh RM, et al. The association of smoking and alcohol abuse on anxiety and depression in patients with recurrent acute or chronic pancreatitis undergoing Total Pancreatectomy and islet autotransplantation: a report from the prospective observational study of TPIAT cohort. Pancreas. 2021;50(6):852–8. https://doi.org/10.1097/mpa.0000000000001850.

12. Yadav D, Palermo TM, Phillips AE, Bellin MD, Conwell DL. Painful chronic pancreatitis - new approaches for evaluation and management. Curr Opin Gastroenterol. 2021;37(5):504–11. https://doi.org/10.1097/mog.0000000000000769.
13. Scott A, Khoruts A, Freeman ML, Beilman G, Ramanathan K, Bellin MD, et al. Successful use of fecal microbiota transplantation in management of nonobstructive recurrent cholangitis following total pancreatectomy and islet autotransplant. ACG Case Rep J. 2024;11(10):e01527. https://doi.org/10.14309/crj.0000000000001527.
14. Coluzzi M, Takita M, Saracino G, Rub Hakim Mohammed A, Darden CM, Testa G, et al. Improved quality of life among chronic pancreatitis patients undergoing total pancreatectomy with islet autotransplantation-single center experience with large cohort of patients. Transpl Int. 2023;36:11409. https://doi.org/10.3389/ti.2023.11409.
15. Darden CM, Mohammed ARH, Kirkland J, Kuncha J, Lawrence MC, Danobeitia JS, et al. Total pancreatectomy with islet autotransplantation outcomes in patients with pancreatitis of genetic etiology: a single-center experience with a large cohort of patients. J Gastrointest Surg. 2024;28(8):1309–18. https://doi.org/10.1016/j.gassur.2024.05.034.
16. Pollard CA, Chung WY, Garcea G, Dennison AR. Assessment of long-term graft function following total pancreatectomy and autologous islet transplantation: the Leicester experience. Hepatobiliary Surg Nutr. 2023;12(5):682–91. https://doi.org/10.21037/hbsn-21-558.
17. Bellin MD, Eaton A, Ramanathan K, Beilman G, Downs E, Schwarzenberg SJ, et al. Long-term islet graft functional assessments in more than 500 patients undergoing total pancreatectomy with Intraportal islet autotransplantation. J Am Coll Surg. 2025;240(4):405–13. https://doi.org/10.1097/xcs.0000000000001294.
18. Chinnakotla S, Beilman GJ, Vock D, Freeman ML, Kirchner V, Dunn TB, et al. Intraportal islet autotransplantation independently improves quality of life after Total Pancreatectomy in patients with chronic refractory pancreatitis. Ann Surg. 2022;276(3):441–9. https://doi.org/10.1097/sla.0000000000005553.
19. Wilson GC, Ahmad SA, Schauer DP, Eckman MH, Abbott DE. Cost-effectiveness of total pancreatectomy and islet cell autotransplantation for the treatment of minimal change chronic pancreatitis. J Gastrointest Surg. 2015;19(1):46–54.; discussion –5. https://doi.org/10.1007/s11605-014-2612-3.
20. Bellin MD, Kerdsirichairat T, Beilman GJ, Dunn TB, Chinnakotla S, Pruett TL, et al. Total Pancreatectomy with islet autotransplantation improves quality of life in patients with refractory recurrent acute pancreatitis. Clin Gastroenterol Hepatol. 2016;14(9):1317–23. https://doi.org/10.1016/j.cgh.2016.02.027.
21. Nanno Y, Hodges JS, Freeman ML, Trikudanathan G, Schwarzenberg SJ, Downs EM, et al. Early metabolic measures predict long-term insulin Independence in recipients of Total Pancreatectomy and islet autotransplantation. Transplant Direct. 2024;10(1):e1561. https://doi.org/10.1097/txd.0000000000001561.
22. Nanno Y, Wilhelm JJ, Heller D, Schat R, Freeman ML, Trikudanathan G, et al. Combination of pancreas volume and HbA1c level predicts islet yield in patients undergoing total pancreatectomy and islet autotransplantation. Clin Transpl. 2020;34(8):e14008. https://doi.org/10.1111/ctr.14008.
23. Bellin MD, Forlenza GP, Majumder K, Berger M, Freeman ML, Beilman GJ, et al. Total Pancreatectomy with islet autotransplantation resolves pain in young children with severe chronic pancreatitis. J Pediatr Gastroenterol Nutr. 2017;64(3):440–5. https://doi.org/10.1097/mpg.0000000000001314.
24. Lane A, Hodges JS, Ptacek P, Louise Berry K, Beilman GJ, Dunn TB, et al. Low prevalence of diabetes distress following total pancreatectomy with islet autotransplantation. Clin Transpl. 2018;32(5):e13237. https://doi.org/10.1111/ctr.13237.
25. Bellin MD, Balamurugan AN, Pruett TL, Sutherland DE. No islets left behind: islet autotransplantation for surgery-induced diabetes. Curr Diab Rep. 2012;12(5):580–6. https://doi.org/10.1007/s11892-012-0296-1.
26. Nanno Y, Wastvedt S, Freeman ML, Trikudanathan G, Schwarzenberg SJ, Downs EM, et al. Metabolic measures before surgery and long-term diabetes outcomes in recipients of total

pancreatectomy and islet autotransplantation. Am J Transplant. 2021;21(10):3411–20. https://doi.org/10.1111/ajt.16573.
27. Bellin MD, Prokhoda P, Hodges JS, Schwarzenberg SJ, Freeman ML, Dunn TB, et al. Age and disease duration impact outcomes of Total Pancreatectomy and islet autotransplant for PRSS1 hereditary pancreatitis. Pancreas. 2018;47(4):466–70. https://doi.org/10.1097/mpa.0000000000001028.
28. Bellin MD, Beilman GJ, Dunn TB, Pruett TL, Chinnakotla S, Wilhelm JJ, et al. Islet autotransplantation to preserve beta cell mass in selected patients with chronic pancreatitis and diabetes mellitus undergoing total pancreatectomy. Pancreas. 2013;42(2):317–21. https://doi.org/10.1097/MPA.0b013e3182681182.
29. Bellin MD, Freeman ML, Schwarzenberg SJ, Dunn TB, Beilman GJ, Vickers SM, et al. Quality of life improves for pediatric patients after total pancreatectomy and islet autotransplant for chronic pancreatitis. Clin Gastroenterol Hepatol. 2011;9(9):793–9. https://doi.org/10.1016/j.cgh.2011.04.024.
30. Bellin MD, Schwarzenberg SJ, Cook M, Sutherland DE, Chinnakotla S. Pediatric autologous islet transplantation. Curr Diab Rep. 2015;15(10):67. https://doi.org/10.1007/s11892-015-0639-9.
31. Gnikpingo T, Benson S, Hodges JS, Downs E, Cook M, Schwarzenberg SJ, et al. Islet graft function by mixed meal tolerance testing is sustained over 4 years in young children undergoing total pancreatectomy with islet autotransplantation. Clin Transpl. 2023;37(12):e15106. https://doi.org/10.1111/ctr.15106.
32. KR ME, Skube ME, Yang Y, Hodges JS, Wilhelm J, Beilman G, et al. Utility of arginine stimulation testing in preoperative assessment of children undergoing total pancreatectomy with islet autotransplantation. Clin Transpl. 2019;33(8):e13647. https://doi.org/10.1111/ctr.13647.
33. Robertson RP, Bogachus LD, Oseid E, Parazzoli S, Patti ME, Rickels MR, et al. Assessment of β-cell mass and α- and β-cell survival and function by arginine stimulation in human autologous islet recipients. Diabetes. 2015;64(2):565–72. https://doi.org/10.2337/db14-0690.
34. Bellin MD, Sutherland DE, Beilman GJ, Hong-McAtee I, Balamurugan AN, Hering BJ, et al. Similar islet function in islet allotransplant and autotransplant recipients, despite lower islet mass in autotransplants. Transplantation. 2011;91(3):367–72. https://doi.org/10.1097/TP.0b013e318203fd09.
35. Sutherland DE, Radosevich DM, Bellin MD, Hering BJ, Beilman GJ, Dunn TB, et al. Total pancreatectomy and islet autotransplantation for chronic pancreatitis. J Am Coll Surg. 2012;214(4):409–24.; discussion 24–6. https://doi.org/10.1016/j.jamcollsurg.2011.12.040.
36. Taylor PN, Collins KS, Lam A, Karpen SR, Greeno B, Walker F, et al. C-peptide and metabolic outcomes in trials of disease modifying therapy in new-onset type 1 diabetes: an individual participant meta-analysis. Lancet Diabetes Endocrinol. 2023;11(12):915–25. https://doi.org/10.1016/s2213-8587(23)00267-x.
37. Downs EM, Brun A, Bellin MD. Nutrition support in the pediatric total pancreatectomy with islet autotransplantation recipient. Nutr Clin Pract. 2024;39(1):100–8. https://doi.org/10.1002/ncp.11101.
38. Downs EM, Eaton A, Witkowski P, Wijkstrom M, Walsh M, Trikudanathan G, et al. Nutritional risks in patients undergoing Total Pancreatectomy islet AutoTransplantation in the POST consortium. J Gastrointest Surg. 2023;27(9):1893–902. https://doi.org/10.1007/s11605-023-05770-1.
39. Wothe JK, Aidoo R, KR ME, Harindhanavudhi T, Trikudanathan G, Freeman ML, et al. Reduced bone mineral density in the first year after total pancreatectomy with islet autotransplantation (TPIAT). Pancreatology. 2021;21(8):1491–7. https://doi.org/10.1016/j.pan.2021.08.013.
40. Avula N, Hodges JS, Beilman G, Chinnakotla S, Freeman ML, Ramanathan K, et al. Increased kidney stone risk following total pancreatectomy with islet autotransplantation. Pancreatology. 2024; https://doi.org/10.1016/j.pan.2024.09.004.

GPSR Compliance

The European Union's (EU) General Product Safety Regulation (GPSR) is a set of rules that requires consumer products to be safe and our obligations to ensure this.

If you have any concerns about our products, you can contact us on ProductSafety@springernature.com

In case Publisher is established outside the EU, the EU authorized representative is:

Springer Nature Customer Service Center GmbH
Europaplatz 3
69115 Heidelberg, Germany

Batch number: 10732090

Printed by Printforce, the Netherlands